Differential Diagnosis
in Dermatology

Commissioning Editor: Belinda Kuhn
Project Development Manager: Hilary Hewitt
Project Manager: Isobel Black; Cheryl Brant
Design Manager: Andy Chapman
Marketing Manager(s): Amy Hey (UK); Meghan Carr (USA)

Differential Diagnosis in Dermatology

Boni E. Elewski MD
Professor of Dermatology
Department of Dermatology
University of Alabama at Birmingham
Birmingham, Alabama
USA

Lauren C. Hughey MD
Assistant Professor of Dermatology
Department of Dermatology
University of Alabama at Birmingham
Birmingham, Alabama
USA

Margaret E. Parsons MD
Assistant Clinical Professor
Department of Dermatology
University of California at Davis Medical Center
Dermatology Consultants of Sacramento
Sacramento, California
USA

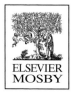

ELSEVIER
MOSBY

MOSBY
An affiliate of Elsevier Inc

First published 2005

ISBN 0 3230 3017 3

British Library Cataloguing in Publication Data
A catalogue record for this book is available from the British Library

Library of Congress Cataloging in Publication Data
A catalog record for this book is available from the Library of Congress

Notice
Medical knowledge is constantly changing. Standard safety precautions must be followed, but as new research and clinical experience broaden our knowledge, changes in treatment and drug therapy may become necessary or appropriate. Readers are advised to check the most current product information provided by the manufacturer of each drug to be administered to verify the recommended dose, the method and duration of administration, and contraindications. It is the responsibility of the practitioner, relying on experience and knowledge of the patient, to determine dosages and the best treatment for each individual patient. Neither the Publisher nor the authors assume any liability for any injury and/or damage to persons or property arising from this publication.
The Publisher

Printed in China
Last digit is the print number: 9 8 7 6 5 4 3 2 1

CONTENTS

PREFACE

This text provides a user-friendly approach to the differential diagnosis of skin disease and is geared to the dermatologist as well as to the primary care physician who treats cutaneous disorders. It is not intended to be an encyclopedia of dermatology, but rather a starting point for diagnosing dermatologic disease. The field of dermatology is rich with many disease entities. Some of these entities are reflective of systemic diseases, an indication of other conditions, and some are just a single lesion to be understood. In learning about these many diseases, most dermatologists are trained to first identify and describe the lesion, then to think through a list of possible entities – the differential diagnosis process.

Divided into three sections, the text begins with a definition list to aid in the understanding and the description of lesion morphology. Correct categorization of lesion morphology, including the subtle features of patterns and distribution, is the first step a skilled dermatologist utilizes in properly identifying a cutaneous disorder. Numerous photographs illustrate salient points and provide a visual image to reinforce the nuances of dermatology terminology.

The second and major section of the text contains the compilation of many lists of possible diagnoses based upon clinical features and morphology. Lists are weighted starting with the most severe and common entities and include a myriad of possible diagnoses for that lesion's morphology, pattern and distribution. Select disorders are further detailed in template form to assist in sorting through the possible diagnoses. These templates include:
1. a description of the lesion
2. regional distribution and location
3. characteristics, symptoms and associations
4. diagnostic pearls and/or dermatopathology specifics
5. possible associated systemic diseases
6. treatment pearls, if applicable.

Photographs are shown to assist the clinician with the correct diagnosis.

The third section of the text is a compendium of specific syndromes and medical conditions with unique dermatologic features.

Although the text does not include every possible diagnosis, it certainly provides a strong starting point for all clinicians who treat patients with skin disease.

BEE
LCH
MEP

DEDICATION

We thank our teachers and mentors who have taught us over the years in the art and science of dermatology.

Our deep appreciation goes to our family, friends, and colleagues who have supported us while working on this project.

ACKNOWLEDGEMENTS

We are grateful to Rebecca Kissel for proofreading the manuscript and to Kristin Ziel for her help in organizing and preparing the illustrations.

We are grateful to Lawrence J. Bass, Craig Elmets, Conway Huang, Michael Jacobs, Jenny Sobera, Amy Theos, Catherine Toms and Jeff Weeks for providing illustrations for the various sections of this book, as follows:

Section I:
Courtesy of Craig Elmets: Furuncle.

Section II:
Courtesy of Lawrence J. Bass: Photoallergic, Phototoxic, and Inverse psoriasis (groin).

Courtesy of Craig Elmets: Acquired digital fibroma, Alopecia areata, Amyloidosis, Anetoderma, Aplasia cutis, Arsenical keratoses, Atopic dermatitis, Behçet's syndrome, Contact dermatitis (lips), Dental sinus, Dermatographism, Elastosis perforans serpiginosa, Favre–Racouchot syndrome, Folliculitis, Foreign body, Gestational pemphigoid/herpes gestationis, Granular cell tumor, Hailey–Hailey disease (axilla), Hand, foot and mouth disease, Lichen planopilaris, Lichen planus, Lichen sclerosus et atrophicus, Lips (perlèche), Liquid nitrogen-induced bulla, Lymphangioma circumscriptum, Maculae cerulae, Myxedema, Nails (koilonychia), Nails (leukonychia), Pilar cyst, Poikiloderma vasculare atrophicans, Primary syphilis, Prurigo nodularis, Prurigo of pregnancy, Pseudoxanthoma elasticum, Psoriasis, Relapsing polychondritis, Scurvy/vitamin C deficiency, Seborrheic dermatitis, Seborrheic keratosis, Seborrheic keratosis (eruptive), Subcorneal pustular dermatoses, Tinea manuum, Trichotillomania.

Courtesy of Michael Jacobs: Erythema multiforme, Hailey–Hailey disease (trunk), Hypomelanosis of Ito, Papular mucinosis, Porokeratosis, Secondary syphilis, Syphilis (oral).

Courtesy of Jenny Sobera: Discoid lupus.

Courtesy of Amy Theos: Angiofibroma, Ash leaf macule, Confluent and reticulated papillomatoses of Gougerot and Carteaud, Connective tissue nevus, Contact dermatitis, Cutaneous T-cell lymphoma, Dermoid cyst, Diaper dermatitis, Eosinophilic folliculitis, Gianotti–Crosti syndrome, Hemangioma, Herpes zoster virus, Infantile hemangioma, Involuting infantile hemangioma, Juvenile xanthogranuloma, Lentigo/freckle, Morphea, Nevus, Nevus of Ota/Ito, Non-bullous congenital ichthyosiform erythroderma, Pigmentary mosaicism, Pigmented purpuric eruption, Psoriasis (Koebner), Verruca planae.

Courtesy of Catherine Toms: Atypical mycobacteria.

Courtesy of Jeff Weeks: Branchial cleft cyst, Erythrasma, Impetigo.

Section III:

Courtesy of Craig Elmets: McCune–Albright syndrome, Neurofibromatosis, Wiskott–Aldrich syndrome.

Courtesy of Conway Huang: Xeroderma pigmentosum.

Courtesy of Michael Jacobs: Hypomelanosis of Ito.

Courtesy of Amy Theos: Cutis laxa, Netherton's syndrome, Nevus of Ito.

PRIMARY LESIONS

Macule – flat lesion up to 1 cm in size

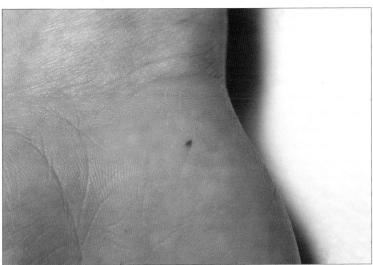

Patch – flat lesion greater than 1 cm in size

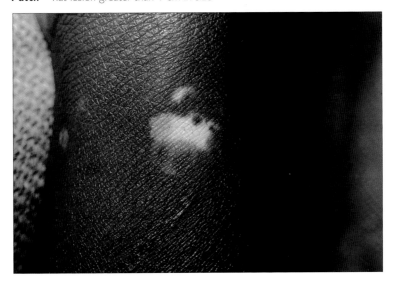

Papule – raised lesion up to 1 cm in size

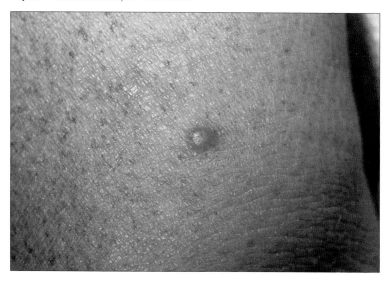

Plaque – raised lesion greater than 1 cm in size

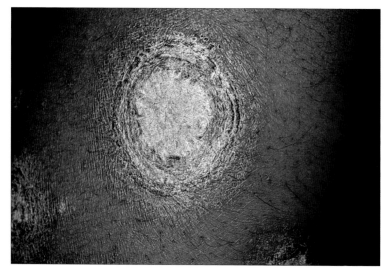

Nodule – solid, firm lesion up to 1 cm in size

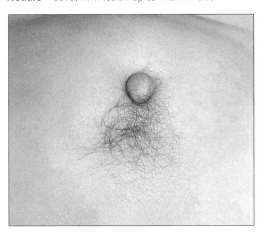

Tumor – solid, firm lesion greater than 1 cm in size

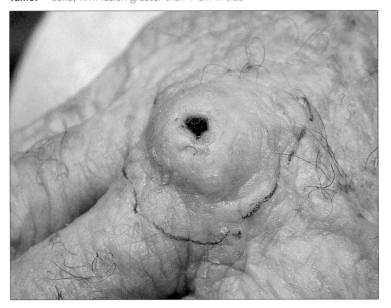

Cyst – fluid- or substance-filled subcutaneous lesion

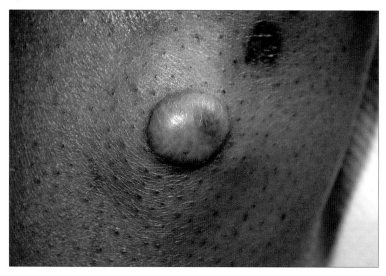

Vesicle – blister up to 1 cm in size

Bulla – blister greater than 1 cm in size

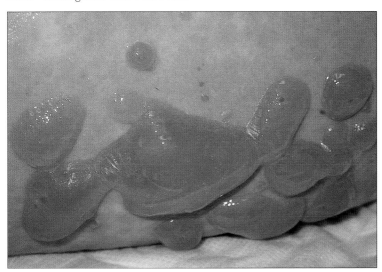

Pustule – raised lesion containing purulent exudate

Furuncle – inflamed follicle with area of central pus and necrosis

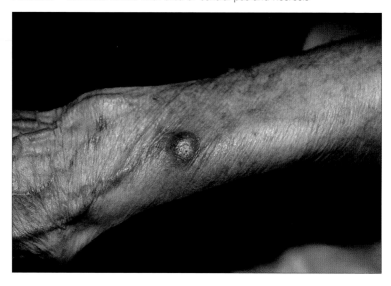

Carbuncle – a collection of several inflammed follicles with pus and necrosis

Wheal/hive – urticarial papule or plaque, usually pink with white area at edge

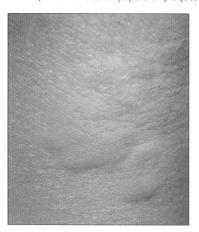

Comedo (closed) – follicular papule that has intact epidermis (acne – 'whitehead')

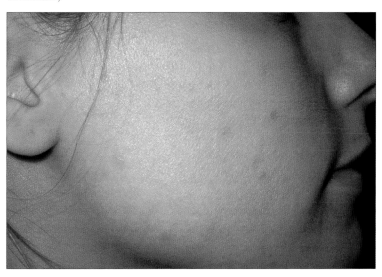

Comedo (open) – follicular structure, open to air, such that fatty acids oxidize and turn a dark color (acne – 'blackhead')

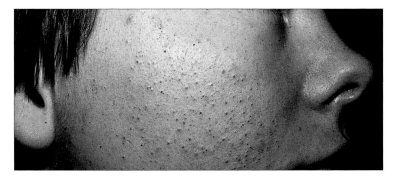

SECONDARY FEATURES

Atrophy – thinning of the epidermis giving a shiny white appearance and/or 'cigarette paper' wrinkling of the epidermis

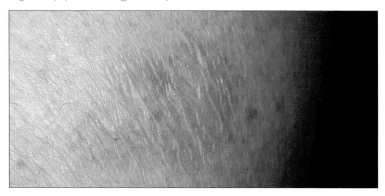

Crust – thickened epidermis with overlying dried exudate

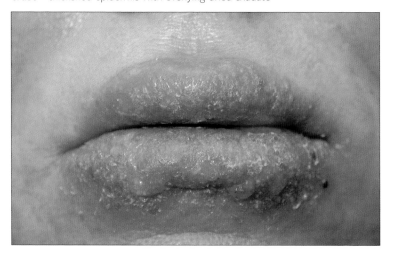

Desquamation – peeling epidermis

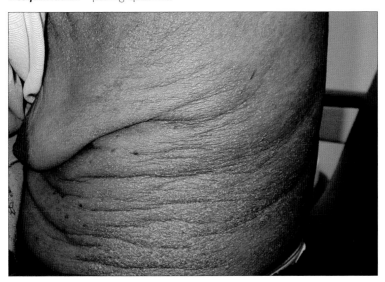

Eczematous – scaling, erythematous, and crusty changes

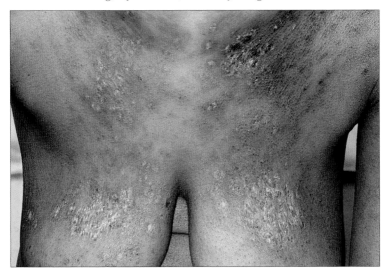

Edema – swollen, fluid-filled subcutaneous tissue

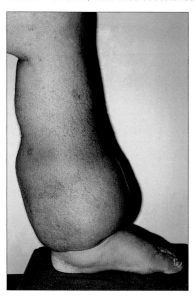

Erosion – shallow, abraded area of the epidermis/mucosa

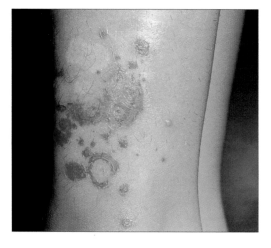

Excoriation – disruption of the epidermis/dermis made by scratching

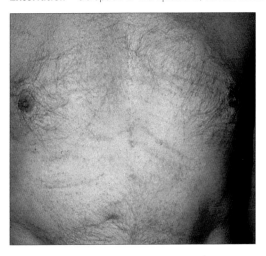

Fissure – crack in the epidermis and possibly the dermis

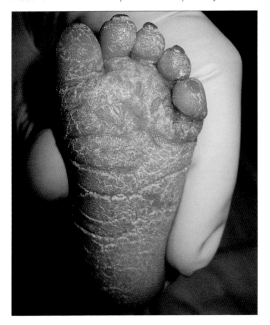

Guttate – tear-drop lesions in a 'splashed on' pattern

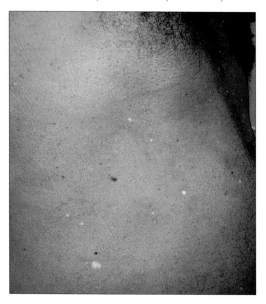

Hyperkeratotic – thickened upper layers of the epidermis

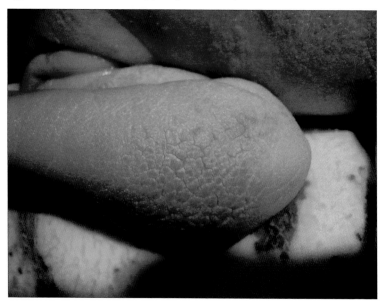

Indurated – firm, solid texture

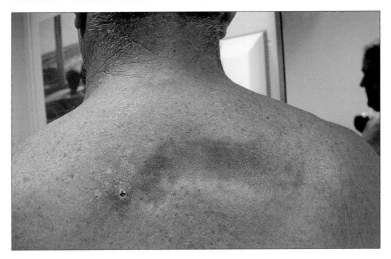

Lichenified – thick texture with increased skin markings resembling tree bark

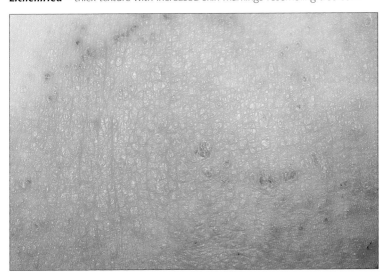

Scale – loose upper epidermal layers

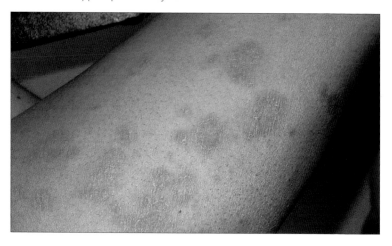

Targetoid – lesion occurs like a bull's-eye target

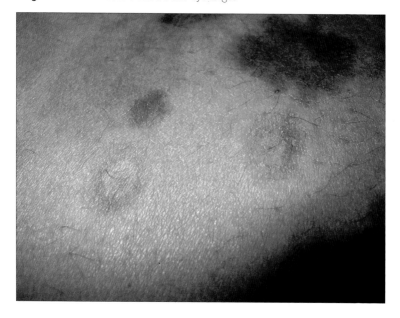

Ulcer – open area of epidermis, and often dermis

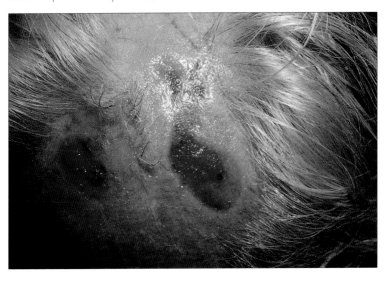

Umbilicated – lesion has a central dell, like an umbilicus

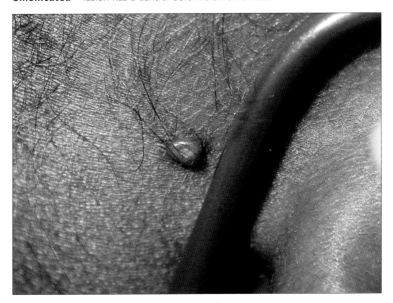

Verrucous – thick, bumpy, wart-like changes

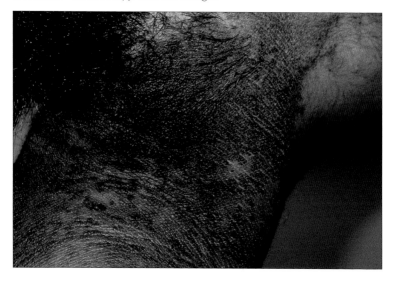

PATTERNS

Acral – relating to hands and feet

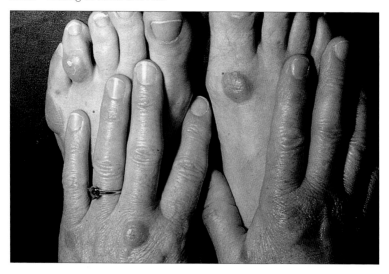

Annular – ring-shaped with central clearing

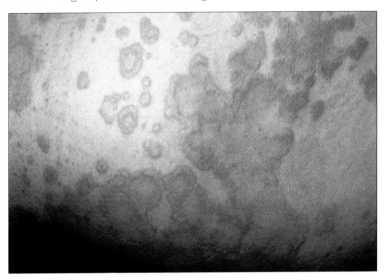

Arcuate – pattern of lesions or single lesion that is arc-shaped

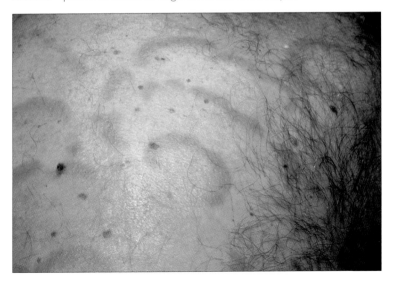

Circinate – pattern of lesions that are circular or somewhat circular in pattern

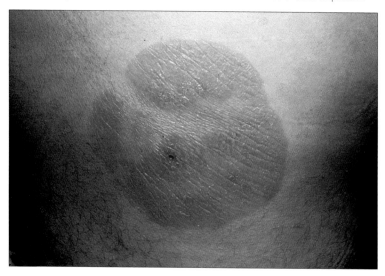

Confluent – lesions coalesce into one another

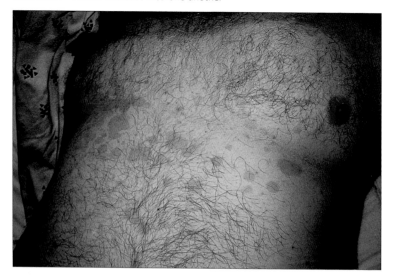

Discrete – lesions occur singly and do not run into each other or coalesce

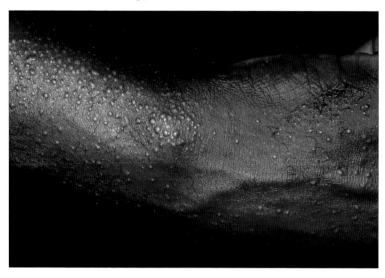

Follicular – pattern of lesions occurs in hair follicles

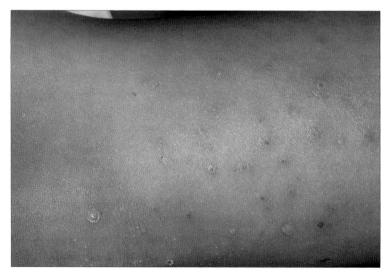

Generalized – lesions that extend over most of the body surface area

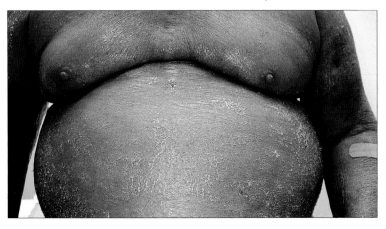

Gyrate – lesions have varied circular and serpiginous patterns

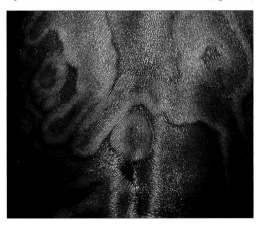

Linear – occurring in a line

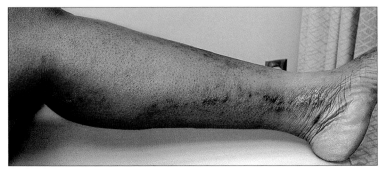

Livedo – net-like, lacy pattern

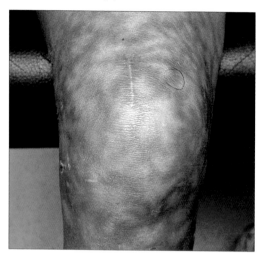

Localized – lesion/lesions limited to one area of body

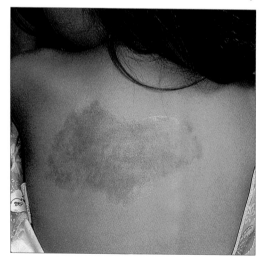

Monomorphous – all lesions are in the same stage of development and look similar

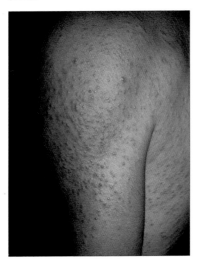

Morbilliform – pattern of lesions that has both macules and papules

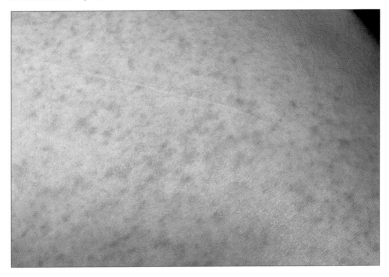

Nummular – coin-shaped

Papulosquamous – pattern of lesions that have scaly papules

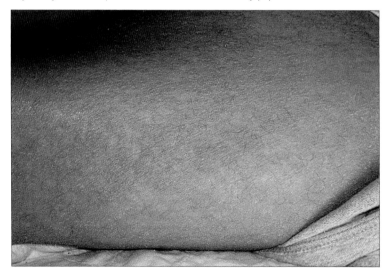

Photodermatosis/photodistribution – lesions confined to sun-exposed areas with sparing of covered areas, under nose, around eyes, and sometimes submental

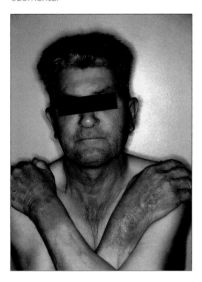

Polymorphous – lesions are of many shapes and types

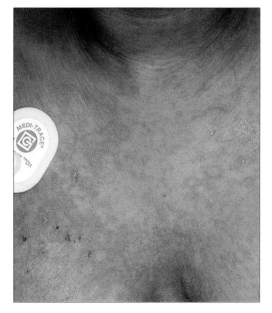

Regional – lesions distributed over a limited area of the body

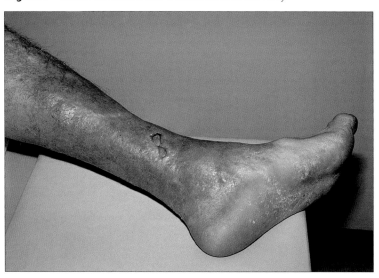

Reticulate – pattern of lesions that is net-like/lacy

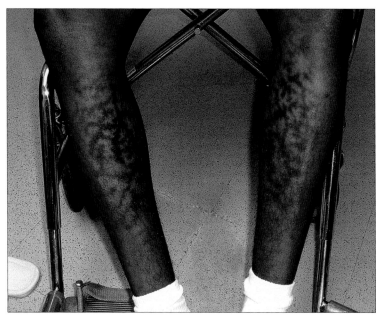

Segmental – lesion/lesions occurring along a body part

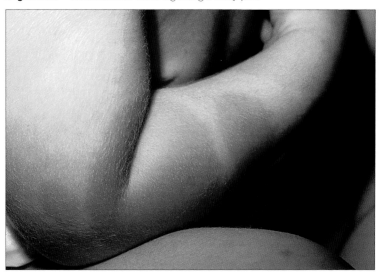

Serpiginous – twisting or snake-like pattern

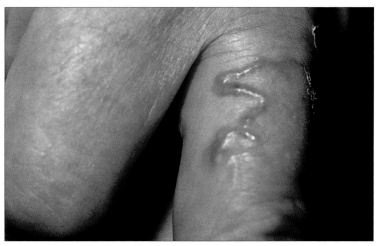

Sporotrichoid – lesions follow the course of lymphatics in a somewhat linear progression, usually up an extremity

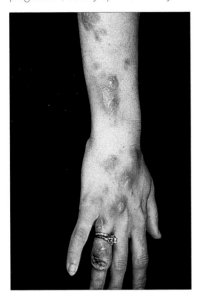

Universal – lesions and disease that include skin, hair and nails

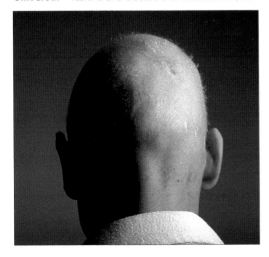

Zosteriform/dermatomal – occurring in a dermatome

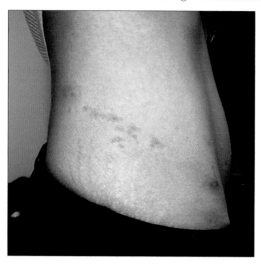

OTHER TERMS

Auspitz sign – pinpoint bleeding dots due to capillaries at surface when a psoriatic plaque is removed

Burrow – tunneling under the superficial skin that causes a raised linear or serpiginous plaque

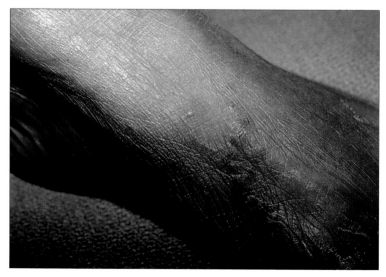

Circumscribed – lesion with well-defined borders

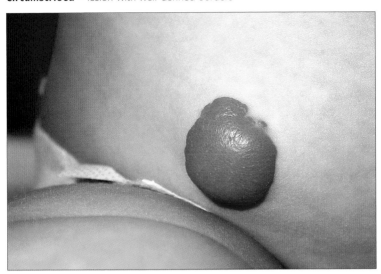

Depigmented – total lack of pigment, also termed amelanotic (use of Wood's light helps to accentuate areas of depigmentation)

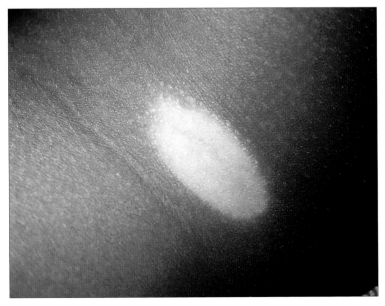

Dimpling – when pressured from sides, the lesion indents in the middle (e.g. dermatofibroma)

Erythema – red ('*red' is a synonym for erythematous*)

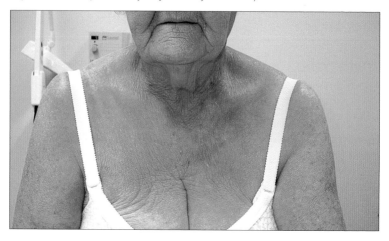

Erythroderma – generalized (> 90% body surface area), red, scaling, swollen skin

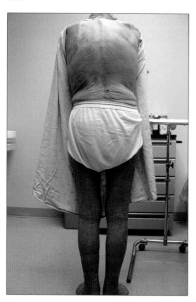

Exfoliative – desquamation (scale) and erythema

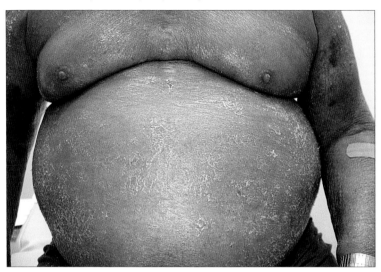

Frambesiform – 'raspberry-like' (e.g. yaws)

Halo – a ring (usually lighter) around a primary lesion of a different color

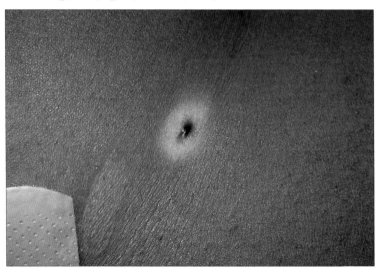

Hyperpigmented – area of increased pigment, darker than actual skin color

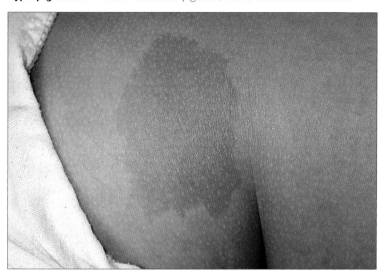

Hypopigmented – area of decreased pigment, lighter than actual skin color

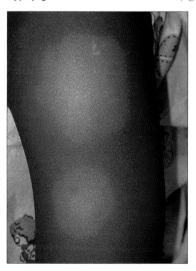

Keratosis – general term for a well-demarcated, elevated cutaneous lesion

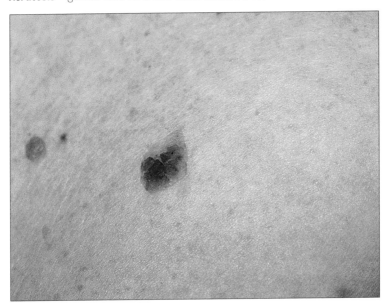

Koebner phenomenon – lesions occur in areas of trauma, often extending in a linear fashion along areas of excoriation

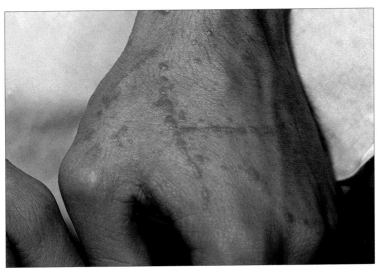

Lichenoid – 'lichen planus-like', purple/pink, flat, firm papules

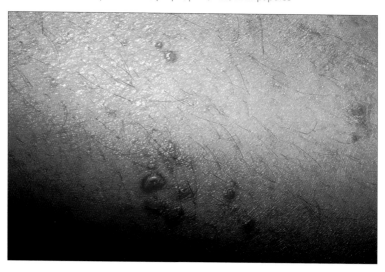

Pedunculated – hanging from a base stalk

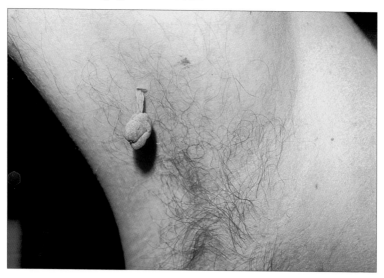

Petechiae – tiny, fine, red macules and papules

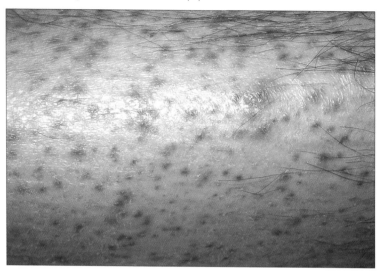

Pit – small, 'ice pick-like' depression in surface

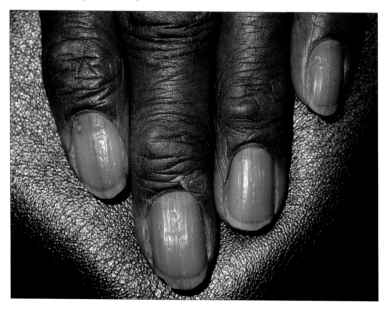

Poikiloderma – areas of mottled pigmentation with atrophy and telangiectasias

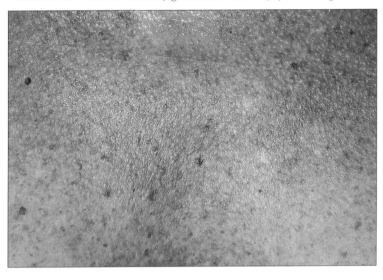

Pruritus – itch

Punctate – small, well-demarcated lesion

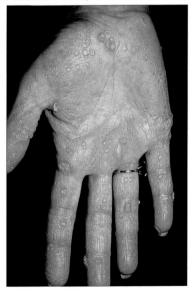

Purpura – erythematous to violaceous macules, papules, patches or plaques

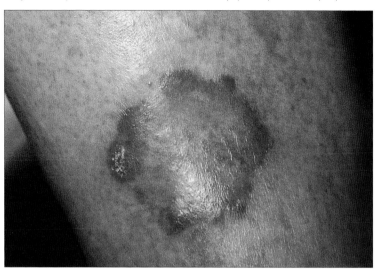

Scar – alteration in the skin secondary to trauma/surgery; may be pink early in course of healing or hypo- or hyperpigmented with older scars

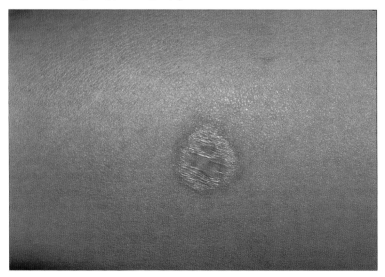

Telangiectasia – small blood vessels visible on the skin surface

Trailing scale – scale on the interior edge of a centrifugally expanding annular lesion

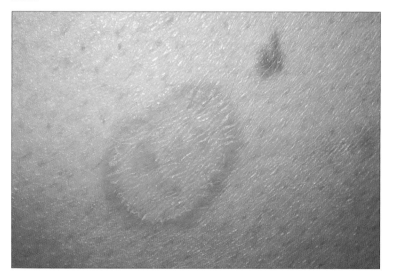

ACNE-LIKE LESIONS

Acne vulgaris

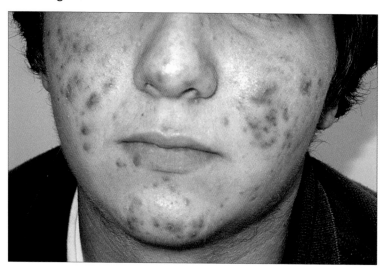

Description erythematous papules, nodules and pustules
(see p. 22, monomorphous)

Location face and upper trunk

Characteristics adolescents most commonly, but can occur through adult years; can be exacerbated by drugs (see box), cosmetics, tars, oils, sun or occlusion as in acne mechanica (cell phone, chin pad)

Tests Histopathology: dilated follicle packed with keratin debris, small to no sebaceous glands and surrounded by inflammation; may progress to follicle rupture with intense neutrophilic and granulomatous reaction

Associated systemic disease none

Treatment pearls topical and/or oral retinoids, topical and/or oral antibiotics, benzoyl peroxide, salicylic acid, azelaic acid, oral contraceptive pills, spironolactone

CAUSES OF DRUG-INDUCED ACNE*

- Anabolic steroids and corticosteroids
- Oral contraceptive pills
- Vitamin B_{12}
- Anticonvulsants (dilantin, phenobarbital)
- Iodides, bromides
- Lithium
- Tetracyclines (if given to a patient on lithium)
- Isoniazid
- Chloral hydrate
- Scopolamine
- Parenteral nutrition (secondary to heavy metal)
- Cyclosporine
- Azathioprine
- Disulfiram
- Quinidine
- Thiouracil

* Drug-induced acne is usually abrupt in onset and monomorphous.

Perioral dermatitis

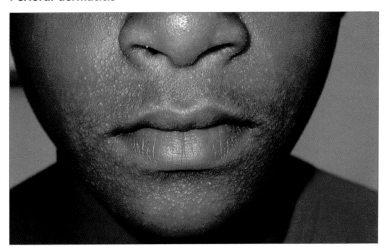

Description erythematous papules and pustules ± associated scale
Location periorificial distribution (which may include periorbital and perioral),
may spare the immediate border surrounding the vermilion lip
Characteristics young females>males usually 20–35 years old, no pruritus
Tests Histopathology: resembles rosacea
Associated systemic disease none
Treatment pearls oral tetracycline, topical clindamycin, topical metronidazole,
avoid topical corticosteroids

Rosacea

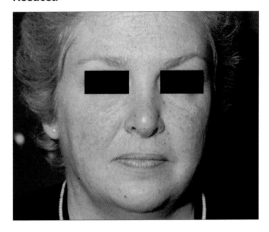

Description erythematous macules, papules and pustules
Location face

Characteristics adults, chronic, exacerbated by many factors including exercise, spicy food, hot drinks, alcohol intake (especially red wine), drugs, Parkinson's disease and connective tissue diseases
Tests Histopathology: telangiectasias, ± edema, perifollicular and perivascular inflammatory infiltrate, sebaceous hyperplasia, ± granulomas
Associated systemic disease none
Treatment pearls topical metronidazole, azelaic acid, sodium sulfacetamide, oral antibiotics

Folliculitis
See page 333

Pseudofolliculitis

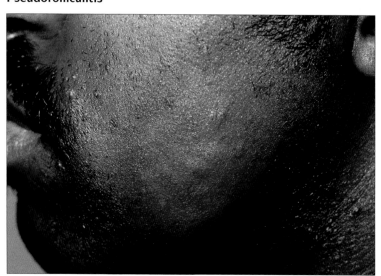

Description perifollicular erythematous papules and pustules, may progress to hyperpigmented areas with keloidal nodules
Location beard distribution or any body area shaved or plucked
Characteristics dark-skinned men typically, but may occur in females who shave or pluck hairs, or in others with tight curly hair
Tests clinical diagnosis
Associated systemic disease none
Treatment pearls stop shaving or decrease frequency of shaving, daily inspection with magnifying mirror to release ingrown hairs with a sterile needle/toothpick which can be followed with 1% hydrocortisone lotion to reduce inflammation, glycolic acid lotions, topical retinoids, topical antibiotics, topical benzoyl peroxide, chemical depilatories, laser hair removal

Pityrosporum folliculitis
See page 334

Milia

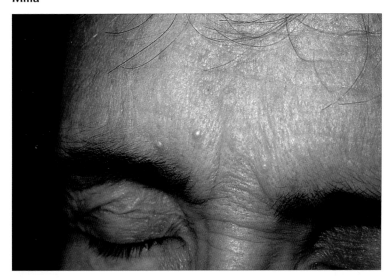

Description firm, pearly white papules 1–4 mm

Location most common on face, milia en plaque may occur pre- and postauricular

Characteristics middle-aged women>men, up to 50% of newborns, may be familial, may occur in response to trauma or after inflammatory conditions

Tests clinical diagnosis; Histopathology: small epidermoid cyst

Associated systemic disease associated with several syndromes and inflammatory disorders, e.g. epidermolysis bullosa acquisita, bullous pemphigoid, porphyria cutanea tarda, varicella zoster virus, Bazex syndrome, Rombo syndrome, basal cell carcinoma syndrome and several genodermatoses including Marie–Unna hypotrichosis syndrome, oral–facial–digital syndrome type I, Naegeli–Franceschetti–Jadassohn syndrome and congenital ectodermal defects

Treatment pearls incision and expression of contents with 11 blade, topical retinoids, oral minocycline for milia en plaque

Favre–Racouchot syndrome

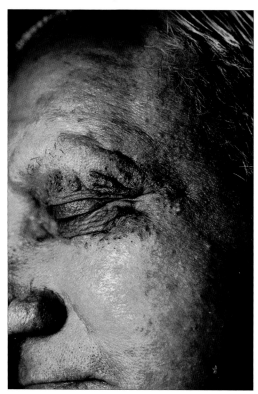

Description multiple, large black open comedones
Location sun-exposed distribution especially on temples and lateral cheeks (periorbital)
Characteristics older adult men, chronic
Tests Histopathology: dilated follicular orifice filled with keratin in association with solar elastosis
Associated systemic disease none
Treatment pearls topical retinoids, topical antibiotics, manual extraction

Chloracne
Description oily skin with recurrent crops of numerous, large open comedones which progress to milia and inflammatory papules and yellow cysts which may scar
Location retroauricular and malar distribution, may progress to buttocks, neck, thighs

Characteristics older adult men, ± increase in dark body hair, usually improves with time

Tests Histopathology: dilated follicles with keratin plugs and multiple small epidermal inclusion cysts

Associated systemic disease associated with exposure to chlorinated aromatic hydrocarbons found in some insulators, insecticides, fungicides and preservatives

Treatment pearls oral and topical retinoids and antibiotics, but often refractory to typical acne treatments

Syringoma
See page 344

Drug reaction
See page 286

Rhinophyma

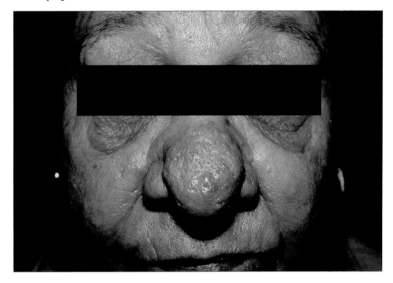

Adenoma sebaceum
See page 590

Trichostasis spinulosa

Lupus miliaris disseminatus faciei

Nevus comedonicus

Sebaceous hyperplasia

Hidradenitis suppurativa

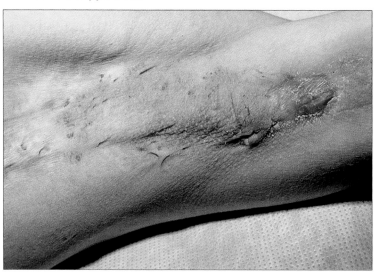

ACRAL BULLA

Friction blister

Description erythematous macule that progresses to a bulla (clear fluid or hemorrhagic), may progress to 'talon noire' while healing on the sole of the foot secondary to oxidation of hemosiderin

Location hands and feet (areas of trauma) most commonly

Characteristics any age, spontaneously heals, painful

Tests Histopathology: pauci-immune intraepidermal bulla

Associated systemic disease none

Treatment pearls small slit in roof of blister to relieve fluid, topical antibiotic, protective bandage

Dyshidrosis

See page 57

Porphyria cutanea tarda (PCT)

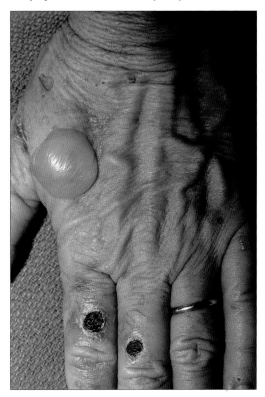

Description large tense bullae and erosions with crust often seen with sclerodermoid changes, hypertrichosis and hyperpigmentation

Location sun-exposed areas especially dorsal hands, face and scalp

Characteristics male>female, middle-aged, chronic, autosomal dominant 20% vs. acquired 80%, Nikolsky sign–, exacerbations in summer

Tests 24-h urine porphyrins, HIV test, hepatitis panel, CBC, LFTs, ferritin level; Histopathology: subepidermal bulla with festooning of dermis, very scant inflammatory infiltrate, pink globules in epidermis termed 'caterpillar bodies'; DIF: IgG and C3 around dermal vessels and some at BMZ

Associated systemic disease associated with hepatitis C virus, HIV, alcoholism, high estrogen states and iron overload states (renal failure, hemochromatosis)

Treatment pearls phlebotomy, no alcohol, avoid estrogens, treat any underlying disease, low dose hydroxychloroquine (Plaquenil)

COMMON DRUGS THAT UNMASK OR AGGRAVATE PCT

- Alcohol*
- Barbiturates
- Chlorinated hydrocarbons (including hexachlorobenzene)
- Estrogens (including OCPs)*
- Griseofulvin
- Iron*
- Nalidixic acid
- NSAIDs
- Phenytoin
- Rifampin
- Sulfa drugs
- Tetracyclines

* Indicates the most common.

Pseudoporphyria

Description large tense bulla that may progress to erosions with crust
Location sun-exposed areas, especially dorsal hands, face and scalp
Characteristics adults, resolves with discontinuation of offending drug
Tests normal urine porphyrins; Histopathology: subepidermal bulla, necrotic keratinocytes, lymphocytic infiltrate
Associated systemic disease none
Treatment pearls discontinuation of drug, sunscreen, topical corticosteroids

PSEUDOPORPHYRIA-CAUSING DRUGS

- Amiodarone
- Barbiturates
- Dapsone
- Diuretics (including furosemide, bumetanide and thiazides)*
- Estrogens (including OCPs)*
- Griseofulvin
- Nalidixic acid
- NSAIDs (especially naproxen)*
- Pyridoxine
- Sulfonamides and sulfonylureas
- Tetracycline

* Indicates the most common.

Epidermolysis bullosa acquisita (EBA)

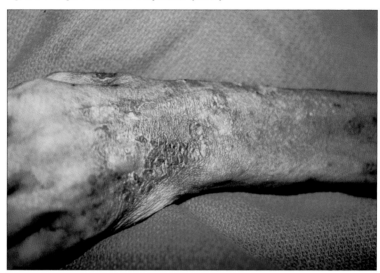

Description non-inflammatory tense bullae that progress to areas of scarring with milia; can be deforming

Location acral and extensor surfaces (sites of trauma), rarely involves mucous membranes

Characteristics any age, increased incidence in Asians and African–Americans, chronic course, autoimmune, may be exacerbated by furosemide [frusemide], tetracycline, nalidixic acid

Tests +pathergy; Histopathology: subepidermal bullae, commonly very mild mixed infiltrate; DIF: IgG at BMZ, IIF +50%

Associated systemic disease inflammatory bowel disease, SLE, RA, dermatomyositis, hematologic malignancies

Treatment pearls often minimal response to therapy; oral and topical corticosteroids, azathioprine, methotrexate, cyclophosphamide, colchicine, dapsone, cyclosporine, IVIG

Contact/irritant dermatitis
See page 189

Photoallergic reaction
See page 423

Polymorphous light eruption (PMLE)
See page 422

Bullous impetigo
See page 121, Impetigo

Bullous bite reaction
See page 120, Bites

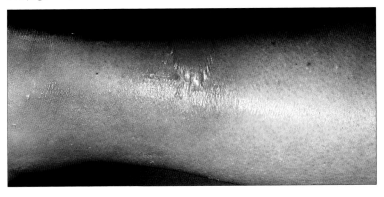

Plant dermatitis (Rhus)
See page 123

Bullous lichen planus

Bullous systemic lupus erythematosus (SLE)

Drug reaction

Hand, foot and mouth disease – Coxsackie virus

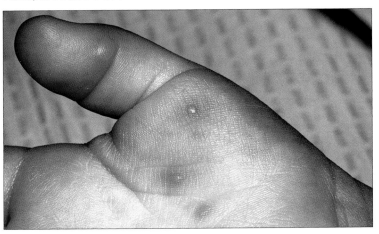

Staphylococcal scalded skin syndrome

Bullous tinea (dermatophytosis)

Herpes simplex virus (herpetic whitlow) or herpes zoster virus

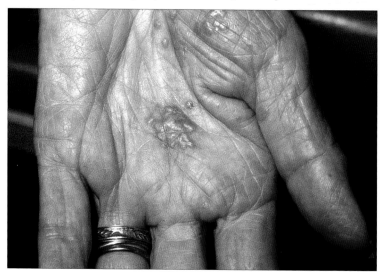

Scabies

Sweet's syndrome

Burn

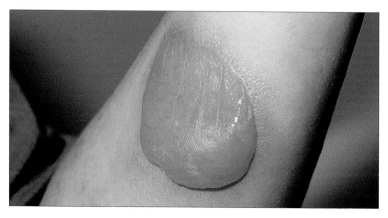

Stevens–Johnson syndrome (SJS)/toxic epidermal necrolysis (TEN)

Bullous pemphigoid

Erythema elevatum diutinum (EED)
See page 16 – Acral

Id reaction

Erythema multiforme

Synovial cyst

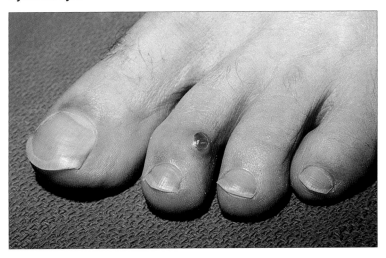

ACRAL ECZEMATOUS DERMATOSES

See page 189, Hand dermatitis

ACRAL EXFOLIATION

See page 163, Exfoliative dermatitis – acral

ACRAL PAPULES AND PLAQUES

Bites

See page 120

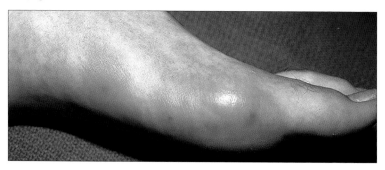

Scabies

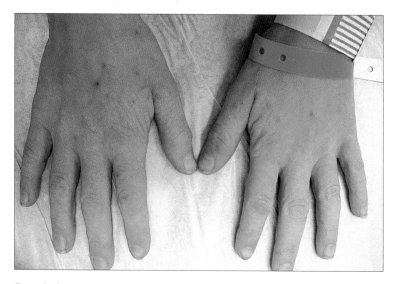

Description erythematous papules, pustules or bullae with surrounding erythema ± crust, ± linear tiny thread-like burrows extending from papules
Location papules usually clustered in groups, in web spaces of digits, on flexor wrists, axillae, around waist, buttocks, genital area, or diffusely over body; can present as scaly, crusted palms

Characteristics resolves with treatment, intense pruritus, ± pain
Tests mineral oil smear of vesicle/papule to see scabies mite, eggs or scybala (feces); Histopathology: parts of scabies mite can often be seen within the stratum corneum, perivascular infiltrate with interstitial eosinophils, +spongiosis, ± papillary dermal edema
Associated systemic disease none
Treatment pearls orally: ivermectin; topically: permethrin, sulfur ointment or lindane (*note:* lindane has been discontinued in some countries and states)

Foreign body reaction
See page 183

Lichen planus
See page 259

Lichen nitidus
See page 386

Granuloma annulare
See page 87

Pustular psoriasis
See page 58

Squamous cell carcinoma
See page 367

Basal cell carcinoma
See page 366

Melanoma
See page 380

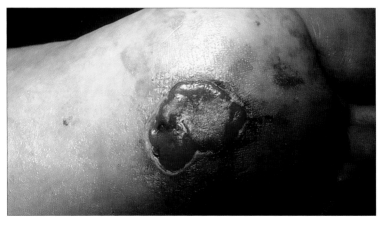

Dermatomyositis

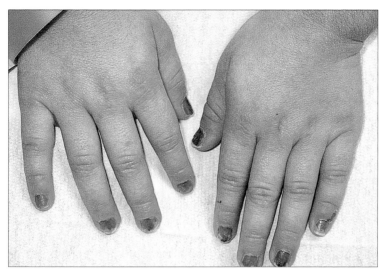

Acrodermatitis enteropathica

Gianotti–Crosti syndrome

Eccrine poroma

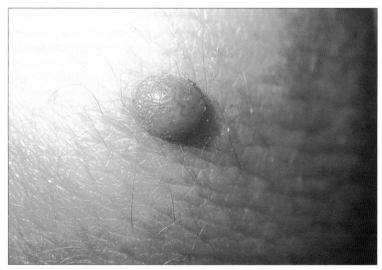

Vaccinia

Molluscum contagiosum

Parvovirus B19 (erythrovirus) (papular–purpuric gloves and socks syndrome)

Herpes simplex virus/herpes zoster virus
See page 50

Anthrax

Acrodermatitis continua of Hallopeau

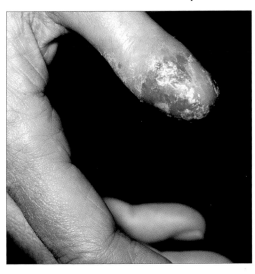

Perforating disorders
Kyrle's disease
Reactive perforating collagenosis

Elastosis perforans serpiginosa

Drug reaction

Pityriasis lichenoides et varioliformis acuta (PLEVA)

Erythema multiforme

Eruptive xanthomas

Acral angiodermatitis

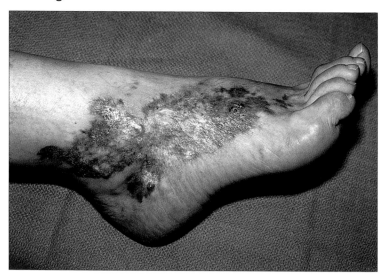

Bywater's lesions (rheumatoid arthritis)

Elephantiasis nostra verrucosa

Vasculitis

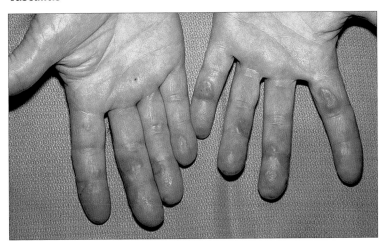

Sarcoid

ACRAL PUSTULES
Dyshidrosis

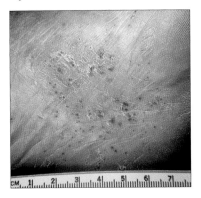

Description deep-seated vesicles on erythematous base
Location lateral fingers, palms and soles
Characteristics chronic, waxes and wanes, pruritic, exacerbated by heat and irritants
Tests Histopathology: acute spongiotic dermatitis
Associated systemic disease none
Treatment pearls topical corticosteroids, UVA, immunosuppressives if very severe and resistant to other therapies

Pustular psoriasis

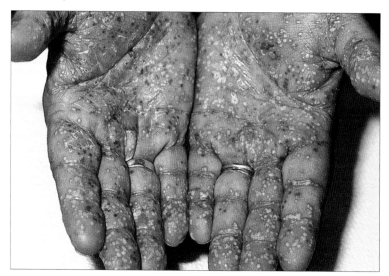

Description deep-seated pustules on an erythematous base with scale
Location can occur diffusely, but more common symmetrically on palms and soles only
Characteristics middle-age onset typical, chronic, may be exacerbated by stress, cigarette smoking and drugs such as lithium
Tests +nail involvement; Histopathology: parakeratosis, acanthosis, neutrophilic pustules within stratum corneum and epidermis
Associated systemic disease none
Treatment pearls topical corticosteroids, oral retinoids, light therapy

Palmoplantar pustulosis

Acropustulosis of infancy

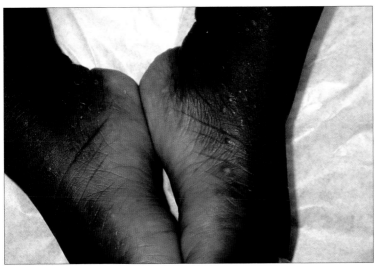

Acrodermatitis continua of Hallopeau
See page 55

Bacterial infection

Tinea (dermatophytosis)

Scabies

Orf

Milker's nodules

Secondary syphilis

Gonoccocemia

ACRAL TUMORS

Verruca vulgaris, verruca planae (wart)

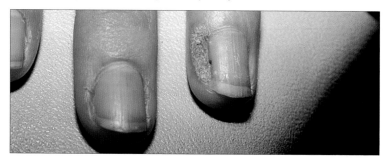

Description verrucous, hyperkeratotic, flat-topped papules
Location anywhere (periungual, fingers, palms, soles)
Characteristics any age, may spontaneously resolve in a child, usually chronic in an adult, asymptomatic
Tests pare with blade to note 'black dots' and disruption of dermatoglyphics unlike a callous; Histopathology: compact hyperkeratosis, papillomatosis, acanthosis, parakeratosis, hypergranulosis, viral inclusions and koilocytic changes in epidermal cells, increased capillaries in dermal papilla
Associated systemic disease may be associated with immunosuppression (HIV, transplant patients)
Treatment pearls cryotherapy, podophyllin, salicylic acid, topical imiquimod, intralesional bleomycin, intralesional antigen therapy, laser, oral cimetidine

Mucous cyst

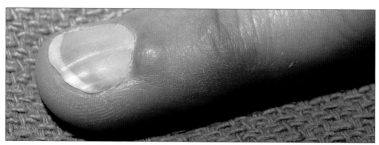

Description skin-colored to pink or blue soft papule, can appear somewhat translucent
Location distal digits often near proximal nail fold or may overlie joints (fingers>toes)
Characteristics female>male, middle-aged, asymptomatic
Tests stringy, clear, mucinous discharge if punctured, may have depressed nail plate distal to cyst; Histopathology: clefts/sparse areas in dermis that stain for mucin
Associated systemic disease osteoarthritis
Treatment pearls no treatment necessary, initial draining may not cure as often cysts are connected to joint space, can try intralesional corticosteroids or repeated incision and drainage

Acquired digital fibroma (acral fibrokeratoma)

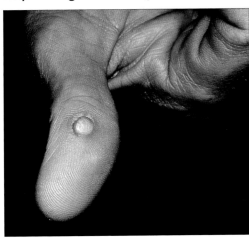

Description skin-colored to pink, firm, solitary papule surrounded by hyperkeratotic, elevated skin
Location any digit (fingers>toes), can be differentiated from supernumerary digits which usually occur on ulnar side of fifth digit
Characteristics middle-aged adults, asymptomatic
Tests Histopathology: thick collagen bundles and vertically oriented blood vessels in the dermis (no nerves in papule as seen in supernumerary digit)
Associated systemic disease none
Treatment pearls no treatment necessary, shave excision

Foreign body
Description erythematous to brown inflamed papule
Location usually occurs at exposed sites
Characteristics asymptomatic or tender
Tests Histopathology: granulomatous inflammation with 'foreign body' giant cells
Associated systemic disease none
Treatment pearls removal of foreign body if possible, intralesional kenalog injection

Pyogenic granuloma
See page 372

Dermatofibroma
See page 381

Molluscum contagiosum
See page 355

Keratoacanthoma

Cutaneous horn

Periungual fibroma (angiofibroma)

Leiomyoma

Hemangioma

Neuroma

Glomus tumor

Exostosis

Supernumerary digit

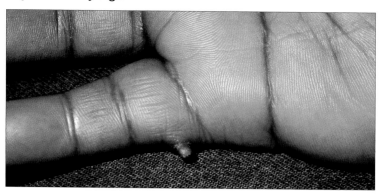

Neurofibroma

Keloid

Dermatofibrosarcoma protuberans (DFSP)

Neurofibrosarcoma

Orf

Milker's nodule

ACUTELY ILL, RASH AND FEVER – MORBILLIFORM (MACULES AND PAPULES)

Drug reaction
See page 286

Stevens–Johnson syndrome (SJS, erythema multiforme major)
See page 64

Erythema multiforme (erythema multiforme minor)
See page 484

Varicella (chicken pox)
See page 67

Meningococcemia
See page 289

Scarlet fever

Enterovirus – echo, Coxsackie

Early Rocky Mountain spotted fever (RMSF)

Parvovirus B19 (erythrovirus) (erythema infectiosum – Fifth disease)

Measles (rubeola)

German measles (rubella)

Toxic shock syndrome

Secondary syphilis (lues)

Endemic typhus

Erythema marginatum (Strep)

Typhoid fever (epidemic)

Leptospirosis

Toxoplasmosis – acquired

Systemic lupus erythematosus (SLE)

'Serum sickness' (wheals)

Dermatomyositis

Pityriasis rosea

ACUTELY ILL, RASH AND FEVER – PURPURA

Drug reaction
See page 286

Bacteremia
Meningococcemia (see p. 289)
Gonococcemia
Staphylococcemia
Pseudomonas bacteremia

Viral (enterovirus)
Echovirus
Coxsackie virus

Rickettsial diseases
Rocky Mountain spotted fever (RMSF) (see p. 291)
Endemic typhus
Epidemic typhus

Vasculitis

ACUTELY ILL, RASH AND FEVER – VESICLES, BULLAE OR PUSTULES

Drug reaction
See page 286

Stevens–Johnson syndrome (SJS, erythema multiforme major)

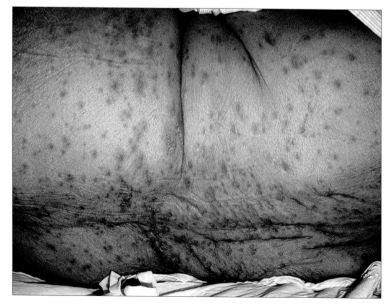

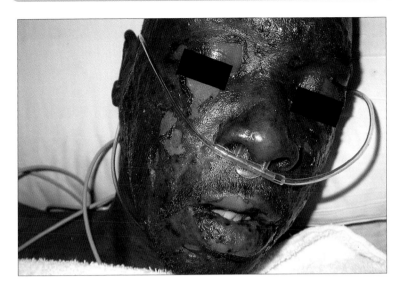

Stevens–Johnson syndrome

Description targetoid erythematous and/or purpuric macules and papules that may progress to bullae, erosions and ulcerations

Location dorsal hands, palms and soles, two or more mucosal surfaces involved and diffusely over body

Characteristics prodrome of fever and respiratory symptoms followed by abrupt onset of painful lesions in adults as well as children, +LAD, +hepatosplenomegaly, +history of drug (NSAIDs, TCN, penicillin, sulfa, anticonvulsants), possible HSV association, long disease course lasting several weeks

Tests elevated ESR, ± elevated LFTs, leukopenia or leukocytosis, anemia, eosinophilia, proteinuria; Histopathology: epidermal necrosis with necrotic keratinocytes, little inflammatory response, ± bulla

Associated systemic disease increased incidence in HIV population

Treatment pearls discontinue drug, supportive care, ± oral corticosteroids, IVIG if severe

Toxic epidermal necrolysis (TEN)

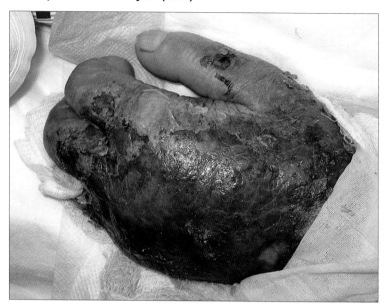

Description erythematous, dusky patches that rapidly progress to large bullae and then to large areas of erosion as skin sloughs

Location entire body including mucosal surfaces (most often oral and conjunctival)

Characteristics female>male, increased incidence with age, HIV+; painful skin and oral mucosa, dysphagia, fever and malaise can precede other findings, can be complicated by sepsis, usually occurs in first 1–3 weeks after starting the new drug

Tests Nikolsky sign+; Histopathology: subepidermal bulla with necrosis of entire epidermis and a mild lymphocytic inflammatory infiltrate

Associated systemic disease none

Treatment pearls discontinue offending drug immediately (commonly sulfa drugs, antibiotics, anticonvulsants, NSAIDs and allopurinol), supportive care in a burn unit, ± IVIG (controversial), systemic corticosteroids are *not* recommended, mortality may approach 35%

Varicella (chicken pox)

Varicella

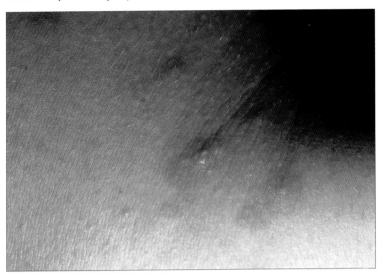

Description pink macules that progress to 'dewdrop' vesicles on an erythematous base
Location starts on trunk, face and oral mucosa and progresses to extremities
Characteristics abrupt onset, recurrent crops for a few days, associated with prodromal malaise, fever, headache, lesions resolve spontaneously in 2 weeks sometimes with scarring; can be associated with pneumonitis or meningitis as a complication or with secondary systemic bacterial infections
Tests Tzanck smear from vesicle to see multinucleate giant cells with viral inclusions, DFA, viral culture; Histopathology: ballooning degeneration of epidermal cells, multinucleate cells within epidermis with viral inclusions, molding of nuclei and marginization of chromatin
Associated systemic disease none
Treatment pearls supportive care, oral antivirals, I.V. acyclovir if started within 24 h of eruption in immunosuppressed

Herpes zoster

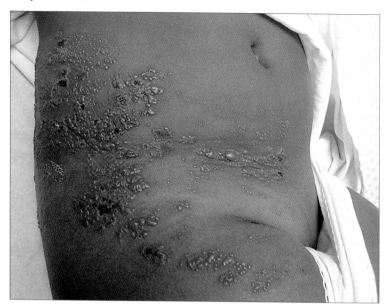

Description linear grouped erythematous vesicles with many erosions

Location eruption occurs within a sensory dermatome and does not usually cross midline unless disseminated

Characteristics prodrome of tingling, pain and pruritus; resolves in weeks, may be associated with chronic pain (postherpetic neuralgia) and may be more severe in elderly

Tests DFA, Tzanck smear, VZV is difficult to culture; Histopathology: epidermal cells with viral inclusions, multinucleate epidermal cells with marginization of chromatin and molding of nuclei and ballooning degeneration of epidermis

Associated systemic disease may be associated with immunosuppression (HIV, transplant patients)

Treatment pearls antivirals (higher dose for zoster) within 72 h of onset, gabapentin for patients with severe pain

Herpes simplex (disseminated)

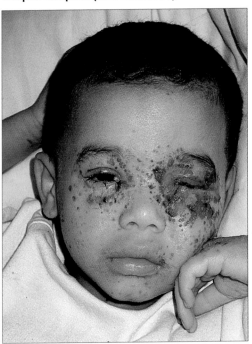

Herpes simplex

Description grouped vesicles on an erythematous base with frequent erosions
Location disseminated over body, can affect visceral organs in young children
Characteristics usually in children (newborn to 3 years old), atopics, immunosuppressed
Tests Tzanck smear, DFA, viral culture; Histopathology: epidermal cells with viral inclusions, multinucleate epidermal cells with marginization of chromatin and molding of nuclei, and ballooning degeneration of epidermis
Associated systemic disease immunosuppression, atopic dermatitis, ichthyosis (*see* Kaposi's varicelliform eruption, p. 238)
Treatment pearls I.V. antivirals

Enterovirus (echo; Coxsackie; hand, foot and mouth disease)

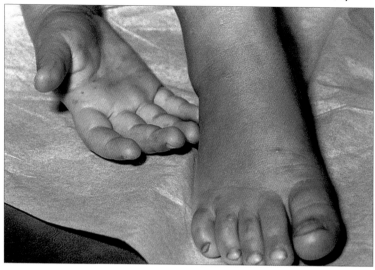

Vaccinia (disseminated)

Variola

Rickettsial pox

Gonoccocemia

Erythema multiforme

ALOPECIA – DIFFUSE

Telogen effluvium

Drug reaction

Anagen effluvium

Trichotillomania

ALOPECIA – LOCALIZED (DISCRETE PATCHES)

Alopecia areata

Tinea capitis

Trichotillomania

Secondary syphilis (lues – alopecia)

ALOPECIA – NON-SCARRING

Androgenetic (male pattern baldness and female pattern baldness)

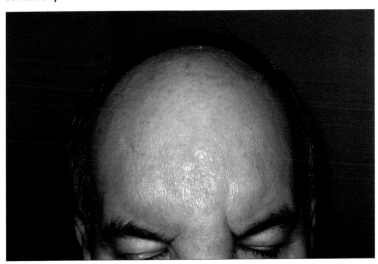

Description thinning hair
Location males: vertex of scalp, frontotemporal and frontoparietal with recession of anterior hairline; females: pattern similar to males or localized loss to top of scalp with widened part width and retention of frontal hair
Characteristics males>females, adults, chronic and progressive, asymptomatic
Tests Histopathology: increased percentage of miniaturized hair follicles, decrease in total number of terminal hair follicles
Associated systemic disease polygenetic inheritance; females: may be associated with hyperandrogenemia, thyroid disease or iron deficiency
Treatment pearls topical minoxidil, oral finasteride, hair transplantation

Telogen effluvium
Description diffuse thinning of hair that falls out with club-shaped root
Location diffusely on scalp
Characteristics usually self-limited and may occur 2–6 months after triggering event (severe illness, stress, rapid weight loss, postpartum, drug exposure, iron deficiency, thyroid disease or others; *see box*) or rarely chronic duration with or without chronic illness
Tests +hair pull test: >6 club hairs when pulling on approximately 40–50 hairs; Histopathology: increased amount of telogen hairs (>15%), no inflammation or scarring
Associated systemic disease may be associated with malignancy, iron deficiency or thyroid disease
Treatment pearls treat underlying disease or avoid triggering event

CAUSES OF TELOGEN EFFLUVIUM

- Fever
- Parturition
- Chronic systemic disease (renal, anemia)
- Emotional or physical stress
- Drugs (ACE inhibitors, allopurinol, amphetamines, anticoagulants, azathioprine, beta-blockers especially propranolol, boric acid mouthwashes, chloroquine, iodides, lithium, methysergide, OCPs, oral retinoids)
- Psychogenic
- Hypothyroidism/hyperthyroidism
- Sudden or severe weight loss
- Discontinuation of oral contraceptive pills
- Hypervitaminosis A
- Iron deficiency
- Cancer chemotherapy (anagen effluvium usually)
- Thallium (anagen effluvium usually)
- Kwashiorkor, marasmus (anagen or telogen effluvium)

Endocrine
Description diffuse thinning of hair with dry, brittle texture
Location diffuse over scalp
Characteristics asymptomatic or pruritic
Tests lab tests: thyroid panel, PTH, calcium, calcitonin, glucose, DHEAS, LH:FSH ratio, total and free testosterone; Histopathology: increase in telogen hairs
Associated systemic disease associated endocrine disorders include hypopituitary, hypo/hyperthyroid, hypoparathyroid, diabetes mellitus, hormonal changes during pregnancy, postpartum or with OCP use
Treatment pearls treat underlying endocrine disorder

Anagen effluvium
Description almost total hair loss, asymptomatic
Location diffuse over scalp
Characteristics resolves when chemotherapeutics stop
Tests clinical diagnosis
Associated systemic disease malignancy treated with chemotherapeutics
Treatment pearls no treatment necessary

Alopecia areata

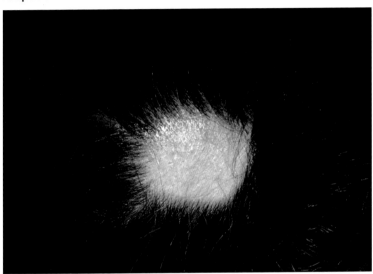

Description solitary or multiple round, well-demarcated bald areas with exclamation hairs at the periphery which may progress to total hair loss
Location usually on scalp but may affect beard, genital or any other non-glabrous skin
Characteristics children to elderly, rapid onset, usually resolves but may be chronic (more likely if prepubertal onset, atopic, +nail changes, ophiasis pattern or universalis loss), asymptomatic or pruritic
Tests may have nail changes (pitting, ridging, onycholysis); Histopathology: lymphocytic infiltrate around the bulb of the hair follicle 'swarm of bees', increased percentage of miniaturized and telogen follicles, ± eosinophils, no scarring
Associated systemic disease can be associated with other autoimmune diseases, postpartum, atopy or Down's syndrome
Treatment pearls oral, intralesional and topical corticosteroids, topical tacrolimus, topical squaric acid, DNCB or anthralin, topical imiquimod, topical minoxidil, PUVA

Traction alopecia

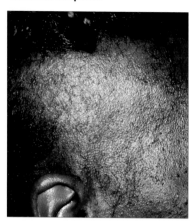

Description patchy areas of hair loss
Location most pronounced in temporal areas of scalp
Characteristics females, children to adults, dark-skinned>light-skinned, chronic, asymptomatic; will worsen with continued traction to the area and may eventually scar
Tests Histopathology: non-scarring to scarring alopecia depending on time course
Associated systemic disease none
Treatment pearls avoid hairstyles that put traction on scalp, topical corticosteroids

Tinea capitis

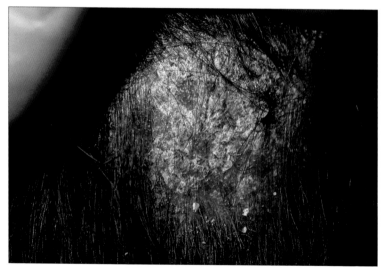

Description well-demarcated erythematous, scaly, crusted patches and plaques with broken off hairs, ± black dots within the patches; can progress to swollen areas that exude pus

Location scalp
Characteristics males>females, children>adults, resolves with treatment, +pruritus
Tests posterior cervical lymphadenopathy, ± green/yellow fluorescence with Wood's light, KOH of pulled hair roots, fungal culture (swab or pulled hairs); Histopathology: fungal elements seen within the epidermis and follicle
Associated systemic disease none
Treatment pearls oral antifungals and adjunct topical antifungals and shampoos, should treat family members with antifungal shampoo

Systemic lupus erythematosus (SLE alopecia)

Description non-scarring diffuse hair thinning with fragile broken hairs, 'lupus hairs', around periphery of scalp (lupus can also cause scarring alopecia – *see below*)
Location diffusely on scalp
Characteristics females>males, young adult to adult onset, chronic, ± pruritus
Tests ANA, anti-ds DNA, anti-Smith; Histopathology: interface change, superficial and deep perivascular and perifollicular lymphocytic infiltrate ± plasma cells, ± follicular plugging, increased mucin
Associated systemic disease SLE patients also at higher risk for alopecia areata
Treatment pearls topical and intralesional corticosteroids, hydroxychloroquine (Plaquenil)

Psoriasis

See page 397

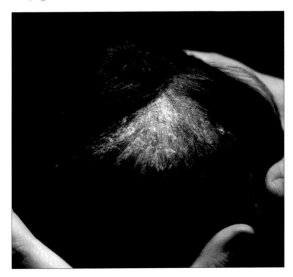

Seborrheic dermatitis
See page 398

Trichotillomania

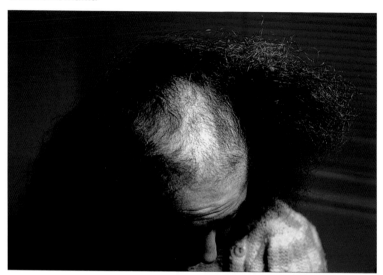

Description areas of hair loss with jagged borders, remaining hairs are broken off at different lengths
Location scalp, eyebrows or any other non-glabrous skin
Characteristics females>males, children>adults, patient pulls or plucks hair themselves, asymptomatic, may be exacerbated by stress
Tests Histopathology: increased percentage of catagen hairs, pigment casts in follicles, hemorrhage
Associated systemic disease depression
Treatment pearls antidepressant, counseling

Secondary syphilis (lues – alopecia)
Description small, scattered hairless areas with irregular borders ± scale, 'moth-eaten'
Location occipital area common but often diffuse over scalp
Characteristics any age, ± local lymphadenopathy
Tests serology: RPR/VDRL and confirmatory MHA-TP/FTA-ABS; Histopathology: lymphocytic and plasma cell perivascular infiltrate with normal epidermis or psoriasiform and lichenoid changes, ± granulomas
Associated systemic disease syphilis is a multisystem infection which can affect the kidneys, brain, GI tract, eyes and joints
Treatment pearls I.M. penicillin G, azithromycin or PCN desensitization if PCN allergic

Chemical/drug
Vitamin A, isotretinoin, acitretin
Methotrexate

Chemotherapy drugs (cytotoxic and antimitotic agents)
Corticosteroids
Thyroid drugs (PTU)
Anticoagulants (heparin)
Bismuth
Thallium
Cholestyramine
Propranolol

Polycystic tumor (virilizing)

Pressure on posterior scalp during intubation or prolonged hospitalization

Nutritional (especially vitamin B$_{12}$ deficiency/pernicious anemia)

Syndromes
Pili torti
Anhidrotic ectodermal dysplasia
Acrodermatitis enteropathica
Myotonic dystrophy
Monilethrix
Rothmund–Thompson syndrome
Werner's syndrome
Netherton's syndrome
Cronkite–Canada syndrome

Loose anagen syndrome

ALOPECIA – SCARRING

Physical/chemical (central centrifugal cicatricial alopecia, hot comb alopecia)

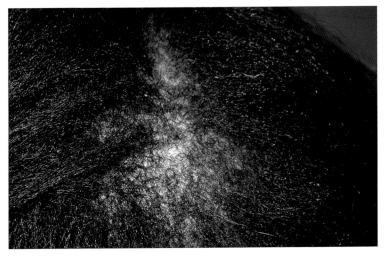

Description small to large areas of white, shiny skin with overlying thinning hair, round or with irregular borders

Location top of scalp progressing onto parietal scalp

Characteristics most common in dark-skinned females, young adult to elderly, slow onset, chronic and progressive, ± pruritus, exacerbated by continued physical trauma

Tests Histopathology: decrease in number of viable follicles leaving fibrous tracts, perifollicular fibrosis and scarring, no inflammatory infiltrate

Associated systemic disease none

Treatment pearls avoid hot irons, perming, relaxing, traction, radiation burns and other trauma

Discoid lupus erythematosus (DLE)

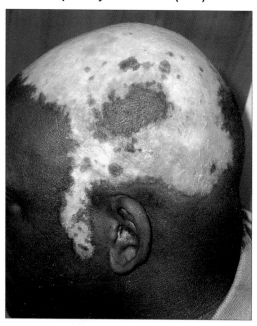

Description well-demarcated, depressed, round areas of pink to white atrophic skin ± surrounding erythema or hyperpigmentation, follicular plugging, ± scarring alopecia of the scalp

Location face, scalp, conchal bowls of ears, other sun-exposed areas

Characteristics females>males, young adult to adult onset, chronic, ± pruritus; 5–10% may progress to systemic lupus erythematosus (SLE)

Tests ± ANA; Histopathology: atrophic epidermis, interface change, superficial and deep perivascular and perifollicular lymphocytic infiltrate ± plasma cells, ± follicular plugging, increased mucin, fibrosis and scarring of follicles

Associated systemic disease SLE in 5–10%, lupus patients also at higher risk for alopecia areata

Treatment pearls daily sunscreen, topical and intralesional corticosteroids, antimalarials, thalidomide

Lichen planopilaris

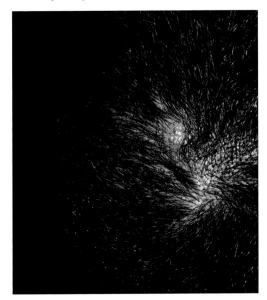

Description pink, hairless scarred areas with irregular borders and with interspersed plugs of normal-appearing hair within the patches, follicular spiny plugs and surrounding erythema
Location frontal scalp common, eyebrows and other non-glabrous skin
Characteristics female>male, adult to elderly onset, can resolve after months to years but scarring is permanent, 50% may also have findings of lichen planus and follicular papules (Graham-Little syndrome)
Tests Histopathology: lichenoid infiltrate with interface change involving the upper portion of follicles, +necrotic keratinocytes, decreased number of viable follicles with perifollicular fibrosis and scarring
Associated systemic disease none
Treatment pearls topical and intralesional corticosteroids, hydroxychloroquine (Plaquenil)

Folliculitis decalvans
Description small pustules, erythema and scale surrounding follicles in areas of scarring alopecia
Location scalp
Characteristics pustules may resolve with treatment, but scarring is permanent, can be recurrent, +pain
Tests bacterial culture; Histopathology: neutrophilic pustules and abscesses within follicles, perifollicular infiltrate of lymphocytes ± plasma cells
Associated systemic disease none
Treatment pearls oral antibiotics, topical corticosteroids

Dissecting cellulitis

Dissecting cellulitis

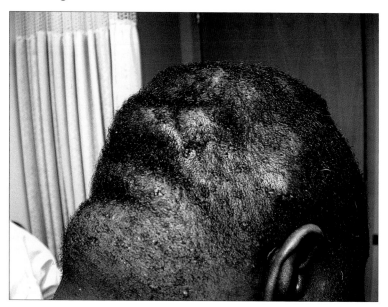

Description erythematous, boggy, inflamed nodules that are connected by sinus tracts, exude pus and progress to areas of scarring hair loss
Location vertex and occiput of scalp most common areas involved
Characteristics dark-skinned males most commonly affected, chronic, severe pain
Tests bacterial culture; Histopathology: dense perifollicular neutrophilic inflammation and abscess formation, ± granulomas, eventual fibrosis and scarring
Associated systemic disease none
Treatment pearls often refractory to treatment, oral antibiotics, intralesional corticosteroids, oral retinoids, surgical excision of severe areas

Infection
Fungus – inflammatory tinea capitis: favus and kerion

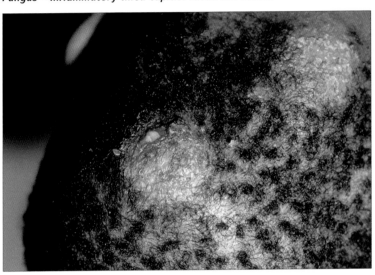

Description *Favus*: malodorous, well-demarcated depressed areas of atrophic alopecia with yellow crust and few 'wiry' hairs; *Kerion*: swollen, boggy areas of alopecia that exude pus and can progress to scarring
Location scalp
Characteristics children>adults; *Favus*: most common in Middle East and Africa, fungal infection resolves with treatment but scarring alopecia is permanent, +pruritus
Tests posterior cervical lymphadenopathy, ± green/yellow fluorescence with Wood's light, KOH of pulled hair roots; fungal culture: swab or pulled hairs; Histopathology: fungal hyphae seen within the epidermis and follicle
Associated systemic disease none
Treatment pearls oral antifungals and adjunct topical antifungals and shampoos, should treat family members with antifungal shampoo, corticosteroids for kerion

Infection

Bacterial
  Pyogenic – carbuncle, furuncle

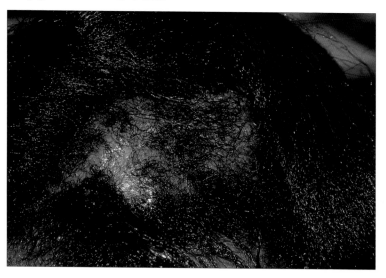

Acne keloidalis nuchae

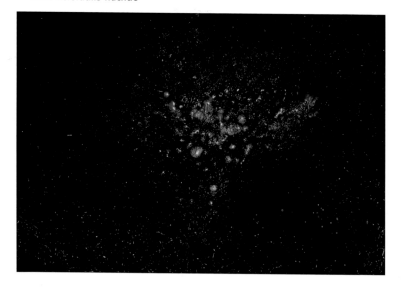

Acne necrotica

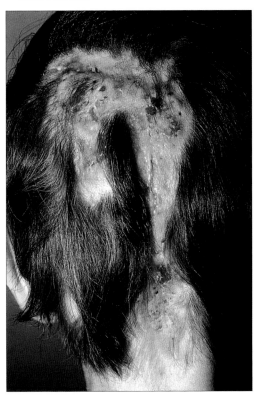

Viral
  Varicella zoster
  Variola
  Varicella
Secondary syphilis (lues)
Atypical mycobacteria
  Tuberculosis
  Leprosy
Yaws
Leishmaniasis

Alopecia mucinosa

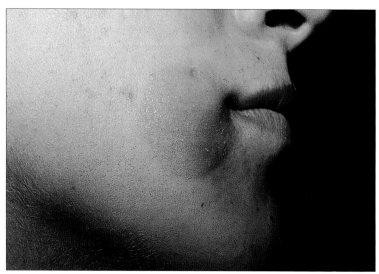

Description solitary or multiple, well-demarcated, erythematous, scaly plaques with follicular prominence ± follicular spiny papules, ± broken off hairs, only scars if severe

Location commonly head and neck or on other non-glabrous skin

Characteristics males>females, children to adult onset, childhood cases usually resolve spontaneously in a few years, adult cases are more chronic, ± pruritus

Tests Histopathology: mucin deposition in follicular epithelium, mixed inflammatory infiltrate, extensive mucin may lead to scarring and follicular destruction

Associated systemic disease up to 30% can progress to cutaneous T-cell lymphoma (CTCL), may be associated with Hodgkin's lymphoma

Treatment pearls oral and topical corticosteroids, dapsone, PUVA

Neoplasm
Basal cell carcinoma
Squamous cell carcinoma
Melanoma
Cutaneous T-cell lymphoma (CTCL)
Lymphoma
Merkel cell
Cutaneous metastases

Developmental
Aplasia cutis

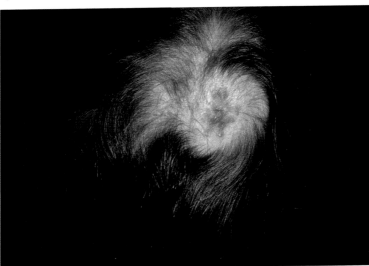

Description solitary, round, hairless 1–5 cm area usually with a surrounding collar of hair, underlying prominent veins and a thin, shiny, membranous covering that progresses with time to a scarred area; may also present as a well-demarcated erosion or ulcer with jagged edge

Location vertex or midline of scalp most common, ± linear arrangement of multiple small lesions, may occur on extremities

Characteristics present at birth, chronic (area will harden and scar with time), asymptomatic

Tests Histopathology: atrophic epidermis, thinning of dermis, loss of adnexa

Associated systemic disease aplasia cutis is a clinical finding with many possible etiologies including fetal ischemia, infection, intrauterine trauma, neural tube defect; can also be associated with Adams–Oliver or Setleis syndrome

Treatment pearls may surgically excise large lesions with imaging first to rule out rare underlying meningeal involvement

Conradi–Hünermann–Happle syndrome
Darier's disease
Epidermal nevi
Ichthyosis
Ichthyosiform erythroderma
Incontinentia pigmenti
Keratosis pilaris atrophicans

Pseudopélade of Brocq is a term used to describe 'burned out', end-stage cicatricial alopecia that can be caused by many entities including hot comb alopecia, lichen planopilaris, SLE/DLE and others.

Tinea corporis

ANGIOKERATOMA-LIKE PAPULES

See page 351, Papules – scaly (angiokeratoma-like)

ANNULAR LESIONS

Tinea corporis (dermatophytosis)

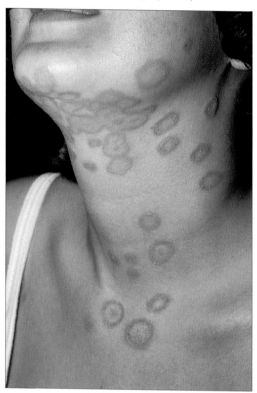

Description annular lesion often with raised, erythematous, scaly border; can be arcuate, circinate or guttate
Location can occur anywhere
Characteristics pruritic
Tests KOH+, fungal culture+; Histopathology: fungal hyphae in stratum corneum
Associated systemic disease none
Treatment pearls topical antifungals, or systemic if diffuse

Granuloma annulare

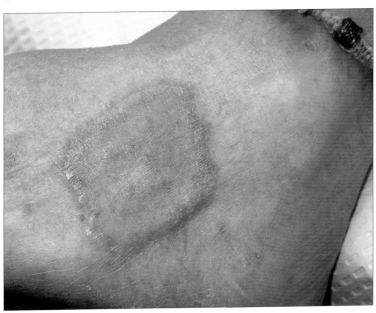

Description annular plaque with raised erythematous border without scale, early and diffuse type lesions can be red papules; deep lesions are subcutaneous skin-colored to red nodules

Location localized (dorsal hands and feet common), generalized (diffuse especially on trunk and proximal extremities), deep (distal legs and arms and scalp), can occur in herpes zoster scars

Characteristics localized form in young adults, generalized form in middle-aged females, deep form in young boys possibly after trauma to the area, usually resolves spontaneously in 2 years but may recur, asymptomatic, rare pruritus

Tests Histopathology: palisading granuloma with degeneration of collagen, +mucin, ± leukocytoclastic vasculitis (LCV) at periphery

Associated systemic disease diabetes, rarely with lymphoma, increased incidence in HIV

Treatment pearls no treatment necessary, biopsy may prompt resolution, topical or intralesional corticosteroids, cryotherapy, excision, dapsone, PUVA, potassium iodide, niacinamide, cyclosporine, antimalarials, systemic retinoids

Urticaria

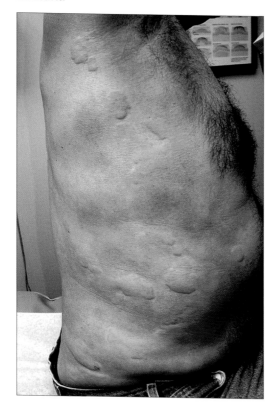

Description erythematous, edematous plaques, some with central clearing, 'wheals/hives'

Location can occur anywhere

Characteristics more common in women, can be triggered by food, drugs, heat, cold, pressure, sunlight, water, infection, or malignancy but most cases idiopathic, lesions last <24 h

Tests Histopathology: normal epidermis, dermal edema, mild perivascular infiltrate with eosinophils

Associated systemic disease none, rarely associated with connective tissue diseases

Treatment pearls daily antihistamines (can combine H_1 and H_2 blockers), leukotriene receptor antagonists, avoid known triggers, biopsy if lesions last >24 h to rule out urticarial vasculitis, workup for chronic vasculitis can include thyroid function, liver enzymes, hepatitis serology, ANA, CBC with differential

Subacute cutaneous lupus erythematosus (SCLE)

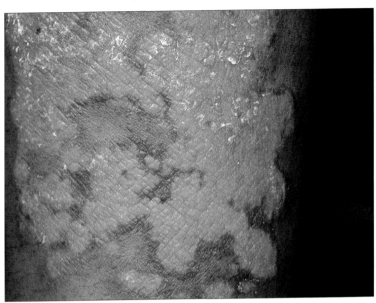

Subacute cutaneous lupus erythematosus

Description polycyclic, erythematous, scaly, annular patches and plaques
Location face, upper chest and back in 'shawl distribution'
Characteristics female predominance, young adult onset, chronic, UV light exacerbates, can be drug induced (*see box*)
Tests ANA+, anti-Ro+; Histopathology: normal epidermis, interface change, superficial and deep perivascular lymphocytic infiltrate, follicular plugging
Associated systemic disease none
Treatment pearls treat with daily sunscreen, antimalarials, topical, intralesional or systemic corticosteroids, thalidomide, discontinue offending drugs

---

COMMON DRUGS THAT CAUSE DRUG-INDUCED SCLE

- ACE inhibitors
- Calcium channel blockers*
- Etanercept
- Griseofulvin
- Hydrochlorothiazide (HCTZ)*
- Interferon-β
- NSAIDs*
- Phenothiazine
- PUVA
- Statins
- Terbinafine

Often Ro antibody positive (SS-A), ± antihistone antibodies.
* Indicates the most common.

Erythema annulare centrifigum

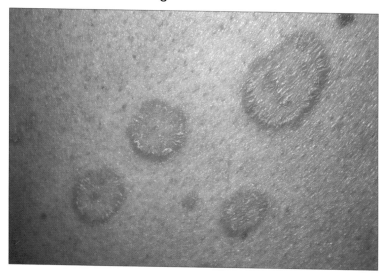

Porokeratosis

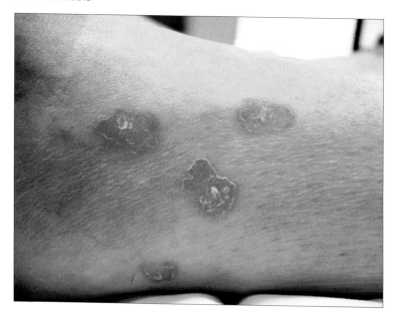

Description disseminated superficial actinic porokeratosis (DSAP): small keratotic papules progress to small, multiple, annular, erythematous patches with

a collarette of scale; porokeratosis of Mibelli (POM): starts as small keratotic papules that progress over years to larger, annular, atrophic plaques surrounded by a raised border with scale ± a depressed groove within the raised border
Location *DSAP*: sun-exposed areas especially legs; *POM*: usually localized to one segment of body often on extremities (dorsal hands and feet), scalp and genital or buccal mucosa
Characteristics *DSAP*: adult female predominance; *POM*: male predominance, early childhood, chronic, rarely progresses to SCC; immunosuppression exacerbates DSAP and POM
Tests monitor for malignant changes; Histopathology: cornoid lamella correlates with collarette of scale seen clinically, hyperkeratosis, mild perivascular infiltrate
Associated systemic disease none
Treatment pearls topical 5-FU, cryotherapy, topical or systemic retinoids

Necrobiosis lipoidica diabeticorum

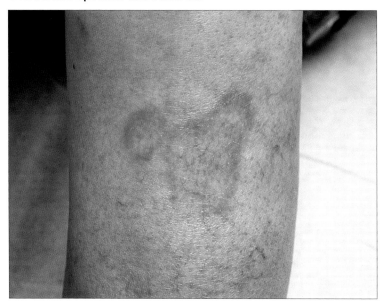

Description yellow, atrophic, annular, indurated plaques with telangiectasias surrounded by violaceous erythema
Location anterior legs most common
Characteristics female predominance, adult onset
Tests Histopathology: dense layers of necrobiosis, fibrosis and granulomas throughout the dermis
Associated systemic disease diabetes
Treatment pearls control diabetes, intralesional or topical corticosteroids, topical retinoids

Erythema multiforme
See page 484

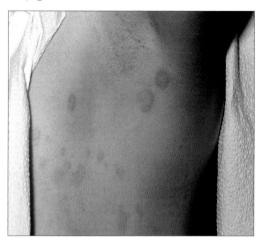

Pityriasis rosea
See page 400

Actinic granuloma

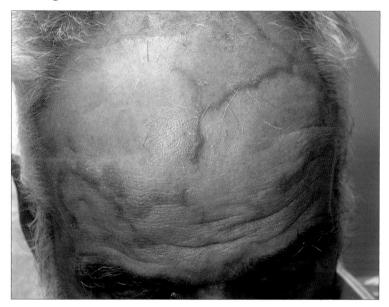

Description large annular erythematous plaque with central atrophy (*some consider this a variant of GA*)

Location sun-exposed areas especially head, neck and dorsal hands
Characteristics female>male, middle-aged adults, resolves in years vs. chronic, asymptomatic
Tests Histopathology: granulomas with elastin within giant cells (elastophagocytosis) absent elastin fibers in the dermis and a sparse lymphocytic infiltrate
Associated systemic disease none
Treatment pearls refractory to treatment, can try PUVA, topical and intralesional corticosteroids

Lichen planus
See page 259

Psoriasis
See page 397

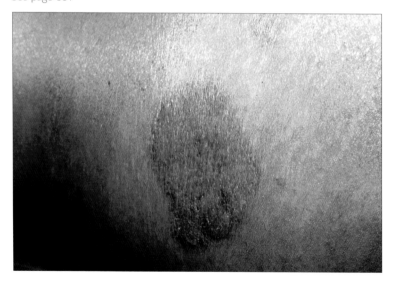

Systemic lupus erythematosus (SLE)
See page 425

Discoid lupus erythematosus (DLE)
See page 78

Sarcoid
See page 443

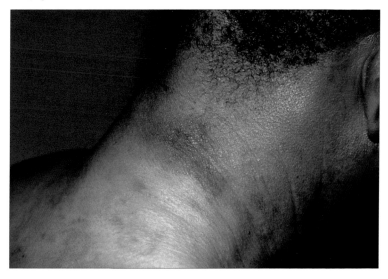

Cutaneous T-cell lymphoma (CTCL)
See page 402

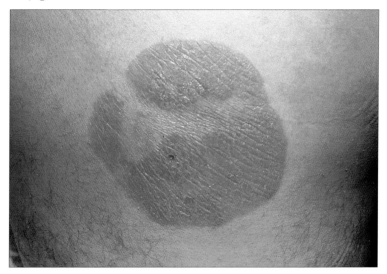

Seborrheic dermatitis
See page 398

Morphea
See page 99

Secondary syphilis (lues)
See page 401

Fixed drug reaction
See page 212

Parapsoriasis

Impetigo
See page 121

Urticarial vasculitis

Erythema chronica migrans (Lyme disease)

Erythema marginatum (Strep)

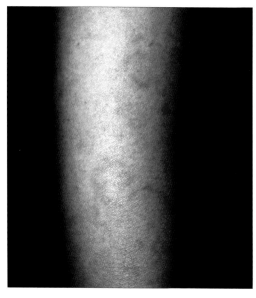

Alopecia mucinosa

Leprosy

Pigmented purpuric eruption (Majocchi's variety)

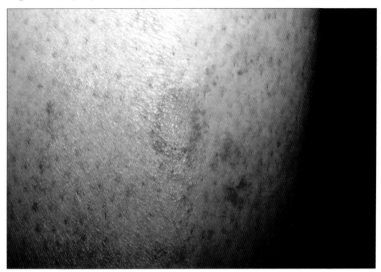

Leishmaniasis

Lupus vulgaris (tuberculosis)

Yaws – tertiary

Subcorneal pustular dermatosis (Sneddon–Wilkinson syndrome)

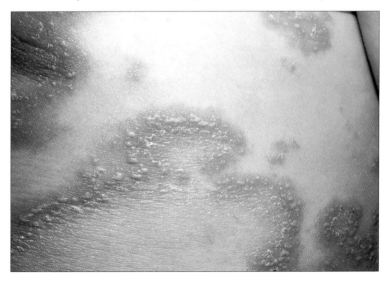

Lymphocytic infiltrate of Jessner

Creeping eruption

Elastosis perforans serpiginosa (EPS)

Sweet's syndrome

Miescher's granuloma

Id reaction

Leukemia/lymphoma cutis

Polymorphous light eruption (PMLE)

Ichthyosis linearis circumflexa

Annular lichenoid dermatosis of youth

ATROPHIC LESIONS
Scar

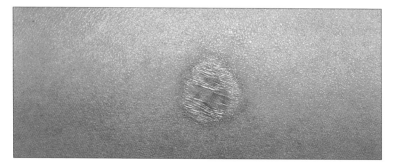

Description pink/violaceous macule or papule usually progresses to white glistening macule or papule with loss of hair
Location in area of previous trauma
Characteristics chronic, asymptomatic
Tests Histopathology: thickened collagen bundles in parallel arrangement, blood vessels can be oriented vertically in the superficial dermis, thin/atrophic epidermis, loss of appendages
Associated systemic disease none
Treatment pearls no treatment necessary

Steroid atrophy

Steroid atrophy (topical or injection)

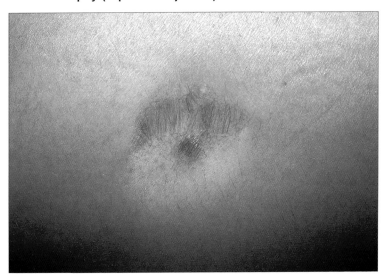

Description thin, white/pink appearing skin with overlying telangiectasias ± a depression if secondary to injected corticosteroids

Location in areas of topical or intralesional corticosteroid use

Characteristics asymptomatic, usually after long-term corticosteroid use, but can occur quickly on the sensitive skin of face, axillae, groin

Tests Histopathology: epidermal atrophy with loss of rete ridges and dilated superficial blood vessels

Associated systemic disease none

Treatment pearls stop corticosteroid use, no treatment is particularly effective after atrophy has occurred

Morphea

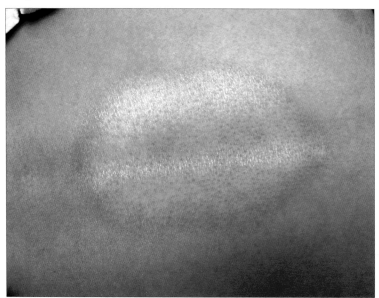

Description skin-colored/pink/light brown/ivory well-demarcated atrophic firm plaque ± telangiectasias and violaceous border, ± follicular prominence

Location asymmetric, can be solitary or diffuse, linear or round, most common on trunk or extremities (en coup de sabre variant occurs midline of scalp extending onto forehead)

Characteristics women>men, any age (linear variant on an extremity most common in first decade of life), may spontaneously resolve in 3–5 years or remain chronic

Tests ± ANA in linear or generalized morphea; Histopathology: normal epidermis, early lesions show perivascular infiltrate with plasma cells, loss of adnexal structures and thickened dermis with increased collagen and with blunt demarcation between dermis and thin subcutaneous fat

Associated systemic disease none (association with *Borrelia burgdorferi* is unlikely)

Treatment pearls topical calcipotriene or oral calcitriol, PUVA or UVA-1 light therapy, physical therapy for linear type extending over a joint to prevent contractures, topical or oral corticosteroids only in early inflammatory phase, methotrexate if severe and rapidly progressive, penicillin, oral retinoids, azithromycin 5-day dose pack once a month

Lichen sclerosus et atrophicus

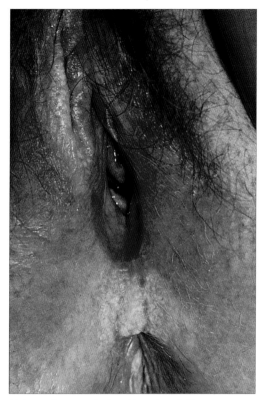

Lichen sclerosus et atrophicus (genital)

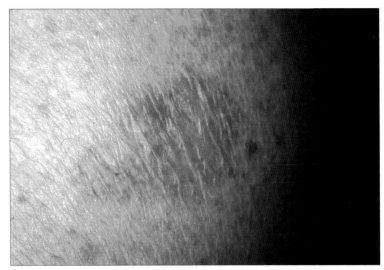

Lichen sclerosus et atrophicus (extragenital)

Lichen sclerosus et atrophicus

Description early blue color progresses to pink/white atrophic macules, ± telangiectasias and follicular plugging
Location primarily in genital mucosa (in females may appear in shape of an hourglass), but can occur in areas of chronic friction extragenitally
Characteristics females>males, any age but peaks bimodally at 8–13 years and 50–60 years, intense pruritus and dryness, may scar the vaginal introitus or lead to phimosis in males
Tests Histopathology: epidermal atrophy with flat epidermal/dermal junction, vacuolar basal layer changes; pink, homogenized collagen and edema of papillary dermis with a band of lymphocytic infiltrate below, loss of elastic fibers
Associated systemic disease none
Treatment pearls high potency topical corticosteroids, topical tacrolimus, PUVA, topical testosterone ointment

Radiation dermatitis

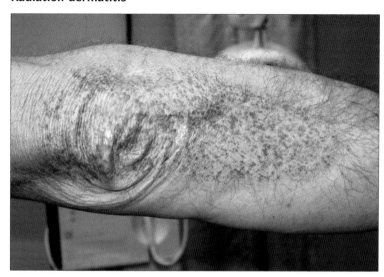

Description hyper- and hypopigmented, pink, mottled atrophic macules ± telangiectasias, ± sclerotic skin, ± ulcerations
Location in the area of previous radiation therapy
Characteristics in patients after radiation therapy, chronic, ± pruritus, ± pain
Tests Histopathology: disordered/irregular epidermis which 'grows around' large, superficial telangiectasias, fibrosis and homogenized collagen in dermis with atypical stellate 'radiation fibroblasts', thick-walled dermal blood vessels; unlike a scar in that skin appendages are present
Associated systemic disease none
Treatment pearls topical corticosteroids

Poikiloderma of Civatte (photoaging)
See page 463

Striae

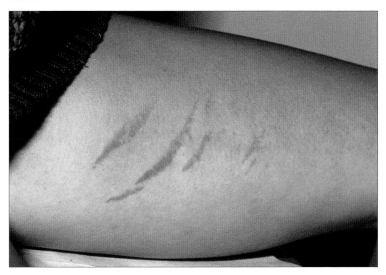

Description linear violaceous macules, depressions or elevations that progress to white/pearly color with time

Location abdomen, flanks/hips, breasts, lumbosacral region and anterior axillary folds most common

Characteristics females>males, light skin>dark skin, any age but common in adolescents after growth spurt, pregnancy or postpartum, or after rapid weight gain; chronic

Tests Histopathology: atrophic (flat) epidermis with loss of rete ridges and appendages

Associated systemic disease can be associated with exogenous or endogenous increases in cortisol

Treatment pearls difficult to treat, can try pulsed dye laser, topical retinoids

Necrobiosis lipoidica diabeticorum (NLD)
See page 91

Morpheaform basal cell carcinoma
See page 366, Basal cell carcinoma

Discoid lupus erythematosus (DLE)
See page 78

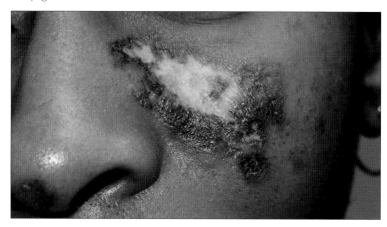

Atrophic lichen planus
See page 259, Lichen planus

Anetoderma (macular atrophy)
See page 108

Atrophoderma of Pasini and Pierini

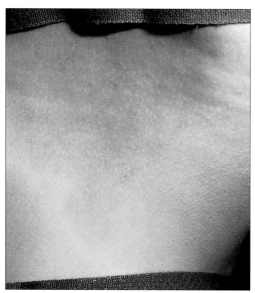

Description single or multiple, small or large skin-colored/light brown, well-demarcated, firm, depressed, atrophic plaque

Location trunk, especially upper back
Characteristics young females, resolves spontaneously in months to years, asymptomatic
Tests Histopathology: thin dermis
Associated systemic disease none
Treatment pearls no effective treatment

Aplasia cutis
See page 85

Sarcoid
See page 443

Secondary syphilis (lues)
See page 401

Involuting infantile hemangioma

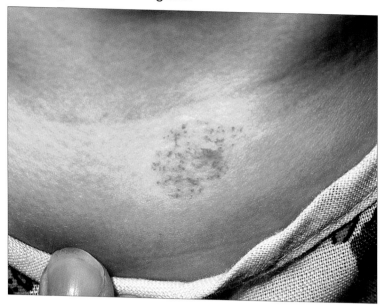

Leprosy

Tuberculosis

Acrodermatitis chronica atrophicans (Lyme disease)

Follicular atrophoderma

Lipoid atrophy

Eosinophilic fasciitis

Focal dermal hypoplasia (Goltz syndrome)

Atrophie blanche

Degos' disease (malignant atrophic papulosis)

ATROPHY WITH CIRCUMSCRIBED PROTRUSION

Scar
See page 97

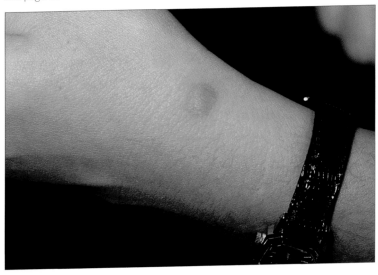

Neurofibroma

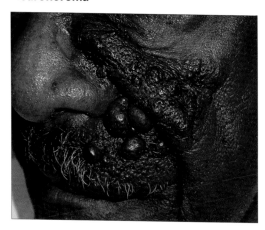

Description can be multiple but more often solitary soft, skin-colored papule; plexiform NF is often larger, subcutaneous nodule with overlying hyperpigmentation
Location can occur anywhere
Characteristics any age, slow growth, chronic, asymptomatic; plexiform NF can undergo malignant transformation
Tests +'buttonhole sign' (can depress neurofibroma into skin); Histopathology: unencapsulated spindle cell proliferation
Associated systemic disease can be associated with neurofibromatosis (usually >6 neurofibromas)
Treatment pearls excision

Nevus lipomatosis
Description groups of small skin-colored to yellow soft papules
Location can occur anywhere but common on hips and thighs ± linear arrangement along skin folds or following Blaschko's lines
Characteristics presents at 0–20 years, chronic, asymptomatic
Tests Histopathology: groups of adipose cells in the dermis among normal skin appendages
Associated systemic disease none
Treatment pearls no treatment necessary, excision

Anetoderma

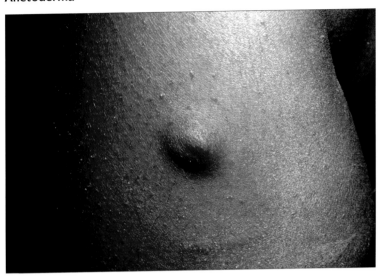

Description pink/brown/skin-colored soft, 'slack', round depressions, macules or elevations
Location trunk and upper extremities most common
Characteristics female>male, peak 15–25 years, asymptomatic, chronic
Tests +'button hole' sign; Histopathology: focal loss of dermal elastic tissue
Associated systemic disease most common primary, but may be secondary to infection, drugs, inflammation or connective tissue disease
Treatment pearls no treatment necessary

Involuting infantile hemangioma

Juvenile elastoma

Connective tissue nevi

Focal dermal hypoplasia (Goltz syndrome)

AXILLARY – PAPULOSQUAMOUS

Contact/irritant dermatitis
See page 189

Inverse psoriasis

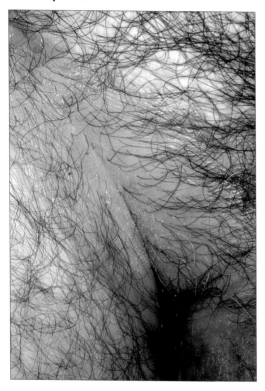

Description moist, erythematous, scaly, well-demarcated patches and plaques of varying size

Location glans penis, groin, axillae, gluteal cleft, inframammary, palms and soles, and/or other flexor or intertriginous areas, ± nail involvement

Characteristics middle-aged onset usually but can occur in infants and children, chronic duration, +Koebner phenomenon, drugs can exacerbate (beta-blockers, lithium, antimalarials, terbinafine, calcium channel blockers, lipid lowering drugs, captopril, glyburide)

Tests Histopathology: parakeratosis, regular acanthosis, small neutrophilic abscesses within epidermis

Associated systemic disease small percentage have associated psoriatic arthritis

Treatment pearls topical tacrolimus/pimecrolimus, topical calcipotriene, low-potency topical corticosteroids

Erythrasma

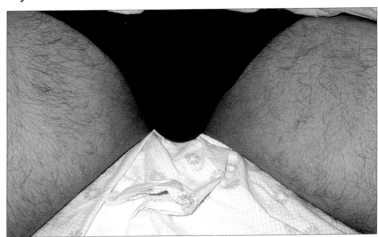

Description brown/red, well-demarcated scaly patches
Location intertriginous areas commonly
Characteristics adults>children, resolves with treatment of *Corynebacterium minutissimum*, asymptomatic vs. mildly pruritic, exacerbated by warm temperature, diabetes, humidity, hyperhidrosis, obesity
Tests fluoresces coral red with Wood's light, gram stain of scale, bacterial culture; Histopathology: numerous gram+ rods seen within the stratum corneum
Associated systemic disease none
Treatment pearls antibacterial soaps, avoid moistness, topical or oral antibiotics such as clindamycin or erythromycin

Pityriasis rosea
See page 400

Tinea versicolor
See page 225

Seborrheic dermatitis
See page 398

AXILLARY – PLAQUES
Acanthosis nigricans

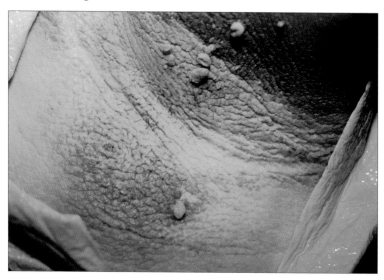

Description hyperpigmented, 'velvety' papules and plaques
Location face, neck, axillae, inguinal/medial thighs, flexor surfaces and palms and lips in malignancy-associated cases
Characteristics rare familial type present at birth, most common after puberty or in adults
Tests Histopathology: papillomatosis, hyperkeratosis, mild hyperpigmentation of basal layer
Associated systemic disease may be idiopathic or associated with obesity, diabetes and other endocrine disorders; drugs (niacinamide, OCPs, glucocorticoids); renal transplant patients; and less likely malignancy (adenocarcinoma)
Treatment pearls treatment of underlying disease, can try keratolytics or topical retinoids

Lichen simplex chronicus (LSC)
See page 201

Contact/irritant dermatitis
See page 189

Fox–Fordyce disease (apocrine miliaria)

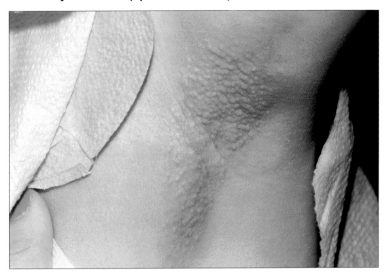

Description skin-colored, follicular papules
Location symmetric in axillae, perineum and areolar regions
Characteristics young females, chronic with possible remission after menopause, extremely pruritic, warm weather may exacerbate, OCPs and pregnancy may improve papules
Tests Histopathology: keratin plug in the duct of the apocrine gland near the follicular ostia with rupture of the duct inducing an inflammatory response
Associated systemic disease none
Treatment pearls OCPs, topical or intralesional kenalog, topical or oral retinoids, topical antibiotics

Hailey–Hailey disease (familial benign pemphigus)

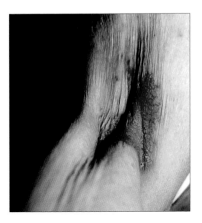

Description vesicles that rupture easily leading to odiferous macerated erythematous patches that often appear vegetative (elevated, fissured and 'velvety') over time
Location axillae, groin, neck, flexor/intertriginous surfaces
Characteristics AD inheritance (defect ATPase 2C1), onset late teens to twenties, chronic but often improves with age, waxes and wanes, worse in warm weather, lesions frequently become secondarily infected, longitudinal leukonychia of nails
Tests Histopathology: intraepidermal vesicles with acantholysis; 'dilapidated brick wall', suprabasilar split, ± dyskeratotic cells, DIF and IIF negative
Associated systemic disease none
Treatment pearls systemic and topical antibiotics, dermabrasion, CO_2 laser, excision with grafts, cyclosporine, dapsone, oral retinoids do not typically help

Pemphigus vegetans
Description flaccid bullae or pustules (Hallopeau type) that erode easily to form macerated vegetative lesions with circinate borders
Location intertriginous, periumbilical, oral and genital mucosa
Characteristics lesions are painful and can be associated with cerebriform changes of the tongue
Tests Histopathology: marked epidermal hyperplasia, suprabasilar split of epidermis, ± intraepidermal eosinophilic abscesses, +DIF: intercellular IgG
Associated systemic disease none
Treatment pearls topical silvadene, topical corticosteroids, oral corticosteroids, azathioprine, cyclophosphamide, methotrexate, mycophenolate mofetil

Epidermal nevus
See page 263

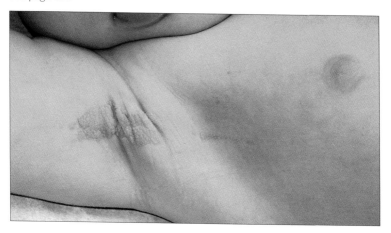

Axillary granular parakeratosis

Description brown/red 'dirty-looking' papules and plaques ± maceration

Location bilateral axillae most commonly, can occur unilaterally and in other intertriginous sites

Characteristics female>male, older adults, spontaneous resolution vs. chronic relapsing and remitting course, pruritic, warm temperature may exacerbate

Tests Histopathology: hyperkeratosis, keratohyaline granules within parakeratosis

Associated systemic disease none

Treatment pearls topical corticosteroids, cryotherapy, oral retinoids, liquid nitrogen, antifungals

Paget's disease
See page 322

Nevus sebaceus (organoid nevus)
See page 494

Pseudoxanthoma elasticum (PXE)
See page 387

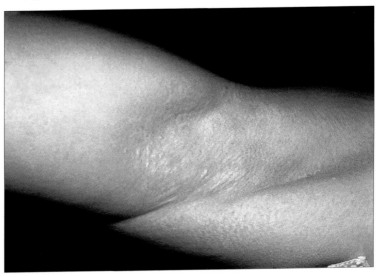

Leukemia/lymphoma cutis
See page 445

Cutaneous T-cell lymphoma (CTCL)
See page 402

Sarcoid
See page 443

Pyoderma vegetans

AXILLARY – RETICULATED
Acanthosis nigricans

Dowling–Degos' disease

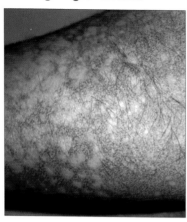

Confluent and reticulated papillomatosis of Gougerot and Carteaud (CARP)

AXILLARY HAIR CHANGES
Trichomycosis axillaris (*Corynebacterium tenuis*)
Description 1–2 mm beaded nodules along the hair shaft ranging in color from yellow, to red, to black
Location axillary or pubic hairs
Characteristics associated with hyperhidrosis and yellow color of the axillary skin
Tests culture Corynebacteria
Associated systemic disease none
Treatment pearls topical antibiotics, shave the affected area

BALANITIS
Trauma (irritant or contact)
Description erythematous patches ± erosion
Location glans penis, usually spares skin crevices
Characteristics males, any age, self-limited
Tests Histopathology: +spongiosis, lymphocytic infiltrate ± eosinophils
Associated systemic disease none
Treatment pearls topical antibiotics, low-potency topical corticosteroids

Candidiasis (balanitis)

Description erythematous, moist (± eroded) patches surrounded by scale and satellite pinpoint papules and pustules, ± fissures
Location glans penis, can extend onto scrotum and inguinal areas including skin crevices
Characteristics male, infant to elderly, more common if uncircumcised, +pain, ± pruritus, exacerbated by moist environment (wet diapers, incontinence), diabetes, immunosuppression or oral antibiotics
Tests fungal culture by scraping area, KOH+ with pseudohyphae and budding yeast
Associated systemic disease topical antifungals (or oral antifungals if severe)

Seborrheic dermatitis

See page 398

Herpes simplex virus (HSV)

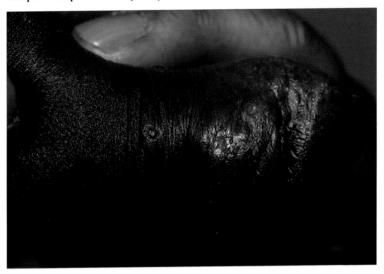

Description small, grouped vesicles on an erythematous base with frequent shallow erosions with scalloped, irregular borders
Location oral, nasal and/or genital mucosa and contiguous skin (can also be disseminated)
Characteristics any age, resolves in 1–2 weeks, +prodrome of pain and burning, exacerbated by stress
Tests Tzanck smear, DFA, viral culture, serology usually not helpful; Histopathology: viral inclusions, multinucleate cells in epidermis, ballooning degeneration leading to intraepidermal vesicle
Associated systemic disease immunosuppression
Treatment pearls oral and topical antivirals started promptly

Inverse psoriasis
See page 109

Lichen planus
See page 259

Plasma cell balanitis (Zoon's balanitis)
Description well-demarcated, moist, erythematous patch with speckled appearance
Location glans penis and prepuce
Characteristics males, middle-aged to elderly onset, occurs in uncircumcised men, asymptomatic vs. pruritic and painful
Tests Histopathology: atrophic epidermis, lichenoid infiltrate with plasma cells, RBC extravasation, hemosiderin deposition and dilated blood vessels
Associated systemic disease none
Treatment pearls circumcision, topical corticosteroids

Erythema multiforme
See page 484

Fixed drug reaction
See page 212

Primary syphilis (chancre)

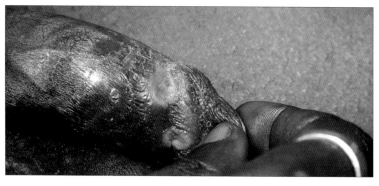

Description solitary erythematous papule that progresses to a larger firm papule with an ulcerated center (chancre)
Location genital most common, can occur on oral mucosa
Characteristics any age, painless, local lymphadenopathy, occurs 2–6 weeks after infection and spontaneously resolves over 1–4 months or faster with treatment
Tests serology: RPR/VDRL and confirmatory MHA-TP/FTA-ABS; Histopathology: ulcer surrounded by lymphocytic and plasma cell infiltrate, endothelial swelling, can stain for spirochetes in primary lesions with Warthin–Starry
Associated systemic disease syphilis is a multisystem infection which can affect the kidneys, brain, GI tract, eyes and joints
Treatment pearls I.M. penicillin G, azithromycin or PCN desensitization if PCN allergic

Secondary syphilis (lues)
See page 401

Behçet's syndrome
See page 328

Cicatricial pemphigoid
See page 128

Erythroplasia of Queyrat
Description well-demarcated, moist, erythematous plaque
Location glans penis
Characteristics male, elderly, usually uncircumcised, progressive to aggressive SCC, asymptomatic
Tests Histopathology: squamous cell carcinoma in situ
Associated systemic disease none
Treatment pearls excision, imiquimod, topical 5-FU

Lichen sclerosus et atrophicus
See page 100

BULLA/VESICLES – ACRAL

See page 45, Acral bulla

BULLA/VESICLES – INFANCY

Impetigo
See page 121

Staphylococcal scalded skin syndrome
See page 156

Herpes simplex virus (HSV)
See page 116

Contact dermatitis

Acrodermatitis enteropathica
See page 151

Bullous congenital ichthyosiform erythroderma (epidermolytic hyperkeratosis)

Congenital porphyria

Congenital syphilis

Epidermolysis bullosa

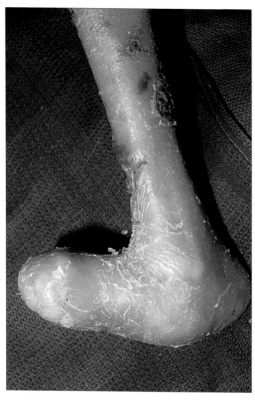

Incontinentia pigmenti

Reiter's syndrome

Toxic epidermal necrolysis (TEN)

Juvenile bullous pemphigoid

Mastocytosis (urticaria pigmentosa)

Epidermolysis bullosa • Incontinentia pigmenti • Reiter's syndrome • Toxic epidermal necrolysis • Juvenile bullous pemphigoid

Bites

BULLA/VESICLES – CHILDHOOD

Bites (papular urticaria)

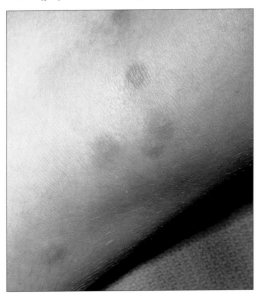

Description red papules pustules or bullae with surrounding erythema ± crust
Location usually grouped on extremities, can occur anywhere
Characteristics children>adults, resolves spontaneously, +pruritus, ± pain
Tests Histopathology: wedge-shaped, usually dense superficial and deep
perivascular infiltrate with interstitial eosinophils, +spongiosis, ± papillary dermal
edema
Associated systemic disease none
Treatment pearls insect repellent, symptomatic treatment: antihistamines,
topical corticosteroids ± topical antibiotics

Impetigo

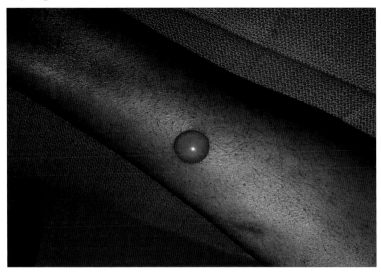

Description erythematous vesicles/bullae that can progress to pustules and then erosions with 'honey-colored' crust (see p. 8 – Crust)
Location common on face, hands and trunk
Characteristics young children>adults, bullous type common in neonates
Tests swab for bacterial culture; Histopathology: subcorneal neutrophils, lymphocytic infiltrate around the superficial portion of the follicle
Associated systemic disease none
Treatment pearls oral antibiotics, topical mupirocin

Varicella (chicken pox)
See page 67

Herpes simplex virus (HSV)
See page 116

Hand, foot and mouth disease (Coxsackie virus)
See page 49

Bullous tinea (dermatophytosis)

Trauma

Erythema multiforme

Bullous drug reaction

Linear IgA disease (chronic bullous disease of childhood)

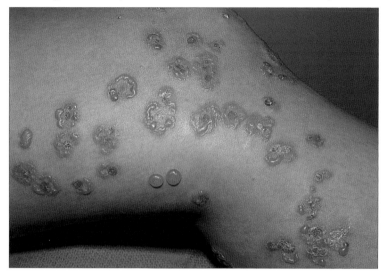

Epidermolysis bullosa

Mastocytosis (urticaria pigmentosa)

Cantharone-induced bulla

Hydroa vacciforme

Lymphangioma circumscriptum

BULLA/VESICLES – ADULT

Bites
See page 120

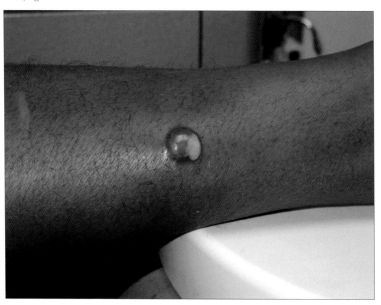

Plant dermatitis (Rhus)

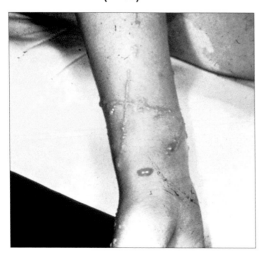

Description erythematous urticarial eruption with vesicles, often linear
Location distributed in exposed areas that came into contact with the plant

Characteristics extremely pruritic
Tests clinical diagnosis
Associated systemic disease none
Treatment pearls prevention of contact, topical corticosteroids, antihistamines

Herpes simplex virus (HSV)
See page 116

Herpes zoster virus (VZV)
See page 68

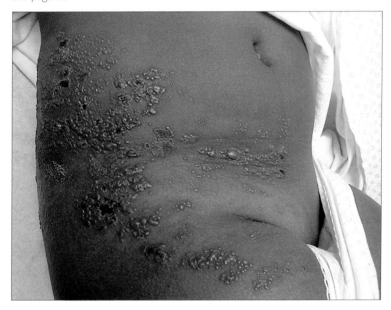

Contact/irritant dermatitis
See page 189

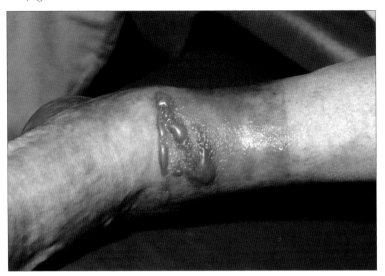

Liquid nitrogen-induced bulla

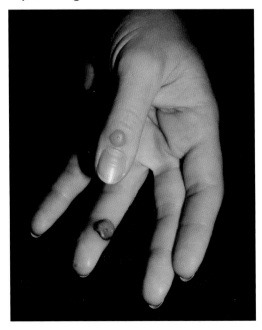

Burn

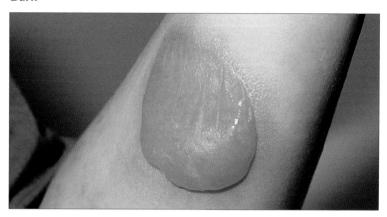

Dermatitis herpetiformis

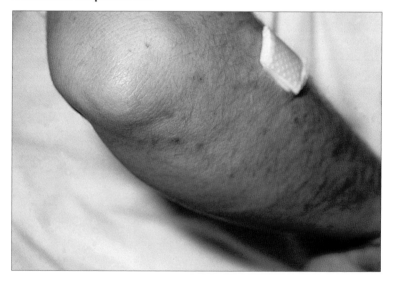

Description symmetrical, grouped, small papules and vesicles on an erythematous base

Location extensor surfaces, scalp, sacrum, buttocks, very rare mucous membrane involvement

Characteristics in adults: male>female, increased incidence in Caucasian populations, peak onset at 40 years, can be familial, chronic waxing and waning course, autoimmune, intense pruritus, menstrual period may induce flare, can heal with hyperpigmentation
Tests antiendomysial antibodies; Histopathology: collection of neutrophils in dermal papillae with edema and subepidermal cleft, DIF: +IgA granular deposits in dermal papillae
Associated systemic disease 90% have evidence of celiac sprue, also less commonly associated with thyroid disease and small bowel lymphoma
Treatment pearls gluten-free diet, dapsone, sulfapyridine, colchicine, tetracycline with niacinamide

Bullous pemphigoid

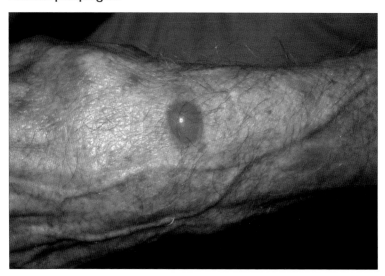

Description large, tense bulla, may have early phase with erythematous macules, papules or urticarial lesions
Location intertriginous and flexor surfaces, may be localized on extremities, 20% may have oral mucosa involvement, usually occurs symmetrically
Characteristics slight male>female, peak onset >65 years, chronic (relapsing and remitting) or self-limited, resolving in 6 years; rare childhood form tends to resolve within 1 year; autoimmune, intense pruritus, can be induced by drugs (penicillamine, diuretics, ACE-I, gold)
Tests Histopathology: subepidermal bulla with scant to dense lymphocytic and eosinophilic infiltrate in dermis, ± eosinophilic spongiosis, DIF: IgG and C3 along BMZ, IIF +70%, up to 50% may have peripheral eosinophilia
Associated systemic disease may be associated with other autoimmune diseases, inflammatory bowel disease, malignancy, neurologic disease or in sites of previous trauma
Treatment pearls oral and topical corticosteroids, azathioprine, colchicine, methotrexate, mycophenolate mofetil, dapsone, tetracycline and niacinamide in combination, IVIG

Cicatricial pemphigoid (mucous membrane pemphigoid)

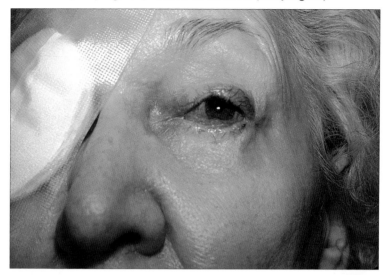

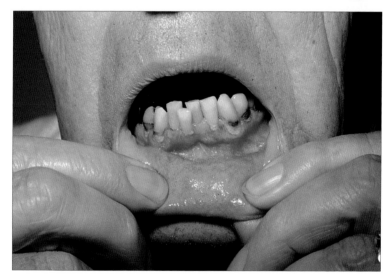

Description mucous membrane erythematous erosions (rare intact bulla) that progress to scar, ± tense bulla on skin that progress to scarred, atrophic plaques
Location mucous membranes especially conjunctiva and oral mucosa (infrequently genital mucosa), ± involvement of skin surfaces (25%)
Characteristics female>male, elderly, chronic course, autoimmune; painful, red, burning; ± epistaxis and dysphagia

Tests Histopathology: subepidermal bulla, mixed infiltrate with eosinophils ± plasma cells, fibrosis of upper dermis; DIF of mucosa: IgG and C3 at BMZ
Associated systemic disease none
Treatment pearls aggressive treatment and referral for regular ophthalmologic examinations to prevent blindness, oral and high-potency topical corticosteroids, dapsone, cyclophosphamide, azathioprine, IVIG

Pemphigus vulgaris

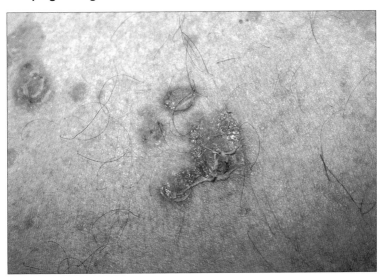

Description erythematous bullae that progress to erosions and heal without scarring
Location oral mucosa almost always involved, common on trunk; conjunctiva and genital mucosa less frequently
Characteristics peak onset 50–60 years, painful
Tests +Nikolsky sign (bulla forms with gentle rubbing on skin of active patients) and +Asboe–Hansen sign (bulla extends laterally when placing pressure on top of bulla); Histopathology: suprabasilar cleft ('tombstone'), perivascular infiltrate, acantholysis; DIF: +intercellular IgG with or without C3; autoantibody titers can be used to follow disease course
Associated systemic disease underlying malignancy can be associated with paraneoplastic pemphigus (skin disease can precede malignancy in up to 30%)
Treatment pearls oral corticosteroids or other systemic immunosuppressants, plasmapheresis

Pemphigus foliaceous

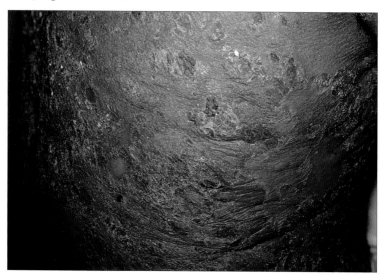

Description flaccid bullae rarely seen as they easily progress to erosions with a collarette of scale

Location trunk, face, scalp (seborrheic dermatitis distribution), no mucosal involvement

Characteristics peak onset 50–60 years, indolent onset

Tests +Nikolsky sign; Histopathology: cleft just below granular layer, acantholysis; DIF: +intercellular IgG with or without C3; autoantibody titers can be used to follow disease course

Associated systemic disease underlying malignancy can be associated with paraneoplastic pemphigus (skin disease can precede malignancy in up to 30%)

Treatment pearls oral corticosteroids or other systemic immunosuppressants, plasmapheresis

COMMON DRUGS THAT INDUCE PEMPHIGUS

- Aspirin
- Captopril and other ACE inhibitors*
- Furosemide
- NSAIDs (including indomethacin)*
- Penicillamine*
- Penicillin
- Phenacetin
- Phenylbutazone
- Propranolol
- Rifampin
- Sulfa drugs
- Thiazides (HCTZ)

* Indicates the most common.

Porphyria cutanea tarda
See page 46

Epidermolysis bullosa acquisita (EBA)
See page 48

Erythema multiforme
See page 484

Bullous drug reaction
See page 286, Drug reaction

Fixed drug reaction
See page 212

Id reaction
See page 142

Miliaria crystallina

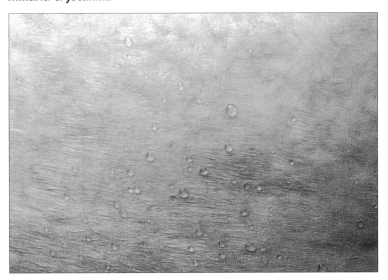

Description pinpoint clear vesicles
Location diaper area, forehead, neck, trunk or anywhere warm and occluded on the body
Characteristics infants to elderly, asymptomatic, resolves spontaneously, exacerbated by heat and occlusion, worse in humid environments
Tests Histopathology: occlusion of the eccrine duct with vesicle formation within the stratum corneum, no dermal inflammation
Associated systemic disease none
Treatment pearls avoid heat and occlusion

Hailey–Hailey disease (benign familial pemphigus)
See page 112

Stevens–Johnson syndrome (SJS, erythema multiforme major)
See page 64

Toxic epidermal necrolysis (TEN)
See page 66

Polymorphous light eruption (PMLE)
See page 422

Urticaria
See page 88

Scabies
See page 52

Sweet's syndrome
See page 447

Mastocytosis (urticaria pigmentosa)
See page 385

Epidermolysis bullosa (EBS, EBJ, EBD)

Bullous eczematous eruptions

Bullae around leg ulcers and fractures

Pressure bulla

Bullous SLE (systemic lupus erythematosus)

Bullous lichen planus

Erythema elevatum diutinum (EED)
See page 16 – Acral

Bullosis diabeticorum

Lymphangioma circumscriptum

Bullous morphea

Lichen sclerosus et atrophicus

Herpes gestationis

Paraneoplastic syndromes (leukemia and cancer bullous eruptions)

Graft-versus-host disease

Radiation dermatitis

BULLA/VESICLES – ELDERLY

Bullous pemphigoid
See page 127

Bullosis diabeticorum

Bullae with cerebral changes

Pemphigus vulgaris

Bullae around leg ulcers

Bullae with edema/stasis changes

Bullous drug reaction

Cicatricial pemphigoid

Liquid nitrogen induced bulla

Coma bulla

BULLA – NON-INFLAMMATORY

Bullous pemphigoid
See page 127

Porphyria cutanea tarda (PCT)
See page 46

Epidermolysis bullosa acquisita (EBA)
See page 48

Trauma (pressure, liquid nitrogen, thermal burn)

Drug reaction

Bullosis amyloid

Lichen sclerosus et atrophicus

Bulla diabeticorum

Bulla secondary to edema or resolving edema

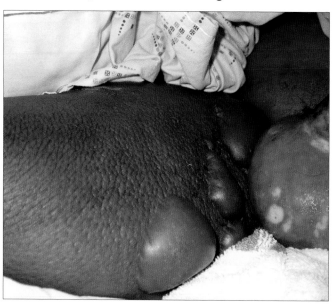

CHANCRE

Primary syphilis
See page 117

Granuloma inguinale (Donovanosis)
Description bright red solitary to multiple papules that can progress to large ulcerated plaques and swollen genitalia
Location genital mucosa or skin, inguinal skin (usually no lymph node involvement)
Characteristics adults, chronic and progressive without treatment, painless, easily bleeds
Tests tissue smear with Giemsa stain+ for bacteria, *Calymmatobacterium granulomatis*; organism very difficult to culture; Histopathology: pseudoepitheliomatous hyperplasia, ulceration and Donovan bodies (bacteria) seen within histiocytes
Associated systemic disease none
Treatment pearls doxycycline and bactrim, or quinolones × 3 weeks; penicillin is ineffective

Lymphogranuloma venereum (LGV)
Description primary lesion is a small erythematous erosion, secondary lesions are large tender lymph nodes that can ulcerate and progress to firm nodules with drainage
Location primary erosion in vagina or on glans penis, secondary lymph node lesions occur unilaterally in inguinal and perirectal area

Characteristics male>female, adults, sexually transmitted; primary lesion is asymptomatic to mildly painful and resolves in 1 week, secondary lymph node lesions are large, painful and progress without treatment; can be associated with proctitis, endemic in Africa, Asia, India and South America
Tests urine test+ for Chlamydia, serology for Chlamydia antibodies; Histopathology: ulceration, mixed infiltrate, organisms are rarely seen
Associated systemic disease none
Treatment pearls doxycycline, macrolide antibiotics

Chancroid

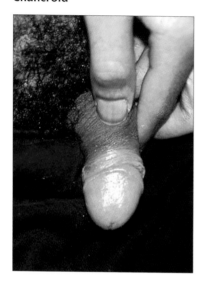

Description erythematous papule or pustule that progresses to one or more soft, dirty ulcerations with irregular, undermined borders
Location genital mucosa and skin with painful inguinal lymphadenopathy (usually unilateral)
Characteristics male>female, adults, painful, sexually transmitted
Tests swab for Gram stain to reveal bacteria, *Haemophilus ducreyi* (+ only 50%), bacterial culture; Histopathology: ulceration with necrosis and neutrophils, granulation tissue, deep mixed infiltrate with plasma cells, organisms rarely seen
Associated systemic disease none
Treatment pearls azithromycin, ceftriaxone, quinolones or erythromycin

Herpes simplex virus (HSV)

Trauma

Bite (human, insect or other)

CYSTS, PSEUDOCYSTS AND FISTULAS OF THE HEAD AND NECK

Epidermal cyst (follicular infundibular cyst, epidermoid cyst)

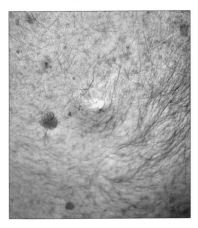

Description usually solitary, soft to firm skin-colored round nodule with or without a punctum
Location anywhere on non-glabrous skin (face and upper trunk especially)
Characteristics asymptomatic, size may wax and wane, ± drainage
Tests Histopathology: epithelium with granular layer surrounds cyst which is filled with loose keratin
Associated systemic disease none
Treatment pearls no treatment necessary, surgical excision of entire cyst wall

Pilar cyst (follicular isthmus cyst, trichilemmal cyst)
Description solitary or multiple firm skin-colored to pink nodule
Location primarily on scalp
Characteristics ± AD inheritance, asymptomatic vs. tender
Tests Histopathology: epithelium without a granular layer surrounds cyst filled with compact homogeneous keratin
Associated systemic disease none
Treatment pearls no treatment necessary, surgical excision of entire cyst wall

Mucocele

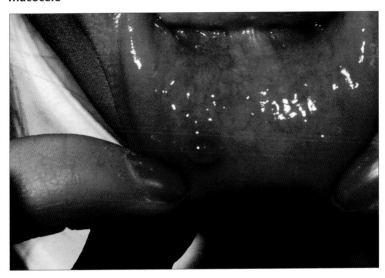

Description small, soft, compressible, translucent to pink/blue papulovesicle ± surrounding erythema
Location oral mucosal surfaces
Characteristics any age, self-limited, recurrent, asymptomatic
Tests Histopathology: mucinous deposition in dermis near salivary ducts surrounded by inflammation and granulation tissue (not a true cyst)
Associated systemic disease none
Treatment pearls no treatment necessary, surgical excision, cryotherapy, electrodessication, intralesional corticosteroids

Thyroglossal duct cyst
Description skin-colored firm nodule
Location anterior midline of neck
Characteristics children, asymptomatic
Tests cyst should move up when patient swallows; Histopathology: thyroid follicles interspersed with a cyst with ciliated epithelial cells
Associated systemic disease none
Treatment pearls surgical excision

Branchial cleft cyst

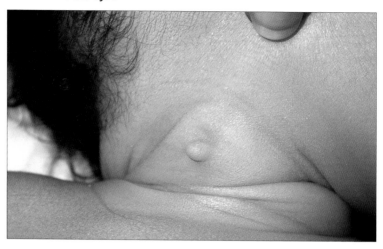

Description usually unilateral skin-colored firm nodule ± mucinous, odiferous drainage
Location preauricular, along the mandible or along the sternocleidomastoid muscle
Characteristics children or young adults, ± AD inheritance, asymptomatic vs. tender and erythematous secondary to infection
Tests Histopathology: lymphoid tissue surrounds cyst
Associated systemic disease none
Treatment pearls surgical excision after imaging to rule out deep extensions

Dermoid cyst

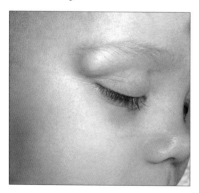

Description large, firm subcutaneous nodule 1–4 cm in diameter
Location occurs along embryonic fusion planes especially midline on head and neck and periorbital
Characteristics infant to childhood, asymptomatic or erythematous if infected

Tests Histopathology: normal adnexal structures surrounding a cyst with stratified squamous epithelial cells
Associated systemic disease none
Treatment pearls surgical excision after imaging to rule out deep intracranial connections or other neural entities

Preauricular cyst (ear pit)
Description small depression in skin ± subcutaneous nodular component
Location unilateral in preauricular area, often on right side
Characteristics infants, young adults, asymptomatic unless infected, ± AD inheritance
Tests Histopathology: epithelial lined cyst with a granular layer
Associated systemic disease rarely associated with hearing loss, can also be associated with several congenital syndromes (Treacher Collins, Naegeli–Franceschetti–Jadassohn, etc.)
Treatment pearls no treatment necessary, surgical excision

Accessory tragus

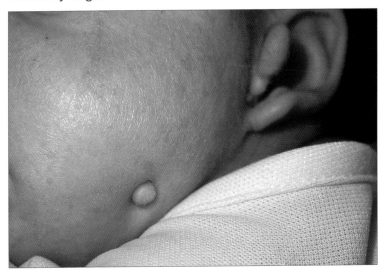

Description usually solitary, unilateral skin-colored nodule ± overlying vellus hair
Location preauricular, along the mandible or along the sternocleidomastoid muscle
Characteristics infant, present at birth or shortly after, asymptomatic
Tests Histopathology: multiple tiny hair follicles, cartilage, connective tissue and fat
Associated systemic disease rarely associated with hearing loss, can also be associated with several congenital syndromes (Goldenhar's, Treacher Collins, Naegeli–Franceschetti–Jadassohn and others)
Treatment pearls no treatment necessary, surgical excision

Dental sinus

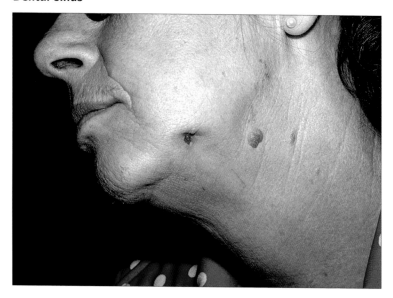

Description usually unilateral fistula opening onto skin with surrounding erythema and induration
Location perioral, along or under mandible
Characteristics any age, resolves with treatment, tender
Tests odontoid x-ray series
Associated systemic disease none
Treatment pearls extraction of infected tooth

Foreign body reaction
See page 183

Pseudocyst of the auricle
Description soft erythematous swollen area
Location unilateral on scaphoid fossa of ear
Characteristics males>females, adults, slow onset, asymptomatic
Tests yellow oily return with aspiration; Histopathology: cavity within cartilage of ear without inflammation (not a true cyst)
Associated systemic disease none
Treatment pearls no treatment necessary, incision and drainage with pressure dressing ± intralesional corticosteroid injection

Tumor

Pyogenic granuloma

Syphilitic osteitis

Fistula of salivary gland

Dacryocystitis

Osteomyelitis

Tuberculosis

Leishmaniasis

Lymphangioma

Actinomycosis

Histoplasmosis

Phaeomycotic cyst (dermatiaceous fungi)

DEPIGMENTED MACULES

See page 222. Hypopigmented macules (hypomelanotic) and depigmented macules (amelanotic)

DERMATITIS – GENERAL
Atopic dermatitis

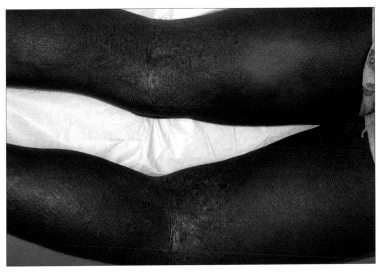

Description scaly erythematous patches, papules and plaques ± crust, ± lichenification

Location *in infants*: face and extensor areas; *in young children*: more diffuse papules and thicker plaques especially in antecubital and popliteal fossae and other flexor surfaces; *in adults*: localized papules and plaques with flexor and face and neck involvement; scaly palms, soles and dorsal hands and feet are commonly present in all age groups

Characteristics children to adults: chronic duration with relapses, intensely pruritic, exacerbated by allergens including contact, airborne and food allergens; can also be exacerbated by immunizations, viral infections and secondary bacterial infections; associated with periorbital hyperpigmentation, hyperlinear palms, xerosis, Dennie–Morgan infraorbital folds and keratosis pilaris; may be worse in winter and with increased stress

Tests ± elevated serum IgE; Histopathology: acute to subacute spongiotic dermatitis with changes of lichen simplex chronicus ± eosinophils

Associated systemic disease atopy

Treatment pearls antihistamines, topical tacrolimus, pimecrolimus or corticosteroids, oral corticosteroids when severe, oral antibiotics, emollients after tub soaks, PUVA, immunosuppressives if very severe (cyclosporine)

Contact dermatitis
See page 189

Polymorphous light eruption (PMLE)
See page 422

Seborrheic dermatitis
See page 398

Photoallergic reaction
See page 423

Id reaction
Description poorly demarcated erythematous patches and papules ± scale and crust

Location symmetric, generalized distribution which can be distant from the original site of the causative dermatitis

Characteristics pruritic

Tests Histopathology: spongiosis of epidermis with perivascular infiltrate ± eosinophils

Associated systemic disease can be associated with allergic contact dermatitis, stasis dermatitis, dyshidrosis and dermatophytosis (tinea)

Treatment pearls topical corticosteroids and antihistamines

Infectious eczematoid dermatitis

Systemic lupus erythematosus (SLE)

Dermatomyositis

Dermatitis associated with internal diseases
Malabsorption
Hypothyroid
Renal disease
Biliary cirrhosis

Carcinoma, lymphoma, leukemia
Pellagra
Wiskott–Aldrich syndrome

DIABETIC SKIN CHANGES

Pruritus

Dermopathy

Sensory loss

Ulceration

Acanthosis nigricans

Candidiasis

Necrobiosis lipoidica diabeticorum

Eruptive xanthoma

Lipodystrophy

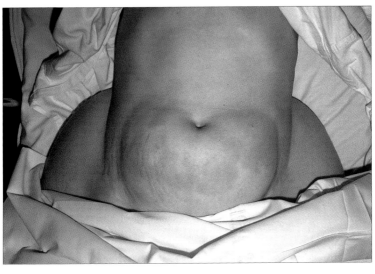

Nephrogenic fibrosing dermopathy

Bullosis diabeticorum

Pyoderma

Arteriosclerotic gangrene

Diabetic drug reactions

DIAPER DERMATITIS

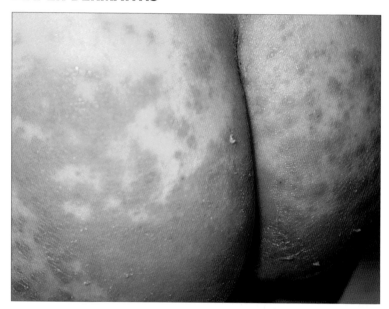

Irritant dermatitis
See page 189, Contact/irritant dermatitis

Candidiasis

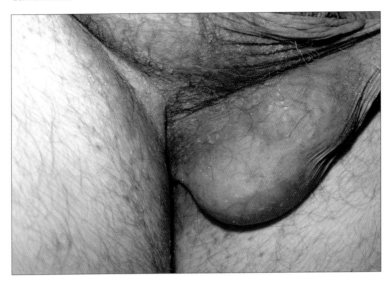

Description moist erythematous confluent macules with fissures, maceration, tiny pustules, white discharge if vaginal and ± satellite pustules and erythema
Location perianal, vaginal, inguinal, diaper area in infants
Characteristics pruritic, can occur after antibiotic therapy
Tests fungal culture, KOH+ for yeast
Associated systemic disease associated with diabetics, immunosuppression, HIV
Treatment pearls systemic, topical or intravaginal antifungals

Seborrheic dermatitis
See page 398

Intertrigo, non-specific
Description well-defined erythematous patches or plaques. Satellite pustules suggest Candida infection
Location inguinal, perianal, perivaginal, axillae, submammary areas, diaper area
Characteristics discomfort with friction. Odor suggests bacterial infection
Tests history for irritants, friction-causing behavior (obesity, sports, tight clothes). Culture for yeast, fungus, bacteria. KOH for yeast, fungal infections
Association systemic disease obesity, immunocompromised, sensitivity to topical products
Treatment decrease friction (petrolatum may help), treat any infection, discontinue irritants, treat moist areas with powder or other drying agent

Contact dermatitis
See page 189, Contact/irritant dermatitis

Inverse psoriasis
See page 109

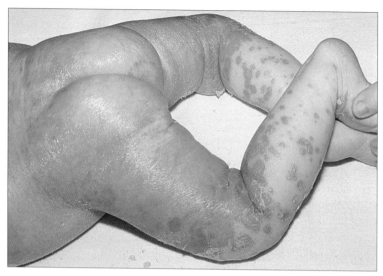

Miliaria (crystallina, rubra and profunda)
See pages 131, 337

Impetigo
See page 121

Herpes simplex
See page 116

Beta-hemolytic Streptococcus (especially perianal)

Perianal dermatitis

Congenital syphilis

Juvenile pemphigoid

Acrodermatitis enteropathica

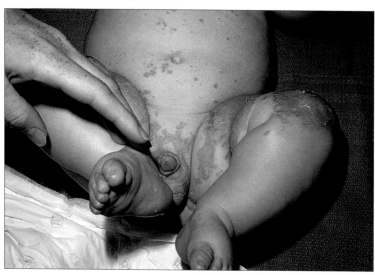

Histiocytosis X (Langerhans' cell histiocytosis, Letterer–Siwe disease)

Jacquet erosive dermatitis

EAR INFILTRATION

Chronic eczema
See page 498, Nummular eczema

Chronic seborrheic dermatitis
See page 398, Seborrheic dermatitis

Squamous cell carcinoma
See page 367

Sarcoid
See page 443

Chronic infection

Relapsing polychondritis

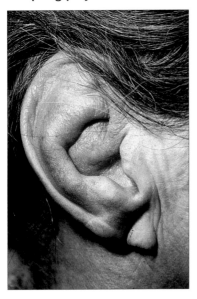

Actinic reticuloid

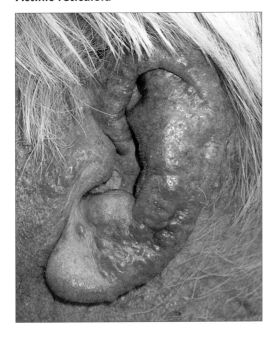

Foreign body reaction

Amyloidosis

Leishmaniasis

Papular mucinosis

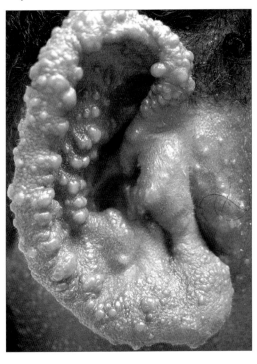

Angiolymphoid hyperplasia with eosinophilia

Leprosy

Gout
See page 182

ECZEMA – CHILDHOOD

Atopic dermatitis
See page 141

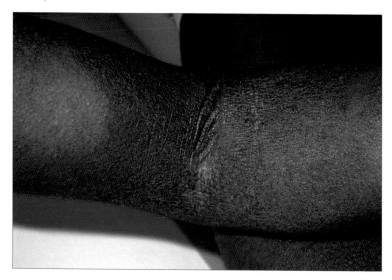

Psoriasis
See page 397

Seborrheic dermatitis
See page 398

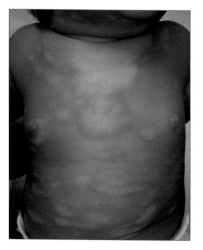

Contact dermatitis
See page 189

Drug reaction
See page 286

Acrodermatitis enteropathica

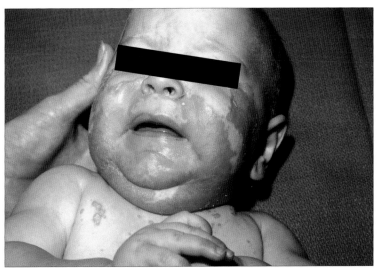

Description well-demarcated erythematous scaling patches with crust, pustules and bulla
Location face especially periorificial, acral
Characteristics premature infants, alcoholics, malabsorption conditions, resolves with treatment, may be associated with angular cheilitis, alopecia, diarrhea, irritability and nail deformities
Tests serum zinc and alkaline phosphatase level; Histopathology: pale epidermis ± intraepidermal bulla, neutrophilic infiltrate
Associated systemic disease zinc deficiency
Treatment pearls zinc replacement

Pityriasis rubra pilaris (PRP)
See page 159

Histiocytosis X

Gluten enteropathy

Immunodeficiency eczema
Leiner's disease (C5 deficiency)
Bruton's agammaglobulinemia
Wiskott–Aldrich syndrome

Aminoacidurias
Job's syndrome
Hartnup's syndrome
Phenylketonuria
Chronic granulomatous disease
Ataxia telangiectasia

EDEMA

Lymphedema

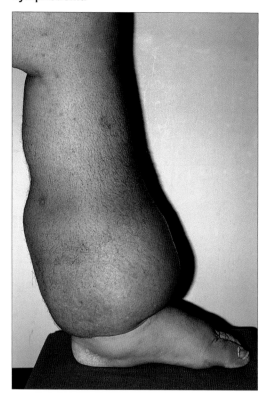

Description swollen, firm skin-colored to pink areas of skin
Location usually dependent areas (lower extremities or sacrum if bedbound), can also occur in other areas if lymph drainage is blocked (arm after mastectomy and node dissection)
Characteristics asymptomatic to tender
Tests exerting pressure with a finger may leave a 'pit' in the skin if acute, chronic lymphedema is usually non-pitting

Associated systemic disease primary lymphedema is associated with lymphatic malformations and can be seen in several syndromes including Milroy, Noonan and Turner; secondary lymphedema is associated with cardiac, liver, heart disease, malignancy, filariasis, amyloidosis, postradiation, post-lymph node excision or post-rosacea

Treatment pearls elevation, compression hose, surgery to repair malformations, treat underlying disease

Myxedema (secondary to hypo- or hyperthyroid)

Connective tissue disease – progressive systemic sclerosis (PSS), mixed connective tissue disease (MCTD)

Scleredema

Eosinophilic fasciitis

Scleromyxedema

Bites

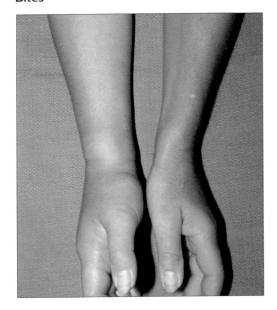

Cellulitis/erysipelas

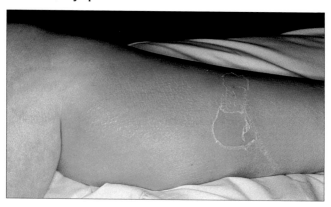

Description erythematous, warm, indurated patch or plaque with ill-defined borders

Location can occur anywhere, often in site of trauma

Characteristics resolves with treatment, painful, ± fever, chills, malaise and regional lymphadenopathy

Tests tissue culture; Histopathology: mixed infiltrate in deep dermis and subcutaneous tissue, blood vessels and lymphatics may be dilated, may see subepidermal bulla if severe

Associated systemic disease none

Treatment pearls oral or I.V. antibiotics, rest, elevation, local wound care to any eroded areas

Plant dermatitis (Rhus)

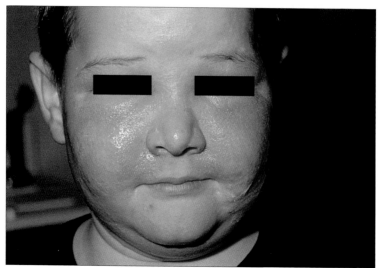

ELBOWS AND KNEES

Psoriasis
See page 397

Lichen simplex chronicus
See page 201

Scabies
See page 52

Erythema multiforme
See page 484

Dermatitis herpetiformis
See page 126

Granuloma annulare
See page 87

Tuberous xanthoma

Eruptive xanthomas

Gout

Juxta-articular nodes

Juvenile pityriasis rubra pilaris (PRP)

Gonococcemia

Rheumatoid nodules

EOSINOPHILIA

Allergic diseases
Asthma
Urticaria
Drug reactions

Cutaneous diseases
Pemphigus
Dermatitis herpetiformis
Erythema multiforme
Bullous pemphigoid
Angiolymphoid hyperplasia with eosinophilia
Eosinophilic folliculitis
Eosinophilic fasciitis (Shulman syndrome)
Well's syndrome
Ofuji's syndrome
Incontinentia pigmenti
Erythema toxicum neonatorum (rarely)

Loeffler's syndrome

Churg–Strauss syndrome

Tropical eosinophilia

Infections
Scarlet fever
Parasites (trichinosis, Echinococcus, filariae, intestinal)

Hematologic diseases
Leukemia
Lymphoma (especially CML)
Polycythemia vera
Pernicious anemia
Hodgkin's lymphoma
Postsplenectomy

Other malignancies

Polyarteritis nodosa (PAN)

Rheumatoid arthritis

Sarcoid

Dilantin hypersensitivity syndrome

Hypereosinophilic syndrome

Eosinophilic myalgia syndrome

Idiopathic

ERYTHRODERMA – INFANCY
Staphylococcal scalded skin syndrome (SSSS)
Description large areas of erythematous tender skin that rapidly progress to flaccid, sterile bulla and then erosions
Location desquamation all over body, also with perioral erosions but mucous membranes spared
Characteristics males>females, infants and children>adults, resolves in 14 days with treatment, occurs with malaise and fever
Tests +Nikolsky's sign; Histopathology: cleft at stratum granulosum, no inflammation in epidermis or dermis (epidermal damage is by staphylococcal toxin, therefore bacteria are not visualized on pathology or culture of bulla), culture of nasopharynx or conjunctiva
Associated systemic disease may be associated with immunosuppression and renal disease in adults
Treatment pearls oral or I.V. antibiotics and topical emollients

Atopic erythroderma
See page 141, Atopic dermatitis

Seborrheic dermatitis
See page 398

Drug reaction/toxic epidermal necrolysis (TEN)
See page 66

Erythrodermic candidiasis

Ichthyosiform erythroderma
Trichothiodystrophy (PIBIDS)
KID syndrome
Conradi–Hünermann–Happle syndrome
Lamellar ichthyosis
Congenital ichthyosiform erythroderma
Ichthyosis bullosa of Siemens

Neonatal lupus

Psoriasis

Pityriasis rubra pilaris (PRP)

ERYTHRODERMA – ADULT (EXFOLIATIVE)

Psoriasis
See page 397

Contact dermatitis
See page 189

Drug reaction
See box and page 286

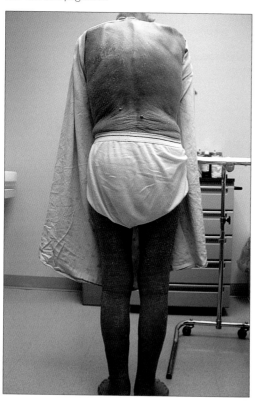

CAUSES OF ERYTHRODERMIC DRUG REACTIONS

- Allopurinol
- Aspirin
- Antibiotics
- Barbiturates
- Carbamazepine
- Codeine
- Dilantin (phenytoin)

- Iodine
- Isoniazid
- Omeprazole
- Penicillin
- Quinidine
- Sulfa drugs
- Vancomycin

Atopic dermatitis
See page 141

Pityriasis rubra pilaris (PRP)

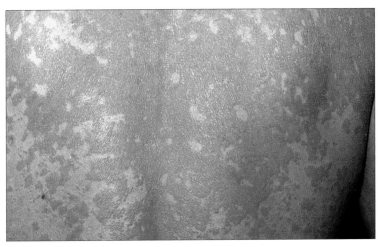

Description orange/red scaling patches confluent in some areas with areas of normal skin interspersed ('islands of sparing') which can progress to erythroderma, hyperkeratotic follicular papules ('nutmeg grater'), hyperkeratotic palms and soles, nail dystrophy
Location usually starts on head and neck and spreads symmetrically in a cephalocaudal direction
Characteristics bimodal peaks: children and adults 50–60 years, usually resolves in 2–3 years, associated with fatigue and malaise, ± pruritus, rarely familial
Tests Histopathology: hyperkeratosis, follicular plugging with perifollicular parakeratosis and alternating horizontal and vertical parakeratosis, mild superficial perivascular lymphocytic infiltrate
Associated systemic disease none
Treatment pearls topical corticosteroids, oral retinoids, methotrexate, cyclosporine, azathioprine

Pemphigus foliaceous
See page 130

Stasis dermatitis
See page 161

Seborrheic dermatitis
See page 398

Ichthyosis

Sézary syndrome/CTCL

Id reaction

Internal malignancy (lymphoma, leukemia)

Tinea (dermatophytosis, especially *Trichophyton violaceum*)

Graft-versus-host disease

Infectious eczematoid dermatitis

Norwegian scabies

Acrodermatitis enteropathica

Lichen planus

ESCHAR – BLACK

Spider bite

Snakes

Anthrax

Clostridium

Pseudomonas infection

Sporotrichosis

Electric burn

Chemical

Ecthyma gangrenosum

Calciphylaxis

EXFOLIATION – LOCALIZED

Contact dermatitis
See page 189

Cellulitis
See page 154

Erysipelas
See page 281

Radiation dermatitis
See page 102

Burn

EXFOLIATIVE DERMATITIS

Atopic dermatitis
See page 141

Psoriasis
See page 397

Contact dermatitis
See page 189

Seborrheic dermatitis
See page 398

Stasis dermatitis

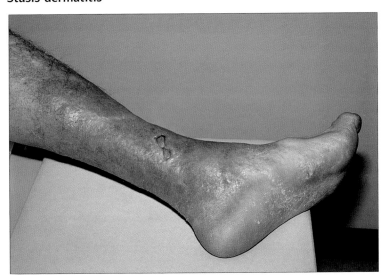

Description 'cayenne pepper' speckled red to brown patches with scaly, eczematous changes
Location bilateral distal lower extremities, usually symmetric
Characteristics females>males, middle-aged to elderly, chronic, asymptomatic to pruritic, may be associated with edema of legs
Tests Histopathology: normal epidermis vs. spongiotic changes with scale, perivascular infiltrate with extravasated RBCs
Associated systemic disease associated with congestive heart failure
Treatment pearls support hose, elevation, topical corticosteroids

Drug reaction
See page 286

Pityriasis rubra pilaris (PRP)
See page 159

Pemphigus foliaceous
See page 130

Id reaction

Ichthyosiform erythroderma

Reiter's syndrome

Cutaneous T-cell lymphoma (CTCL)

Lichen planus

Internal malignancy
Leukemia
Lymphoma
Lung
Rectum
Thyroid
Multiple myeloma

Malabsorption
Pellagra
Kwashiorkor

Norwegian scabies

Tinea (dermatophytosis, especially *Trichophyton violaceum*)

Stevens–Johnson syndrome (SJS)/toxic epidermal necrolysis (TEN)

Staphylococcal scalded skin syndrome

Scarlet fever

Papular pruritic eruption of AIDS

DRUGS WHICH CAUSE AN EXFOLIATIVE DERMATITIS

- Antimalarials
- Arsenic
- Aspirin
- Barbiturates
- Captopril
- Cephalosporins
- Codeine
- Gold
- Iodine
- Isoniazid
- Mercury
- NSAIDs
- Penicillin
- Phenytoin
- Quinidine
- Sulfonamides
- Terbinafine

EXFOLIATIVE DERMATITIS – ACRAL
Keratolysis exfoliativa

Keratolysis exfoliativa

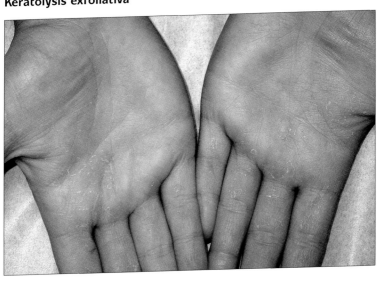

Description non-inflammatory, annular, superficial scaling of palms without preceding vesicles

Location palms and soles

Characteristics any age, self-limited (resolves in days), may recur, asymptomatic, increased incidence in summer months

Tests KOH–

Associated systemic disease none

Treatment pearls no treatment necessary

Contact/irritant dermatitis
See page 189

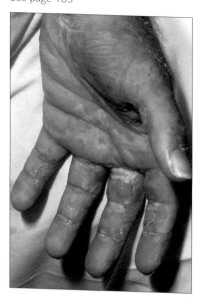

Drug reaction
See page 286

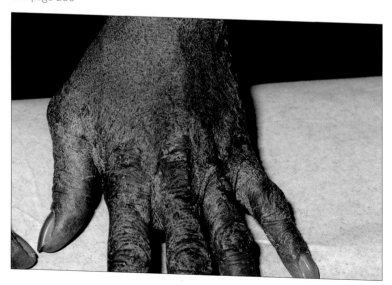

Palmoplantar psoriasis
See page 397

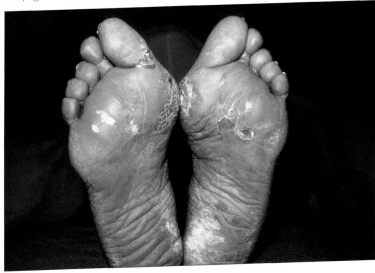

Dyshidrosis
See page 57

Viral exanthem

Acral bulla diabeticorum

Kawasaki's disease

Stevens–Johnson syndrome (SJS)/toxic epidermal necrolysis (TEN)

EYELID EDEMA

Contact dermatitis
See page 189

Atopic dermatitis
See page 141

Cellulitis

Hordeolum (stye)

Chalazion

Erysipelas

Trauma

Bites

Blepharochalasis

Dermatomyositis

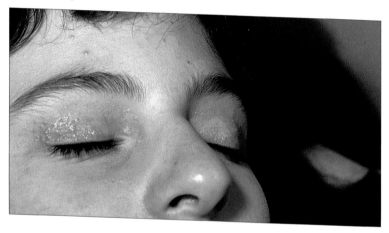

Cutaneous T-cell lymphoma (CTCL)

Anthrax

Cat-scratch disease

Herpes simplex or herpes zoster

Lymphedema

Cavernous sinus thrombosis

Angioedema

Nephritis

Congestive heart failure

Hypo- or hyperthyroidism

Anemia

Leukemia

Sarcoid

Hypoalbuminemia

Trichinosis

Filariasis

Onchocerciasis

EYELID TUMOR

Xanthelasma
Description small, thin yellow/brown oval plaque (see p. 392, Xanthoma)
Location periorbital, usually bilateral and multiple
Characteristics middle-aged adults, chronic, progressive, asymptomatic
Tests Histopathology: collection of foamy histiocytes within the dermis
Associated systemic disease may be associated with liver disease in females, 50% may have hyperlipidemia
Treatment pearls no treatment necessary, scissor excision, CO_2 laser

Hidrocystoma

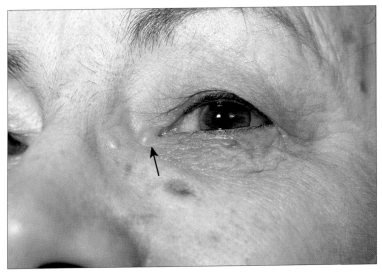

Description solitary or multiple, small clear/translucent or bluish, round, non-inflammatory papulovesicle
Location usually solitary on eyelid and other areas of the face, can occur anywhere

Characteristics any age, may resolve but often chronic, asymptomatic, may be exacerbated by warm temperature

Tests Histopathology: finger-like cystic areas surrounded by apocrine cells (decapitation secretion) and a fibrous stroma

Associated systemic disease rarely associated with Schöpf–Schulz–Passarge syndrome of ectodermal dysplasia

Treatment pearls no treatment necessary, can try aspiration of fluid within vesicle with needle and syringe, surgical excision, electrocautery, laser

Milia
See page 42

Seborrheic keratosis
See page 381

Syringoma
See page 344

Basal cell carcinoma
See page 366

Squamous cell carcinoma
See page 367

Keratoacanthoma
See page 368

Actinic keratosis
See page 501

Meibomian cyst

Lipoma

Nevus

Trichilemmoma (Cowden's syndrome)

Neurofibroma

Melanoma

Kaposi's sarcoma

Necrobiotic xanthogranuloma

Cyst of Mall's gland

Epidermal inclusion cyst

Pilomatrixoma

Trichoepithelioma

Hemangioendothelioma

Pyogenic granuloma

Cylindroma

Lipoid proteinosis

FIGURATE ERYTHEMA

Tinea corporis (dermatophytosis)
See page 86

Urticaria (annular)
See page 88

Subacute cutaneous lupus erythematosus (SCLE)
See page 89

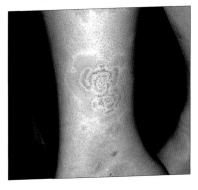

Erythema multiforme
See page 484

Erythema chronica migrans

Erythema marginatum

Necrolytic migratory erythema

Erythema annulare centrifigum

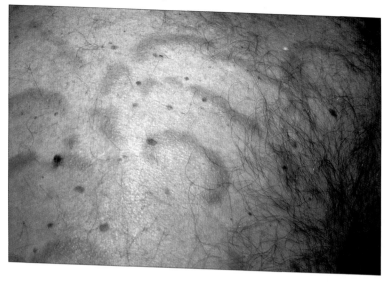

Erythema gyratum repens

Cutaneous T-cell lymphoma (CTCL)

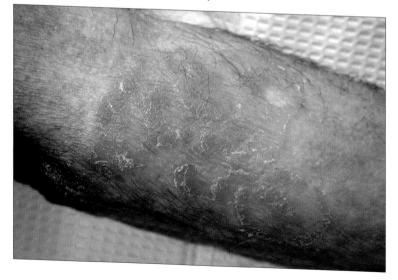

Annular erythema of infancy (rule out neonatal lupus)

Carriers of chronic granulomatous disease (CGD)

Mothers of boys with CGD may have annular rash

Secondary syphilis (lues)

Familial annular erythema (rare)

Psoriasis (annular)

Tinea versicolor

Bullous pemphigoid

FOLLICULAR KERATOSES

Keratosis pilaris

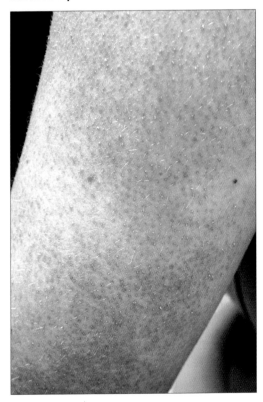

Description hyperkeratotic follicular papules ± surrounding erythema
Location lateral arms and thighs, less frequent on cheeks
Characteristics children and adults, usually improves with age, asymptomatic,
exacerbated in warm weather
Tests Histopathology: hyperkeratosis over follicular ostia and follicular plugging
Associated systemic disease atopy
Treatment pearls keratolytics, emollients/humectants, gentle exfoliation, topical
retinoids

Atrophoderma vermiculatum

Keratosis pilaris atrophicans

Lichen spinulosus

Lichen planopilaris

Pityriasis rubra pilaris

Kyrle's disease

Darier's disease
See page 196

Keratosis pilaris decalvans

Scurvy/vitamin C deficiency

Phrynoderma/vitamin A deficiency

Fiberglass dermatitis

Lichen scrofulosorum

Fox–Fordyce syndrome
See page 112

Id reaction

Sarcoid

Seborrheic dermatitis

Perforating folliculitis

Drug reaction

Tinea versicolor

Pityriasis rosea

Infundibular folliculitis of Hitch and Lund

Follicular cutaneous T-cell lymphoma (CTCL)

Eosinophilic folliculitis

FOOT LESIONS – DARK BROWN TO BLACK

Nevus
See page 379

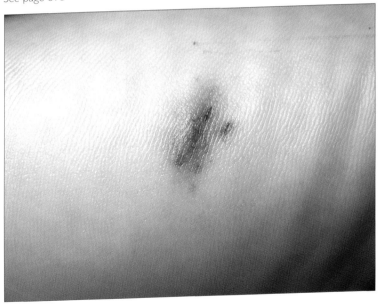

Melanoma
See page 380

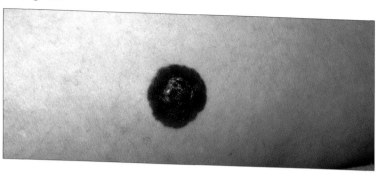

Blue nevus
See page 358

Kaposi's sarcoma
See page 364

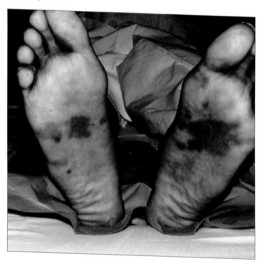

Black heel or talon noire secondary trauma
See page 45, Friction blister

Tinea nigra

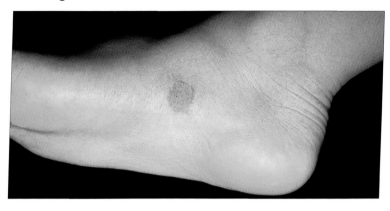

Description well-demarcated brown/gray/black patch ± scale
Location palms most common, also on soles, can occur anywhere
Characteristics common in tropical environment, resolves with treatment, asymptomatic
Tests KOH; Histopathology: hyphae seen within stratum corneum
Associated systemic disease none
Treatment pearls topical keratolytics, topical antifungals

Tennis or sportsman's toe (black toenail)

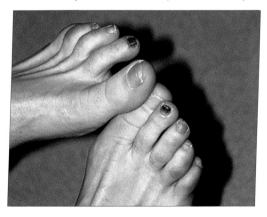

Sarcoid

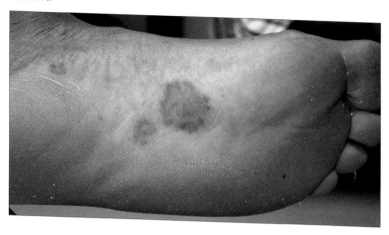

Verruca plantaris

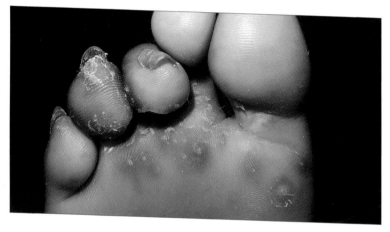

FURUNCULOSIS-LIKE LESIONS

Furuncle

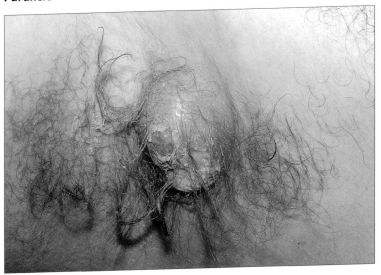

Description erythematous/violaceous deep nodule
Location can occur anywhere
Characteristics any age, resolves with treatment, painful
Tests bacterial culture; Histopathology: dilated follicle with neutrophilic abscess surrounding
Associated systemic disease none
Treatment pearls oral antibiotics

Tuberculosis
See page 184

Atypical mycobacteria
See page 185

Sporotrichosis

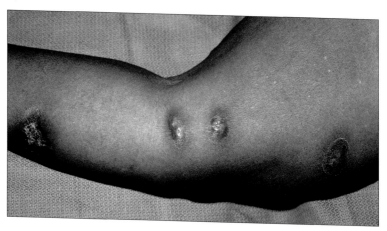

Description erythematous papule at site of inoculation that progresses weeks later to several ulcerated, purulent papules and subcutaneous nodules

Location ulcerated papules extend up an extremity in a linear 'sporotrichoid' distribution

Characteristics adults>children, common in gardeners or those exposed to sphagnum moss, resolves with treatment, painless

Tests tissue culture; Histopathology: deep dermal and subcutaneous granulomas ± necrosis/abscess, cigar-shaped organisms rarely seen

Associated systemic disease none

Treatment pearls oral itraconazole, potassium iodide

Blastomycosis

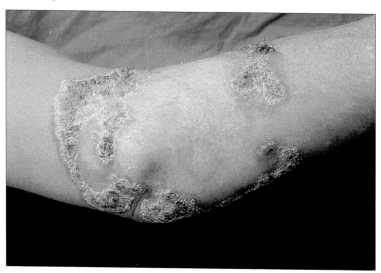

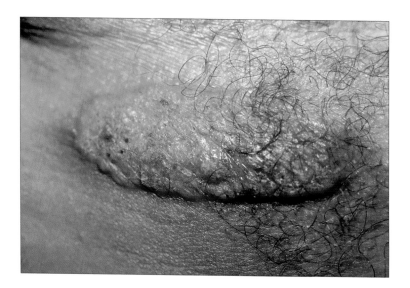

Description well-demarcated, bleeding/crusted verrucous papules or pustules and plaques which may progress to ulceration and heal centrally with cribriform scarring

Location face and exposed skin most common, may affect mucous membranes

Characteristics males>females, resolves with treatment, painful, common in the South-eastern and Midwestern US, may affect many internal organs including lungs

Tests tissue culture, +KOH; Histopathology: pseudoepitheliomatous hyperplasia with 8–15 μm broad-based budding yeast noted in areas of necrosis with PAS stain

Associated systemic disease none

Treatment pearls oral antifungals

Histoplasmosis

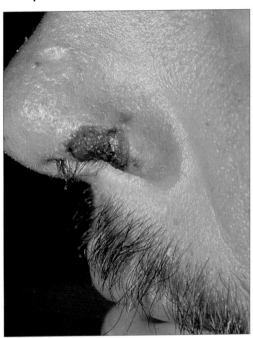

Description cutaneous manifestations rare, may present with mucocutaneous ulcers or erythematous subcutaneous nodules with ulceration and overlying crust

Location oral ulcers or nodules on extremities

Characteristics males>females, usually self-limited, may occur with erythema nodosum, common in the Ohio and Mississippi river valleys especially near caves, bird coops, or near building demolitions

Tests tissue culture, serology, skin test, CXR with lung calcifications and mediastinal lymphadenopathy, +KOH; Histopathology: granulomatous inflammation with 2–4 μm yeasts seen within the histiocytes ('parasitized histiocytes') with PAS stain

Associated systemic disease none

Treatment pearls treatment may not be necessary if self-limited and cutaneous, oral antifungals for systemic disease

Coccidioidomycosis

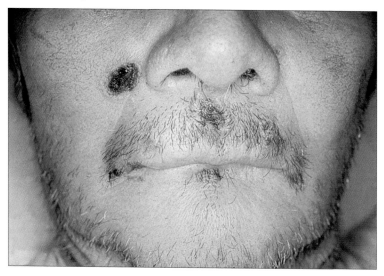

Description erythematous macules, papules, pustules, plaques, or subcutaneous abscesses ± sinus tracts and ulceration, may also be verrucous
Location common on head and neck including face, may also present with a diffuse macular eruption
Characteristics male>female, bimodal; children and elderly, dark skin>light skin, resolves with treatment, initial infection occurs with
flu-like symptoms, may occur with erythema multiforme or erythema nodosum, common in South-western US
Tests tissue culture, serology, skin test, CXR with cavitary lesions, +KOH; Histopathology: granulomas with abscess/necrosis and endospores containing 30–60 μm spherules seen with PAS stain
Associated systemic disease none
Treatment pearls difficult to treat, oral antifungals

Cryptococcosis
See page 356

Spider bite

Phaeohyphomycotic cyst

Leishmaniasis

Nocardia

Yaws

Cutaneous metastases

Tularemia

Syphilis (primary and secondary)

GRANULOMAS – CUTANEOUS

Granuloma annulare
See page 87

Gout

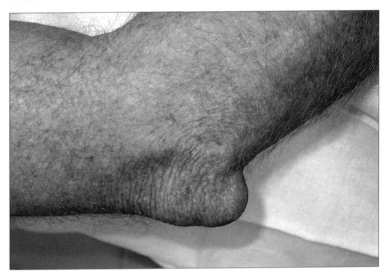

Description skin-colored/yellow to red, firm subcutaneous or dermal nodules ± ulceration and drainage
Location common over joints, helix of ears
Characteristics male>female, >40 years, waxing and waning course, painful, ± fever, +joint pain, exacerbated by drinking alcohol, dehydration, renal insufficiency and medications such as diuretics
Tests elevated ESR, WBC and serum and urine uric acid level, joint aspirations show monosodium urate crystals; Histopathology: palisaded granuloma with clefts and amorphous pink material in center, negative birefringence; abnormal x-ray of joint
Associated systemic disease none
Treatment pearls NSAIDs, colchicine, allopurinol, hydration

Rheumatoid nodule

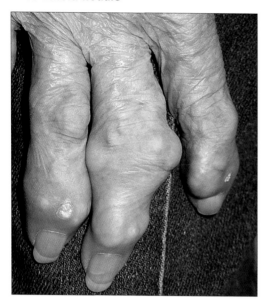

Description skin-colored to erythematous nodules of varying sizes
Location overlying joints or extensor surfaces exposed to trauma
Characteristics can occur at any age but typically in older adults, chronic
Tests Histopathology: palisading granuloma surrounding fibrin
Associated systemic disease associated with severe rheumatoid arthritis
Treatment pearls treat underlying rheumatoid arthritis

Foreign body reaction

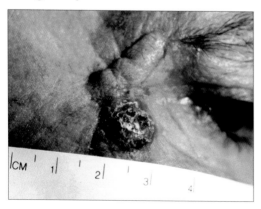

Description erythematous/brown papule, nodule or plaque ± ulceration
Location exposed areas most common
Characteristics chronic, painful

Tests Histopathology: dermal epithelioid granulomas with surrounding mixed infiltrate and giant cells, ± foreign body seen under polarized light
Associated systemic disease none
Treatment pearls excision

Necrobiosis lipoidica diabeticorum
See page 91

Sarcoid
See page 443

Malignant tumors
Basal cell carcinoma
Small cell carcinoma
Metastatic
Keratoacanthoma
Epithelioid sarcoma

Deep fungal
Sporotrichosis
See page 178
Blastomycosis
See page 179
Coccidioidomycosis
See page 181
Cryptococcosis

AFB+ granulomas
Tuberculosis

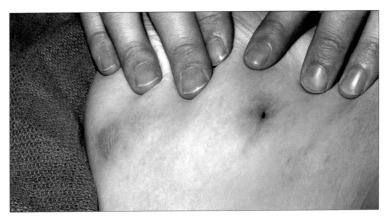

Description erythematous/brown papule, plaque or subcutaneous nodule that progresses to ulceration (gumma) or verrucous lesions which heal with scarring
Location *lupus vulgaris*: TB on the face or ears with 'apple-jelly' appearance of red/brown plaque; *scrofuloderma*: subcutaneous nodular TB with sinus tracts and drainage; *miliary TB*: disseminated diffusely over body with tiny pinpoint papulovesicles

Characteristics cutaneous lesions may resolve spontaneously in several months to years, cutaneous disease may evolve from endogenous infection or from exogenous inoculation, ± pain, regional lymphadenopathy is common
Tests tissue culture and/or PCR; PPD; CXR shows cavitary lesions; Histopathology: caseating dermal granulomas with surrounding lymphocytic inflammation and a +AFB stain
Associated systemic disease tuberculosis is a systemic infection with manifestations in the lungs as well as other organs
Treatment pearls antituberculoid treatment appropriate for region for 6 months (may include isoniazid, ethambutol, streptomycin, rifampin and pyrazinamide)

Atypical mycobacteria

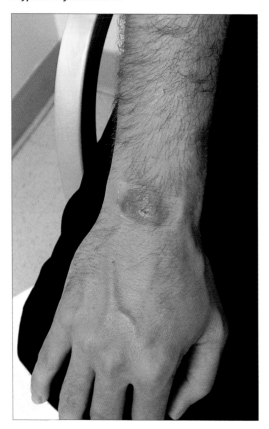

Description erythematous papules, pustules, keratotic plaques or subcutaneous nodules ± necrosis/abscess formation and drainage, can progress to verrucous or ulcerated lesions
Location extremity lesions are most common, may be in a linear 'sporotrichoid' distribution that follows lymphatic drainage

Characteristics resolves with treatment, painful
Tests tissue culture, PCR; Histopathology: dermal caseating granulomas with surrounding lymphocytic inflammation, +AFB stain
Associated systemic disease none
Treatment pearls excision, minocycline, antituberculous drugs based on type of atypical mycobacterium

Leprosy

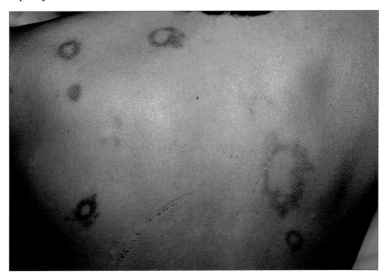

Description *lepromatous*: many, small, symmetric, ill-defined hypopigmented macules that progress to solid or annular erythematous papules and plaques, may progress to leonine facies; *tuberculoid*: few, large, asymmetric well-demarcated, infiltrated, erythematous plaques ± annular configuration
Location face, extremities, buttocks common, and the back in tuberculoid leprosy
Characteristics male>female in lepromatous type but total number of cases is equal, bimodal incidence with peaks at 10–15 years and 30–60 years, ± anhidrosis, anesthesias and alopecia within the plaques, ± palpable peripheral nerves, may be associated with the 'Lucio' phenomenon of necrotizing, cutaneous small vessel vasculitis or with erythema nodosum, resolves with treatment but hypopigmentation may remain
Tests Histopathology: granulomas ± linear arrangement following nerves; *lepromatous*: many organisms within histiocytes (globi) with mild inflammation; *tuberculoid*: few organisms and intense inflammatory infiltrate
Associated systemic disease none
Treatment pearls multidrug therapy may include rifampin, sulfone, clofazimine, ofloxacin, dapsone; may require thalidomide or prednisone for inflammation

Tick bite

Syphilis/yaws

Parasites

Mycetoma (nocardia)

Orf/milker's nodule

Leishmaniasis

Pyoderma

Trauma (burn)

Pyoderma gangrenosum

Vasculitis

Iododerma/bromoderma

Radiation dermatitis

Folliculitis

Lupus miliaris disseminatus faciei

Actinic granuloma (Miescher's granuloma of the face)
See page 92

Pemphigus vegetans
See page 113

HALO LESIONS

Halo nevus

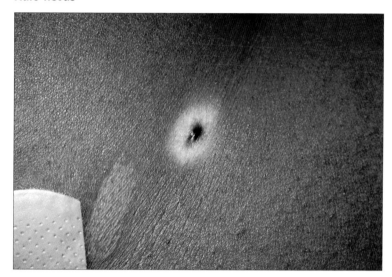

Description well-demarcated, round or oval, pink or brown, macule or papule surrounded by a hypopigmented ring
Location upper back is common
Characteristics light skin>dark skin, children and teenagers>adults, may resolve completely or persist
Tests Histopathology: nests of melanocytes in epidermis and/or dermis with surrounding dense lymphohistiocytic infiltrate within and surrounding nests
Associated systemic disease associated with vitiligo and melanoma
Treatment pearls biopsy if nevus appears atypical

Spitz nevus
See page 368

Melanoma
See page 380

Psoriasis (Woronoff's ring)

Dermatofibroma
See page 381

Neurofibroma

Urticaria
See page 88

Congenital nevus
See page 379, Nevus

Blue nevus
See page 358

Molluscum contagiosum

Verruca planae (flat warts)

Sarcoid

Lichen planus

HAND DERMATITIS
Contact/irritant dermatitis

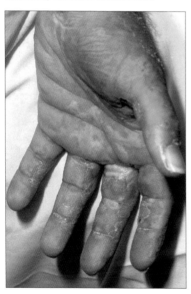

Description erythematous, scaly patches and plaques ± vesicles/bullae, may heal with hyperpigmentation
Location can occur anywhere
Characteristics waxing and waning course, pruritic
Tests Histopathology: spongiotic dermatitis ± eosinophils
Associated systemic disease none
Treatment pearls topical corticosteroids, detergent/soap/deodorant counseling, avoid irritant or contact allergen

CAUSES OF CONTACT DERMATITIS OF HANDS

Household products
- Nickel, copper, gold
- Rubber
- Potassium dichromate
- Topical medications (benzocaine, neomycin, bacitracin, benadryl)
- Balsam of Peru and other fragrances
- Resins
- Antibacterials in soaps and cleansers
- Essential oils (eugenol, clove, anise, spearmint, balsam of Peru, eucalyptus)

Products used by medical personnel
- Benzalkonium Cl (Zephiran)
- Formalin
- Glutaraldehyde
- Latex
- Local anesthetics
- Iodine compounds
- Topical antibiotics (neomycin, bacitracin)
- Alcohol
- Phenothiazine

Products used by dentists
- Acrylic monomer
- Latex

Dyshidrosis
See page 57

Atopic dermatitis
See page 141

Psoriasis
See page 58

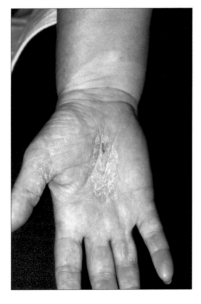

Tinea manuum (dermatophytosis)

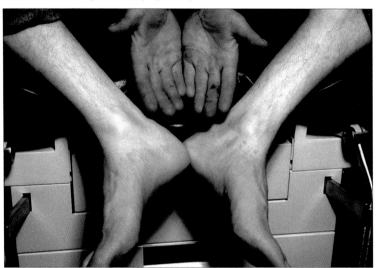

Description diffuse scale ± erythema covering one or both palms
Location palms
Characteristics any age, resolves with treatment, ± pruritus, may be associated with several dystrophic fingernails consistent with onychomycosis, may be associated with moccasin-type tinea pedis on bilateral soles (one hand–two foot disease)
Tests KOH+, fungal culture+; Histopathology: fungal hyphae noted within the stratum corneum
Associated systemic disease none
Treatment pearls topical and/or oral antifungals

Scabies
See page 52

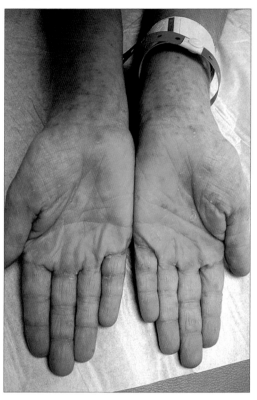

Viral exanthem (HSV, Hand, foot and mouth disease, and others)

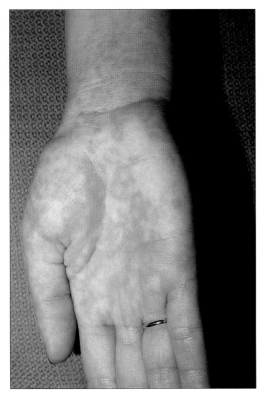

Drug reaction

Bacterial infection

Candidiasis

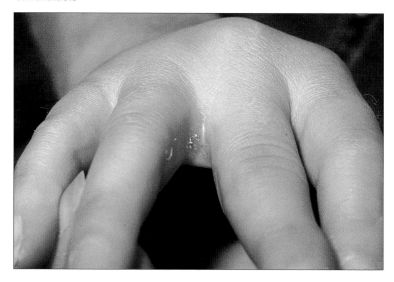

Secondary syphilis (lues)

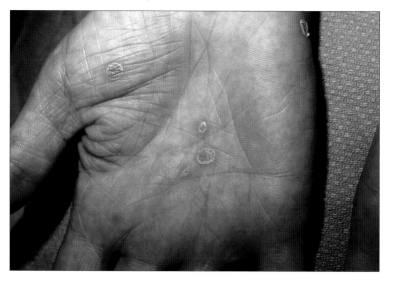

HIRSUTISM

Polycystic ovarian syndrome
Drugs (dilantin, minoxidil)
Testosterone (arrhenoblastoma, hilar cell)
Cortisone
Hurler's syndrome
Mumps
Malnutrition (anorexia)
Acromegaly

HYPERHIDROSIS

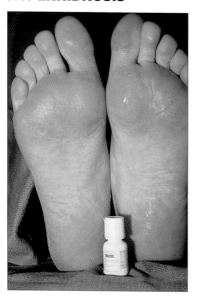

Emotional

Hyperthyroidism

Hyperparathyroidism

Diabetes

Menopause

Pheochromocytoma

Carcinoid syndrome

Drugs
Insulin
Meperidine
Emetics
Antipyretics

Spinal injury

Stroke

Infection
Night sweats secondary to tuberculosis, malaria

Malignancy
Night sweats secondary to lymphoma, leukemia or other malignancy

HYPERKERATOTIC PAPULES

Keratosis pilaris
See page 171

Darier's disease (keratosis follicularis)

Description red papules and plaques, some with central crusty core, that progress to eroded, malodorous and verrucous areas on trunk; flat-topped, skin-colored verrucous lesions on dorsal hands; punctate hyperkeratosis of palms; white papules on oral mucosa
Location flexural folds, intertriginous, face and ears, scalp and trunk
Characteristics onset at puberty, AD inheritance (defect ATPase 2A2), nails with longitudinal red and white stripes and V-shaped notching at distal nail plate, exacerbation in summer and with lithium
Tests Histopathology: superbasilar acantholysis, dyskeratotic cells in epidermis
Associated systemic disease none
Treatment pearls topical and oral retinoids, topical and oral antibiotics for common secondary infection, cyclosporine

Grover's disease (transient acantholytic dermatosis)

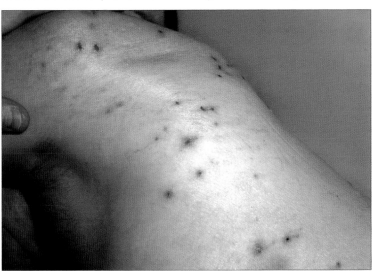

Description red papules and fragile vesicles that erode into scaly patches and plaques
Location symmetric on trunk in sun-exposed areas
Characteristics older males, chronic, pruritic, may be exacerbated by heat
Tests Histopathology: four patterns: intraepidermal acantholysis like Hailey–Hailey; localized dyskeratotic acantholysis like Darier's; spongiotic; or suprabasilar or subcorneal cleft-like pemphigus; all patterns have perivascular lymphocytic infiltrate ± eosinophils and plasma cells.
Associated systemic disease none
Treatment pearls topical corticosteroids, topical or oral retinoids, light therapy, dapsone

Hailey–Hailey disease (familial benign pemphigus)
See page 112

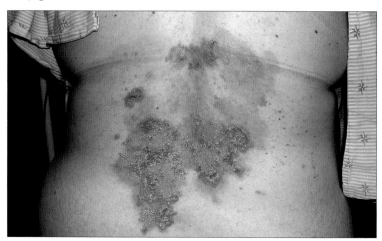

Verruca vulgaris

Prurigo nodularis

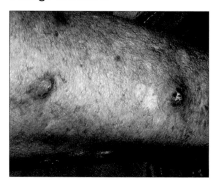

Description hyperkeratotic, firm, scaly papule
Location can occur anywhere within reach of the hands, spares central back ('butterfly sign')
Characteristics female>male, adults, asymptomatic to pruritic
Tests Histopathology: hyperkeratosis, acanthosis, sparse mixed infiltrate
Associated systemic disease none
Treatment pearls topical or intralesional corticosteroids, stop picking, antihistamines, doxepin, cryotherapy, phototherapy

Verruca planae (flat warts)

Chromoblastomycosis

Trichilemmoma

Acrokeratosis verruciformis of Hopf

Angiokeratoma

Pityriasis rubra pilaris

Lichen spinulosus

Cutaneous horn

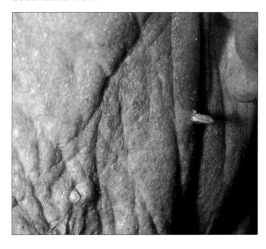

Keratoacanthoma

Squamous cell carcinoma

Hypertrophic actinic keratosis

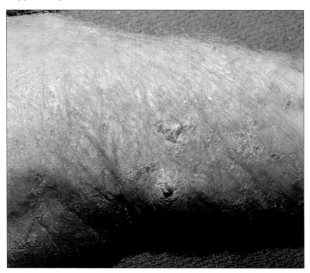

Seborrheic keratosis

Epidermal nevus

Confluent and reticulated papillomatosis of Gougerot and Carteaud (CARP)

Focal epidermolytic hyperkeratosis

Lichen striatus

Perforating diseases (Kyrle's disease)

Elastosis perforans serpiginosa (EPS)

Vitamin A excess or deficiency

HYPERKERATOTIC PLAQUES
Lichen simplex chronicus (LSC)

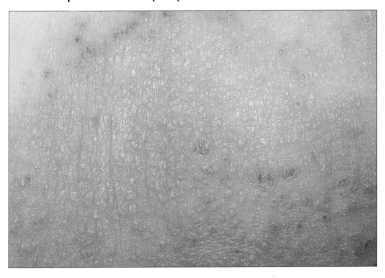

Description hyperpigmented, scaly plaques with accentuated skin markings
Location can occur anywhere
Characteristics patient has a habit of rubbing/scratching the area, lesion present for months
Tests Histopathology: acanthosis and hyperkeratosis
Associated systemic disease none
Treatment pearls avoid rubbing area, topical corticosteroids

Hypertrophic actinic keratosis
See page 501

Hypertrophic discoid lupus erythematosus
See page 78, Discoid lupus erythematosus

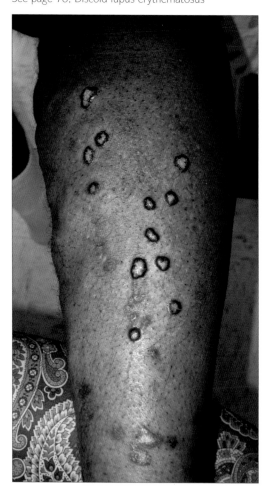

Hypertrophic lichen planus
See page 259, Lichen planus

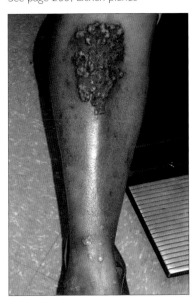

Psoriasis
See page 397

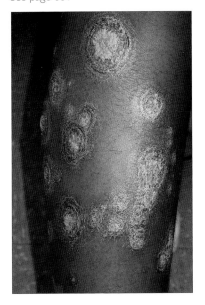

Pemphigus vegetans
See page 113

Norwegian scabies

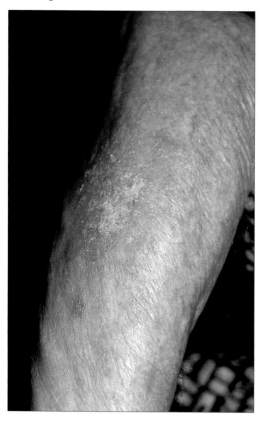

Description hyperkeratotic papules and plaques with thick overlying crust and surrounding erythema, ± linear tiny thread-like burrows extending from peripheral papules, ± pustules or bulla
Location usually in groups, in web spaces of digits, crusted palms, on flexor wrists, axillae, around waist, buttocks, genital area, elbows, or diffusely over body
Characteristics resolves with treatment, intense pruritus, ± pain
Tests mineral oil smear of crusted area to see many scabetic mites, eggs, or scybala (feces); Histopathology: parts of numerous mites seen within the stratum corneum, perivascular infiltrate with interstitial eosinophils, +spongiosis, ± papillary dermal edema
Associated systemic disease none
Treatment pearls orally: ivermectin; topically: permethrin, sulfur ointment or lindane (*note:* lindane has been discontinued in some countries and states)

Chronic stasis dermatitis

Epidermolytic hyperkeratosis

Flegel's syndrome (hyperkeratosis lenticularis perstans)

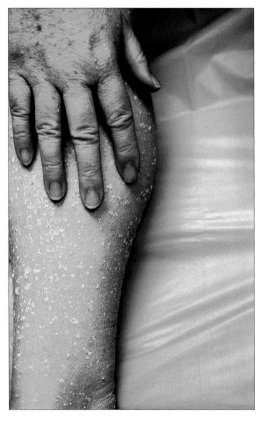

HYPERPIGMENTATION – DIFFUSE

Chronic systemic diseases
Chronic renal failure

Connective tissue diseases
Scleroderma
Dermatomyositis

Drugs
Minocycline
Antimalarials
Phenothiazines

Gold, silver (Au, Ag)
Zidovudine (AZT)
Amiodarone
Psoralens
Dilantin
Busulfan
Clofazimine
Arsenic (inorganic)
ACTH
Pyridium

Endocrine diseases
Addison's disease
Cushing's syndrome (pituitary)
Hyperthyroidism
Acromegaly
Pheochromocytoma
Pregnancy
Nelson's syndrome

Gastrointestinal
Cirrhosis – especially biliary
Malabsorption/malnutrition
Whipple disease (severe)

Postinflammatory pigmentation following a diffuse rash

Metabolic
Porphyria cutanea tarda (PCT)
Folate, B_{12} deficiency
Nutritional deficiency
Hemochromatosis
Vitamin A ($\uparrow$ or $\downarrow$)
Pellagra ($\downarrow$ niacin)
Scurvy ($\downarrow$ vitamin C)
Gaucher's syndrome
Niemann–Pick disease

Neoplastic
Melanosis secondary to metastatic melanoma
ACTH-producing tumor
Hodgkin's lymphoma

Nervous system disease
Schilder's disease

Infections
Malaria
Kala-azar (leishmaniasis)

HYPERPIGMENTATION – LINEAR AND ELEVATED

See page 262, Linear lesions

HYPERPIGMENTATION – LINEAR AND FLAT

See page 269, Linear lesions – flat and hyperpigmented

HYPERPIGMENTED MACULES AND PATCHES (BROWN MACULES)

Post-inflammatory hyperpigmentation

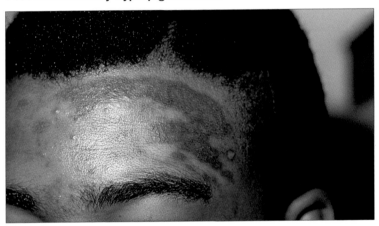

Description brown, poorly demarcated macules/mottled appearance
Location in area of previous inflammation
Characteristics resolves slowly with time, asymptomatic, exacerbated by sunlight
Tests Histopathology: increased melanin in epidermis ± pigment incontinence in dermis
Associated systemic disease none
Treatment pearls sunscreen, topical hydroquinone, topical retinoids, chemical peels, laser for dermal pigment

Post-inflammatory hyperpigmentation

Melasma

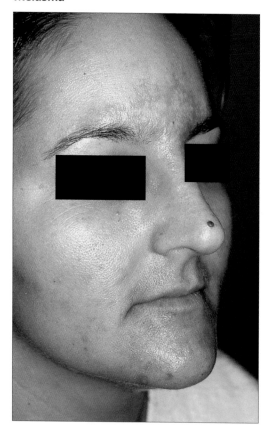

Description well-demarcated brown macules and patches
Location common on face
Characteristics female>male, dark skin>light skin (increased in Hispanic, Asian and Middle-Eastern women), adults, chronic, asymptomatic, exacerbated by sunlight and increased estrogen states (OCPs, pregnancy)
Tests Histopathology: increased epidermal or dermal melanin ± increase in melanocytes
Associated systemic disease none
Treatment pearls sunscreen, topical hydroquinone, topical retinoids, topical azelaic acid, avoid OCPs

Nevus

See page 379

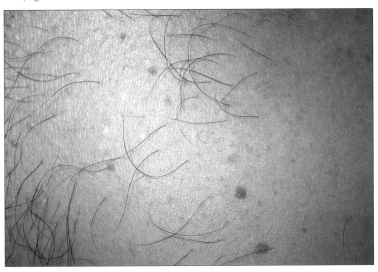

Lentigo/freckle (ephelide)

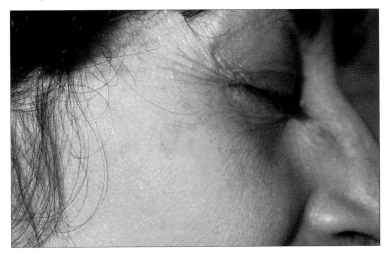

Lentigo

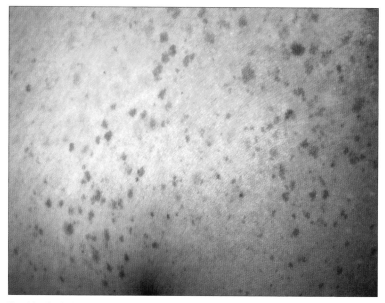

Freckle (ephelide)

Description brown, well-demarcated macules

Location common on face and sun-exposed areas, can occur on mucosa (oral or genital), nailbed, palms, soles

Characteristics lentigines are chronic, freckles may completely fade when sunlight absent, asymptomatic, exacerbated by sunlight

Tests Histopathology: increased melanin ± increased melanocytes

Associated systemic disease may be associated with xeroderma pigmentosum, LEOPARD, LAMB, NAME, Peutz–Jeghers, Laugier–Hunziker, Cantu, Cowden's or Carney syndrome

Treatment pearls no treatment necessary, laser

Café-au-lait spot

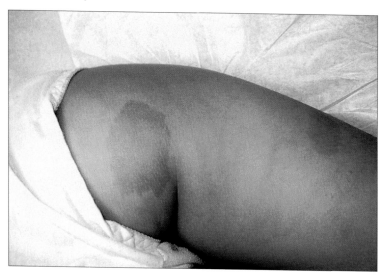

Description single (or multiple), well-demarcated, oval, hyperpigmented macule or patch

Location trunk and proximal extremities most common

Characteristics presents at birth or after in childhood, chronic, asymptomatic, more common in dark skin

Tests Histopathology: normal epidermis with mild increase in melanin content of keratinocytes within the basal layer

Associated systemic disease if >6 in number, may be associated with neurofibromatosis; if large with 'coast of Maine' appearance, may be associated with McCune–Albright syndrome; other syndrome associations include tuberous sclerosis, Russell–Silver, Watson's, Bloom's and Westerhof's

Treatment pearls no treatment necessary

Tinea versicolor
See page 225

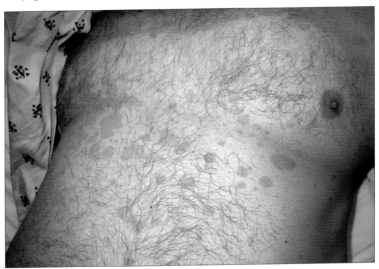

Fixed drug reaction

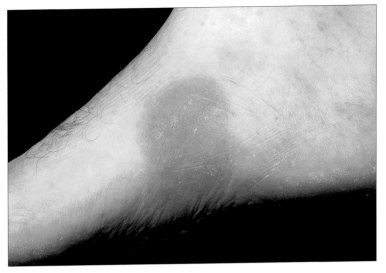

Description brown–red usually solitary well-demarcated macule, may be targetoid, ± erosion
Location 50% on genital and oral mucosa, can occur anywhere on body

Characteristics resolves in weeks to months with postinflammatory hyperpigmentation if drug stopped, asymptomatic, exacerbated by re-exposure to drug (NSAIDs and sulfa drugs most commonly, *see box for additional common drugs*)

Tests Histopathology: necrotic keratinocytes in epidermis, mixed infiltrate, pigment incontinence, ± interface change, usually with eosinophils

Associated systemic disease none

Treatment pearls avoid offending drug, no other treatment necessary

---

COMMON DRUGS CAUSING FIXED DRUG REACTION

- Barbiturates*
- Carbamazepine*
- Ciprofloxacin
- Gold
- Hydrochlorothiazide (HCTZ)
- NSAIDs (including diclofenac, ibuprofen, naproxen and piroxicam)*
- Phenacetin
- Phenolphthalein*
- Phenylbutazone
- Pseudoephedrine
- Quinidine
- Salicylates
- Sulfa drugs*
- Tetracyclines (including doxycycline and minocycline)

* Indicates the most common.

Granuloma faciale

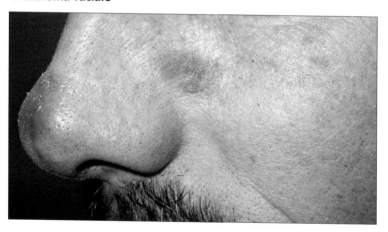

Description brown/red solitary well-demarcated patch or plaque

Location face most common

Characteristics light skin>dark skin, male>female, chronic course, asymptomatic

Tests Histopathology: normal epidermis, grenz zone with dense mixed infiltrate in the dermis including eosinophils especially perifollicular, ± leukocytoclastic vasculitis

Associated systemic disease none

Treatment pearls difficult to treat, can try intralesional corticosteroids, electrocautery, laser, dermabrasion, dapsone, PUVA

Secondary syphilis (lues)
See page 401

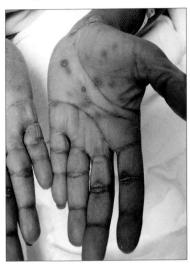

Sarcoid
See page 443

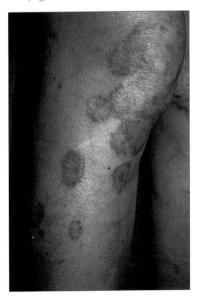

Mastocytoma
See page 384

Drugs
Minocycline
Amiodarone
Psoralen
Gold, silver (Au, Ag)
Phenothiazines
Zidovudine (AZT)
Antimalarials

Arsenic (chronic)

Mongolian spot
See page 435

Nevus of Ota/Ito
See page 434

Labial melanosis

Macular amyloidosis

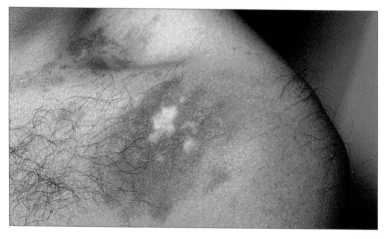

Berloque dermatitis

Phytophotodermatitis

Incontinentia pigmenti

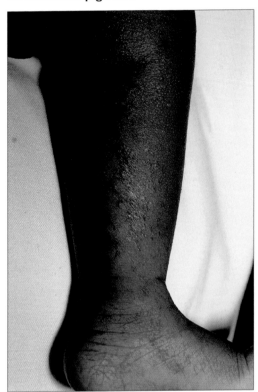

Postradiation pigmentation

Mastocytosis (urticaria pigmentosa)

Erythema dyschromicum perstans (ashy dermatosis)

Maculae cerulae (*after spider bite*)

Acanthosis nigricans

Pinta

Tinea nigra
See page 175

Ochronosis (endogenous and exogenous)

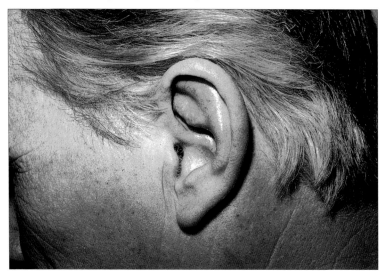

Anetoderma

Leprosy
See page 186

Pityriasis rosea

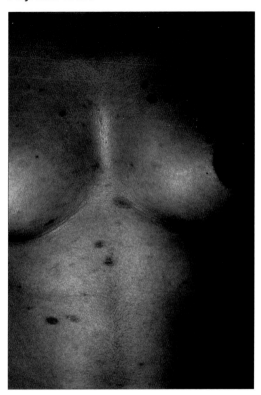

Psoriasis (resolving)

HYPERTRICHOSIS – LOCAL

Hirsutism (androgen excess)

Pregnancy

Drugs (topical minoxidil)

Congenital nevus

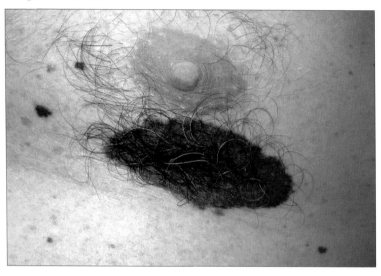

Teratoma or spina bifida

Malnutrition (anorexia)

Trauma

Pretibial myxedema

Topical corticosteroid application

Dermatofibroma

Chronic thrombophlebitis

HYPERTRICHOSIS – GENERALIZED

Porphyria cutanea tarda (PCT)

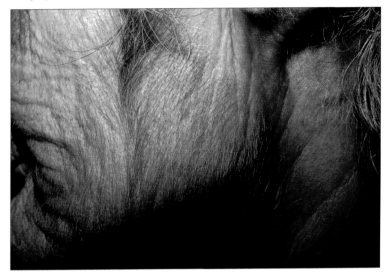

Drugs (minoxidil, oral phenytoin)

Malignancy associated (hypertrichosis lanuginosa acquisita)
See page 285

Polycystic ovary disease

Hurler's syndrome

Dermatomyositis/tumor

Teratoma

Mumps

Malnutrition (anorexia)

Acromegaly

Nervous system disorders
Multiple sclerosis
Post-encephalitis
Chronic meningitis
Schizophrenia
Post-concussion

Thymic tumor

HYPOHIDROSIS

Heat stroke

Dehydration

Drugs
Anticholinergics
Ganglionic blockers

Hypothyroidism

Sjögren syndrome

Systemic sclerosis

Inflammation of skin

Hypothalamic lesion

Horner's syndrome

Hyperkeratosis/ichthyosis (mechanical obstruction)

Peripheral neuropathy

Miliaria profunda

Tropical anhidrotic asthenia

Hereditary anhidrotic and hidrotic ectodermal dysplasia

Angiokeratoma corporis diffusum universale
(Fabry's syndrome)

HYPOPIGMENTATION – LINEAR

See page 271, Linear lesions – hypopigmented or depigmented

HYPOPIGMENTED MACULES (HYPOMELANOTIC) AND DEPIGMENTED MACULES (AMELANOTIC)

Depigmented macules (amelanotic)
Vitiligo

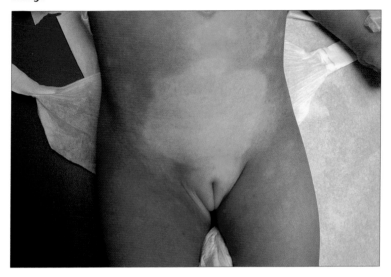

Description depigmented, well-demarcated macules (may be hypopigmented if early or resolving)

Location common on dorsal hands, flexor wrists, face (especially periorificial), genital area, knees, elbows, axillae and groin, vitiligo of scalp may lead to white hair; can be localized to one area of the body, segmental or generalized

Characteristics children and young adults most commonly, self-limited vs. chronic, asymptomatic, ± Koebner phenomenon

Tests Histopathology: absence of melanocytes in the basal layer

Associated systemic disease may be associated with thyroid abnormalities, pernicious anemia, diabetes, mucocutaneous candidiasis, alopecia areata or other autoimmune diseases

Treatment pearls high-potency topical corticosteroids, sunlight, nbUVB, PUVA, tacrolimus, excimer laser

Piebaldism

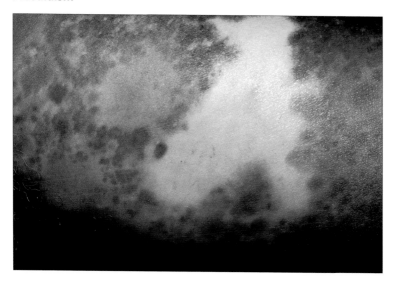

Discoid lupus erythematosus (DLE)

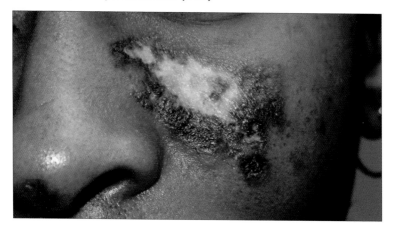

Scleroderma (salt and pepper pattern)

Halo nevus

Chemical leukoderma
Secondary to catechols, phenols or monobenzyl ether of hydroquinone

Melanoma with surrounding associated leukoderma especially after regression

Postinflammatory hypopigmentation
Can sometimes be depigmented

Hypopigmented macules (hypomelanotic)
Postinflammatory hypopigmentation

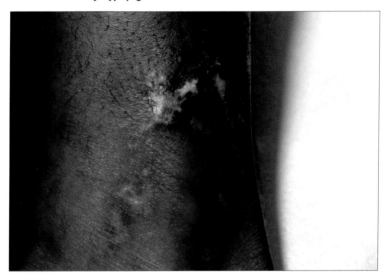

Description light, poorly demarcated macules/mottled appearance
Location in area of previous inflammation
Characteristics resolves slowly with time, asymptomatic
Tests Histopathology: normal epidermis with pigment incontinence in dermis
Associated systemic disease none
Treatment pearls topical retinoids

Tinea versicolor

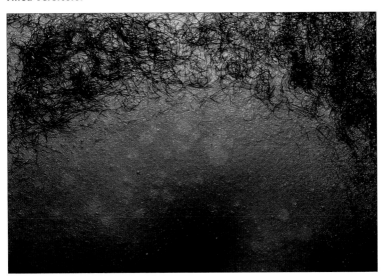

Description hypo- or hyperpigmented macules and confluent patches with brawny scale

Location upper trunk and back most common, can be on face of children or groin in adults

Characteristics self-limited, recurs in hot weather

Tests KOH; Histopathology: 'spaghetti and meatballs', both yeast forms and hyphae seen in the stratum corneum

Associated systemic disease none

Treatment pearls topical antifungals, topical selenium sulfide shampoo, oral antifungals if resistant to therapy or very severe

Seborrheic dermatitis
See page 398

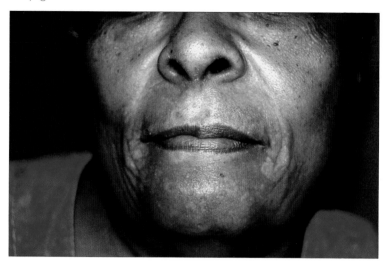

Pityriasis alba

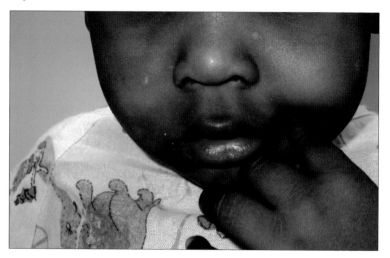

Description hypopigmented macules and patches ± brawny scale
Location common on face in symmetric distribution, upper arms, shoulders
Characteristics young children>adults, dark skin>light skin, considered a subset of atopic dermatitis, resolves with time, worse in summer

Tests Histopathology: subacute spongiotic dermatitis
Associated systemic disease atopy
Treatment pearls no treatment necessary

Idiopathic guttate hypomelanosis

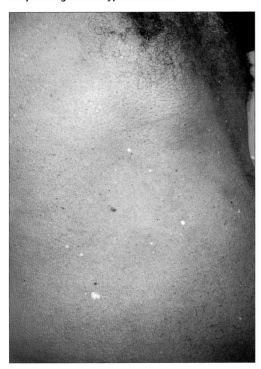

Description very small, round, well-demarcated hypopigmented macules
Location common on lower extremities>upper extremities
Characteristics dark skin>light skin, older age, chronic
Tests Histopathology: flat interface between epidermis and dermis, reduced number of melanocytes in the basal layer
Associated systemic disease none
Treatment pearls no treatment necessary

Corticosteroid induced hypopigmentation (iatrogenic)
Description poorly demarcated hypopigmented macule
Location in area of previous topical or intralesional corticosteroid use, can be linear if previous intralesional injection
Characteristics resolves with time
Tests Histopathology: flattened atrophic epidermis with underlying telangiectasias and pigment incontinence
Associated systemic disease none
Treatment pearls discontinue corticosteroids

Sarcoid
See page 443

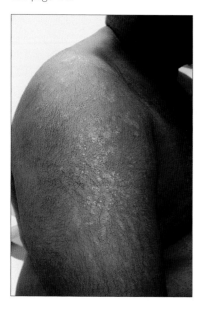

Secondary syphilis
See page 401
Lichen sclerosus et atrophicus
See page 100

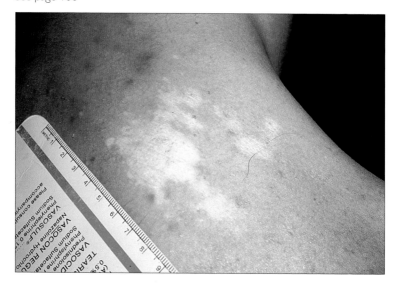

Systemic lupus erythematosus (SLE)
Discoid lupus erythematosus (DLE)
Scleroderma/morphea
Pityriasis lichenoides chronica
Cutaneous T-cell lymphoma (CTCL)

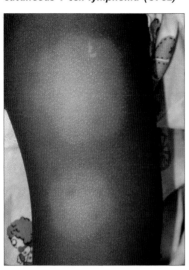

Follicular mucinosis
Parapsoriasis

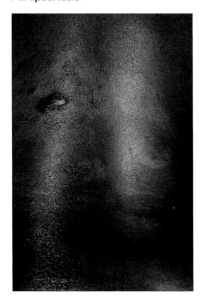

Hypopigmented macules

Psoriasis (post-treatment)
Atrophic lichen planus
Achromic verruca planae (flat warts)

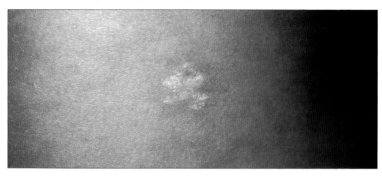

Achromic seborrheic keratosis
Hydroquinone use
Nevus anemicus

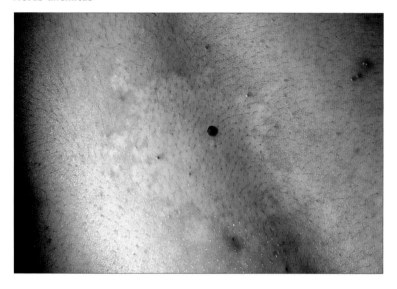

Nevus depigmentosus

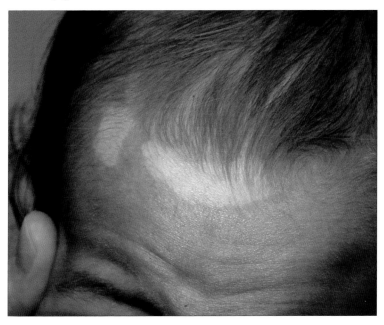

Hypopigmented macules

Hypomelanosis of Ito

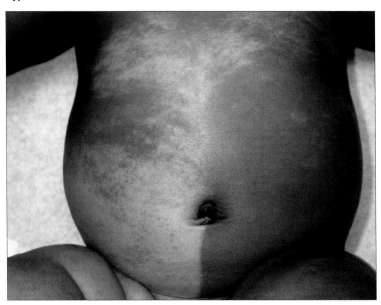

Incontinentia pigmenti
Radiation dermatitis
Sclerosing basal cell carcinoma
Leprosy
Tuberous sclerosus
Phenylketonuria
Regressed melanoma

Ash leaf macule

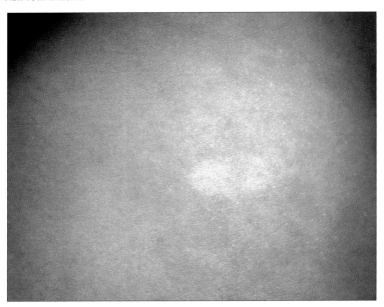

ICHTHYOSIS – CONGENITAL (BORN WITH COLLODION MEMBRANE)

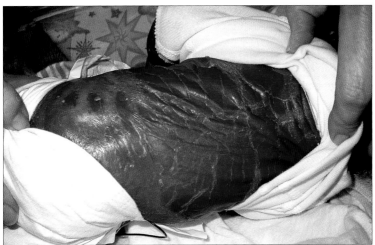

Lamellar ichthyosis

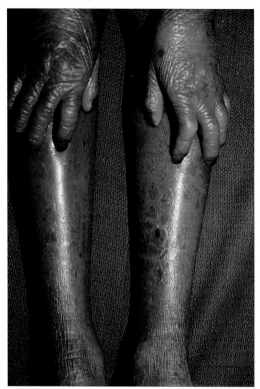

Non-bullous congenital ichthyosiform erythroderma

Sjögren–Larsson syndrome

Trichothiodystrophy

Netherton's syndrome

Ectodermal dysplasia

Neutral lipid storage disease

Idiopathic self-healing ichthyosis

ICHTHYOSIS – CONGENITAL (BORN WITH ERYTHRODERMA)

KID syndrome (keratitis, ichthyosis, deafness)

Trichothiodystrophy (PIBIDS)

Conradi–Hünermann–Happle syndrome

Lamellar ichthyosis

Non-bullous congenital ichthyosiform erythroderma

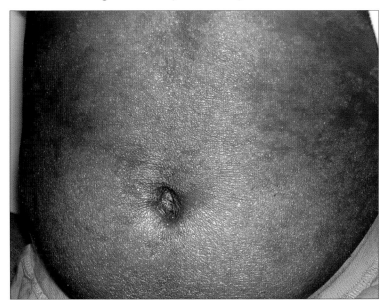

Bullous congenital ichthyosiform erythroderma (epidermolytic hyperkeratosis)

Ichthyosis bullosa of Siemens

ICHTHYOSIS – ACQUIRED

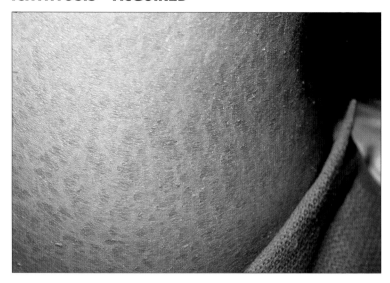

Hypothyroidism

Malnutrition

Sarcoid

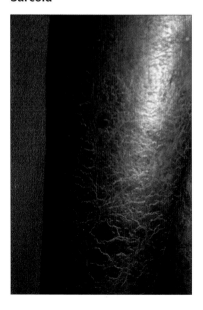

Hyperparathyroidism

Hodgkin's lymphoma

Systemic lupus erythematosus (SLE)

Leprosy

Lymphoproliferative disorders

Kaposi's sarcoma, classic type

Drugs
Clofazimine
Cimetidine
Nicotinic acid
Butyrophenone
Azacosterol hydrochloride

HIV/AIDS

INFANTS – BULLA

See page 118, Bulla/vesicles – infancy

INFANTS – PAPULOSQUAMOUS

See page 405, Papulosquamous – infants

INFANTS – PUSTULES

See page 492, Pustules – newborns

INFLAMMATORY BOWEL DISEASE ASSOCIATED CUTANEOUS MANIFESTATIONS (ULCERATIVE COLITIS AND CROHN'S DISEASE)

Pyoderma gangrenosum

Granulomas

Erythema nodosum

Aphthous ulcers

Malnutrition

Contact/irritant dermatitis at stoma sites

Erythema

Lichen planus

Vascular thrombosis

INGUINAL MASS
Hernia

Ectopic testes

Hydrocele

Arterial aneurysm

Carcinoma

Lymphoma

Mononucleosis

Syphilis (primary, secondary and tertiary)

Lymphogranuloma venereum

Granuloma inguinale

Pyogenic (lymph node enlargement secondary to balanitis)

Gonoccocemia

Chancroid

KAPOSI'S VARICELLIFORM ERUPTION
Disseminated HSV superimposed on underlying skin disease including entities listed below

Atopic dermatitis

Darier's disease

Pemphigus foliaceous

Hailey–Hailey disease

Ichthyosis vulgaris

Congenital ichthyosiform erythroderma (CIE)

Cutaneous T-cell lymphoma (CTCL)

Sézary syndrome

Burns

KERATODERMA – PALMOPLANTAR

Psoriasis
See page 397

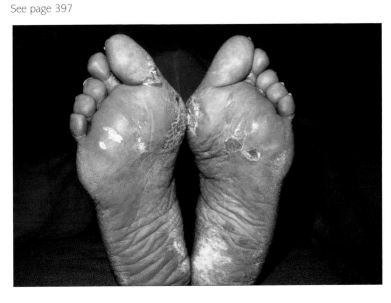

Contact dermatitis
See page 189

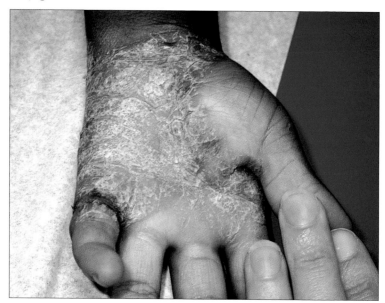

Tinea manuum (dermatophytosis)
See page 191

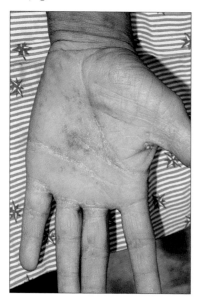

Tinea pedis (dermatophytosis)

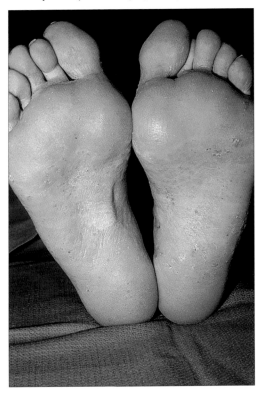

Description three presentations: *moccasin type* with scale and erythema in 'moccasin' pattern on plantar surface (see p. 191); *interdigital type* with erythema, scale, maceration and fissures in the toe webs and contiguous skin; *vesicular type* with vesicles/bulla usually localized to the instep area
Location plantar surface extending onto lateral foot but rarely dorsal foot, ± involvement of toe webs
Characteristics male>female, adults>children, resolves with treatment, ± pruritus, moccasin type may be associated with onychomycosis of several toe nails
Tests KOH, fungal culture; Histopathology: fungal hyphae seen within stratum corneum
Associated systemic disease none
Treatment pearls topical antifungals, or systemic antifungals if resistant to treatment

Norwegian scabies
See page 204

Pityriasis rubra pilaris
See page 159

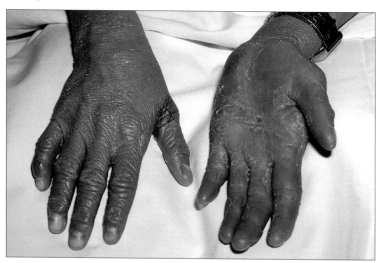

Trauma

Paraneoplastic

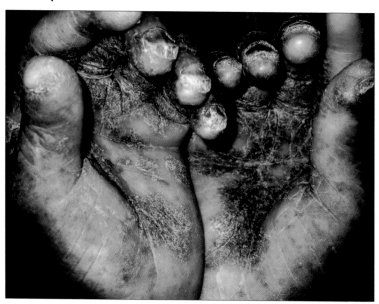

Sézary syndrome

Myxedema associated

Arsenic poisoning (chronic)

Keratoderma climactericum

Lymphedematous associated

Pachyonychia congenita

Dyskeratosis congenita

Epidermolysis bullosa

Progressive keratoderma
Increases until middle age; upper and lower extremity patches

Punctate keratoderma

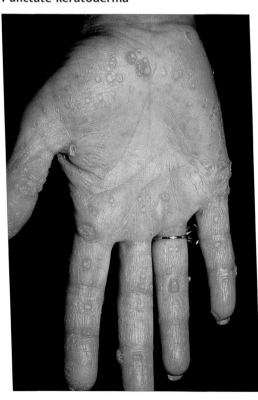

Linear punctate keratoses (striate keratoderma)

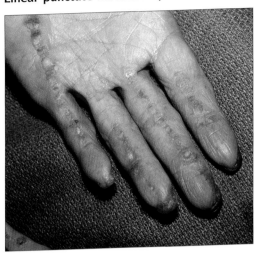

Keratolysis exfoliativa – recurrent involvement of hands/feet Kawasaki's disease

Secondary syphilis

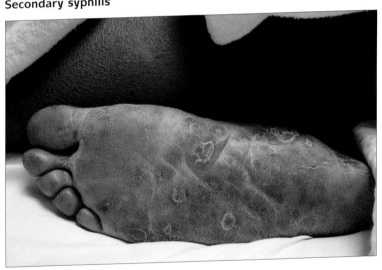

Yaws

Atopic dermatitis

Dyshidrosis

Erythroderma (of various causes)

Reiter's syndrome

Syndromes with keratoderma
Lamellar ichthyosis

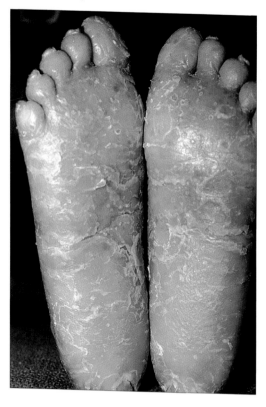

Bullous congenital ichthyosiform erythroderma (epidermolytic hyperkeratosis)
Ichthyosis hystrix (Curth–Macklin syndrome, mutilating palmoplantar keratoderma)
Unna–Thost syndrome
Hidrotic ectodermal dysplasia (Clouston syndrome)
Howell–Evans syndrome (with esophageal cancer)
Naegeli–Franceschetti–Jadassohn syndrome

Striate keratoderma
Linear and radiates from palms with corneal dystrophy, onset 5–20 years
Richner–Hanhart syndrome
Papillon–Lefèvre syndrome
Mal de Meleda syndrome
Olmsted's syndrome

KERATOSIS – PUNCTATE

Darier's disease

Basal cell nevus syndrome

Lichen planus

Arsenic

Punctate keratoderma

KOEBNER PHENOMENON

Psoriasis (Koebner secondary to leg cast)

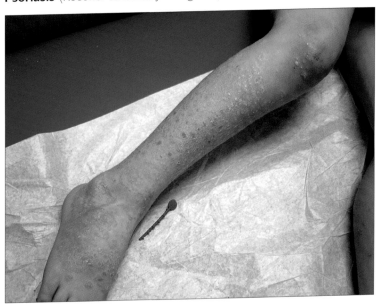

Lichen nitidus

Lichen planus

Verruca

Molluscum contagiosum

Dermatographism

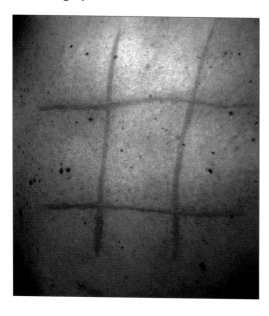

Sarcoid

Vitiligo

Erythema multiforme

Plant dermatitis (Rhus – pseudo-Koebner)

Lichen sclerosus et atrophicus

Darier's disease

Porokeratosis of Mibelli

Reactive perforating collagenosis

Xanthoma (hyperlipidemia associated)

LEG ULCERS

Venous ulcer

Arterial ischemia

Scar

Post-radiation

Necrobiosis lipoidica diabeticorum

Basal cell carcinoma

Squamous cell carcinoma

Melanoma

Systemic lupus erythematosus (SLE)

Discoid lupus erythematosus (DLE)

Polyarteritis nodosa (PAN)

Rheumatoid arthritis (Felty's syndrome)

Diabetic ulcer

Stasis

Atrophie blanche

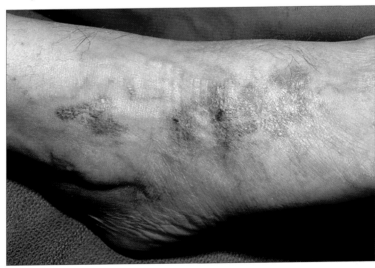

Infections
Deep fungal
Bacterial
Atypical mycobacteria
Viral

Bite (especially spider)

Trauma

Emboli/thrombi

Sickle cell disease

Hemolytic anemia

Thrombocytosis

Pyoderma gangrenosum

Sweet's syndrome

LEGS – EDEMA AND TUMORS

Lymphedema
See page 152

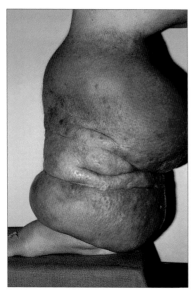

Elephantiasis nostra verrucosa

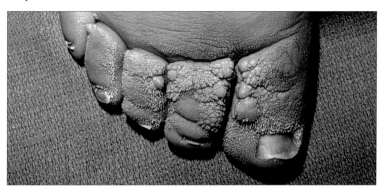

Description skin-colored/pink/brown verrucous papules and plaques
Location lower extremities most common, will occur in any area of chronic edema
Characteristics adults, chronic, asymptomatic, exacerbated by edema
Tests Histopathology: hyperkeratosis, acanthosis, dermal edema
Associated systemic disease usually there is an underlying disease causing chronic edema (congestive heart failure, renal, hepatic, or other)
Treatment pearls treat underlying edema, oral retinoids

Myxedema

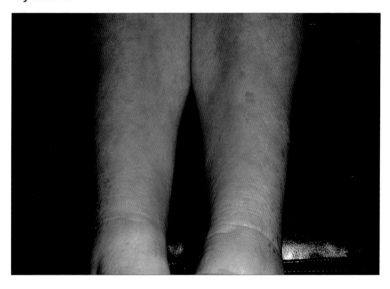

Description skin-colored to yellow/pink indurated skin with 'peau d'orange' appearance
Location pretibial surface most common

Characteristics female>male, adults, asymptomatic, ± pain and pruritus, ± overlying hypertrichosis and hyperhidrosis, myxedema is non-pitting
Tests thyroid panel. Histopathology: increased mucin in dermis, perivascular lymphocytic infiltrate, stellate fibroblasts, hyperkeratosis and papillomatosis
Associated systemic disease hyperthyroidism (can occur after hypothyroidism treatment)
Treatment pearls treatment of underlying thyroid disease usually does not improve myxedema, topical and intralesional corticosteroids, compression hose

Chromoblastomycosis
See page 537

Cutaneous T-cell lymphoma (CTCL)

Kaposi's sarcoma

Verruca vulgaris
See page 60

Lymphangioma

Lymphosarcoma

Lichen amyloidosis
See page 260

Iododerma/bromoderma

Angiokeratoma circumscriptum

LEGS – TENDER NODULES

Erythema nodosum

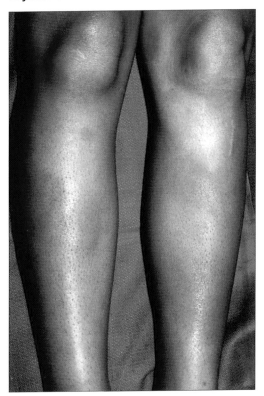

Description deep, erythematous, subcutaneous nodules
Location bilateral shins symmetrically
Characteristics females>males, 20–40 years peak, acute onset, resolves spontaneously in weeks to months but may recur, painful, ± fever and malaise
Tests check ASO titer, CBC, ESR, CXR, PPD; Histopathology: septal panniculitis without vasculitis
Associated systemic disease may be associated with sarcoidosis, inflammatory bowel disease, Behçet's syndrome, infections (Strep, tuberculosis/leprosy, fungal, lymphogranuloma venereum, EBV, tinea capitis), hematologic malignancies, drugs (sulfa, OCPs, aspirin), postvaccination; however, up to 50% of cases are idiopathic
Treatment pearls aspirin, NSAIDs, potassium iodide, treat underlying disease and rest

Subacute nodular migratory panniculitis (erythema nodosum migrans)
Description deep, erythematous, subcutaneous nodules that expand centrifugally to leave central clearing
Location often unilateral
Characteristics females>males, older adults, more chronic course and less painful than classic erythema nodosum, rarely associated with systemic symptoms
Tests Histopathology: similar to erythema nodosum with more granulomas and septal widening
Associated systemic disease usually no associated disease (rarely thyroid disease or Strep infection)
Treatment pearls aspirin, NSAIDs, potassium iodide and rest

Lupus profundus (lupus panniculitis)

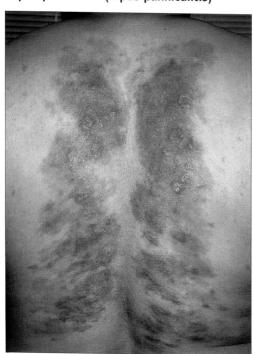

Description erythematous/violaceous, deep, indurated plaques
Location face, trunk and proximal extremities
Characteristics females>males, adults, onset may precede other symptoms of lupus, chronic course, ± pain
Tests ± low titer ANA; Histopathology: normal epidermis, superficial and deep perivascular lymphocytic infiltrate and a lobular panniculitis with hyaline necrosis of the fat ± plasma cells

Associated systemic disease DLE or SCLE>SLE
Treatment pearls antimalarials, oral or intralesional corticosteroids, cyclophosphamide, dapsone, thalidomide

Leukocytoclastic vasculitis

Erythema induratum (nodular vasculitis)

Gumma (tertiary syphilis)

Leprosy

Weber–Christian disease

Polyarteritis nodosa (PAN)

Thrombophlebitis

Emboli
Bacterial
Cholesterol
Tumor
Dysproteinemia

Panniculitis associated with pancreatitis/malignancy

Calcification in vessel secondary to uremia/hyperparathyroidism

α-1 Antitrypsin deficiency

LEONINE FACES

Cutaneous T-cell lymphoma (CTCL)

Leprosy

Leishmaniasis

Actinic reticuloid

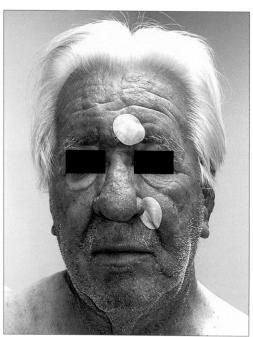

Papular mucinosis

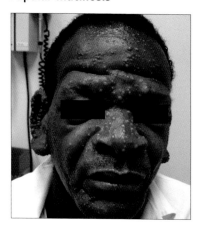

Amyloidosis

Histiocytosis

Scleromyxedema

Setleis syndrome

LEUKOPLAKIA
Leukoplakia

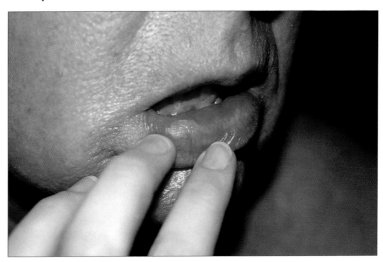

Description well-demarcated white patch or plaque
Location oral mucosa especially tongue, floor of mouth and soft palate
Characteristics men>>women; onset usually after age 40; asymptomatic; exacerbated by smoking and alcohol use, physical irritants, chronic trauma and poor oral hygiene
Tests Histopathology: hyperkeratosis ± dysplasia of epidermis
Associated systemic disease none
Treatment pearls excision if dysplasia as often premalignant for SCC, avoid carcinogenic substances

White sponge nevus
Description 'spongy' white papule
Location oral or perineal mucosa (buccal mucosa most common)
Characteristics AD inheritance (K4 and K13 mutation), progression until puberty, asymptomatic
Tests Histopathology: acanthosis, vacuolated cells in stratum spinosum
Associated systemic disease none
Treatment pearls no treatment necessary, tetracycline can lead to improvement

Lichen planus (mucosal)

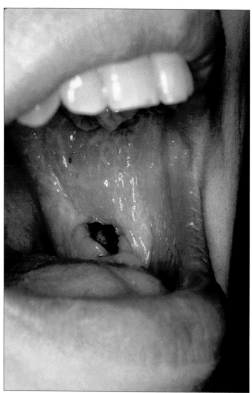

Description white lacy patches or eroded areas
Location oral or genital mucosa
Characteristics usually adult onset, +Koebner phenomenon, can be associated with drugs, may resolve spontaneously in 1–3 years, oral manifestations may be chronic, painful
Tests monitor mucosal lesions for malignant change; Histopathology: wedge-shaped hypergranulosis, saw-toothed rete ridges, lichenoid lymphocytic infiltrate with vacuolar basal layer changes and Civatte bodies
Associated systemic disease hepatitis C virus
Treatment pearls cyclosporine swish and spit, potent topical, intralesional or systemic corticosteroids, oral retinoids, griseofulvin, metronidazole, cyclosporine, dapsone, topical tacrolimus

Oral candidiasis (thrush)

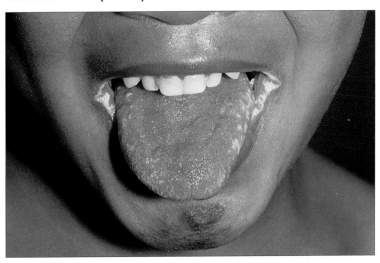

Description grey/white 'cottage cheese-like' plaques with underlying erythema ± maceration, ± perlèche
Location oral or genital mucosa and tongue
Characteristics increased incidence in immunosuppressed, resolves with treatment, associated with a smooth, red tongue
Tests will not scrape off mucosa with a tongue blade
Associated systemic disease immunosuppression, malnutrition
Treatment pearls antifungal troches, oral antifungals

Lichen sclerosus et atrophicus
See page 100

Oral florid papillomatosis

Trauma – physical (bite line) or chemical

Darier's disease

Pachyonychia congenita

Dyskeratosis congenita

LICHENOID PAPULES
Lichen planus

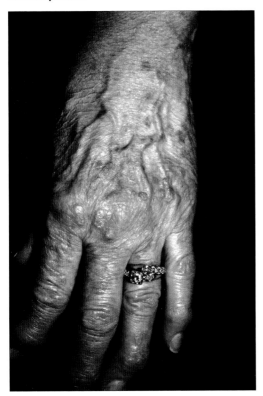

Description pink/purple polygonal flat papules ± tiny overlying white streaks; can be annular, atrophic, bullous, hypertrophic or linear

Location diffuse including flexor wrists, trunk, shins, dorsal hands, also frequently involves nails (pterygium, thickening, onycholysis, longitudinal ridges) and oral and genital mucosa (white lacy or erosive changes)

Characteristics usually adult onset, may resolve spontaneously in 1–3 years, oral and genital manifestations may be chronic, +pruritus, +Koebner phenomenon, can be associated with drugs

Tests Histopathology: wedge-shaped hypergranulosis, saw-toothed rete ridges, lichenoid lymphocytic infiltrate with vacuolar basal layer changes and Civatte bodies

Associated systemic disease hepatitis C virus

Treatment pearls topical, intralesional or systemic corticosteroids, light therapy, oral retinoids, griseofulvin, metronidazole, cyclosporine, dapsone, monitor mucosal lesions for malignant changes

Lichenoid drug reaction (*see box*)

COMMON CAUSES OF LICHENOID DRUG REACTIONS	
• ACE inhibitors*	• NSAIDs
• Allopurinol	• Penicillamine*
• Antimalarials*	• Phenytoin
• Beta-blockers (including timolol ophthalmic solution)	• Proton pump inhibitors (including omeprazole, lansoprazole and pantoprazole)
• Bismuth*	
• Carbamazepine	• Quinine*
• Furosemide	• Quinidine*
• Gold*	• Simvastatin (and other HMG-CoA reductase inhibitors)
• Hydrochlorothiazide (HCTZ)*	
• Hydroxyurea	• Spironolactone
• Interferon-α	• Sulfonylureas (including chlorpropamide and tolbutamide)
• Lithium	
• Lorazepam	• Tetracyclines (including doxycycline and minocycline)
• Methyldopa	

* Indicates the most common.

Lichen striatus
See page 262

Lichen planus-like keratosis

Lichen amyloidosis (LA)/macular amyloidosis (MA)

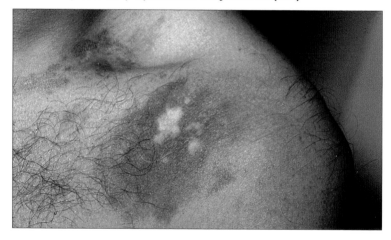

Description *LA*: red/brown papules and verrucous, hyperkeratotic plaques ± scale; *MA*: reticulated red/brown macules and papules
Location *LA*: anterior shins most common; *MA*: upper back most common

Characteristics adults, more common in skin types III and IV (*LA*: Chinese; *MA*: Central and South Americans), chronic, pruritic

Tests Histopathology: pink amorphous material (amyloid derived from keratinocytes) localized to the dermal papilla with epidermis 'cupping' around it in 'ball and claw' formation (+apple-green birefringence)

Associated systemic disease no systemic involvement but can be associated with connective tissue diseases and primary biliary cirrhosis

Treatment pearls avoid friction, high-potency topical corticosteroids, keratolytics, topical DMSO, UVB or UVA phototherapy, dermabrasion, oral retinoids, cryotherapy, excision, laser

Lichen nitidus
See page 386

Lichen aureus

Pityriasis lichenoides chronica (PLC)

Pityriasis lichenoides et varioliformis acuta (PLEVA)

Papular granuloma annulare

Guttate psoriasis

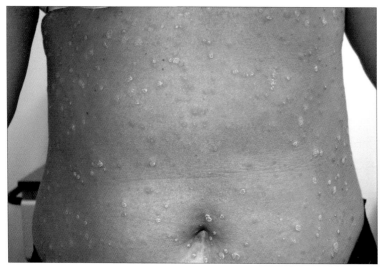

Gottron's papules (dermatomyositis)

Id reaction

Sarcoid

Lichen myxedematosus (papular mucinosis)

Oid-Oid disease

Verruca vulgaris

Secondary syphilis

Bowenoid papulosis

Seborrheic keratosis

LINEAR LESIONS

Lichen striatus

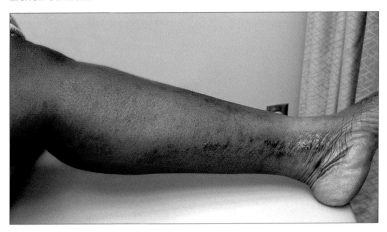

Description inflammatory pink to brown flat papules in a linear distribution which may heal with hypopigmentation

Location follows lines of Blaschko, common on extremities

Characteristics children>adults, self-limited, abrupt onset, resolves in years, asymptomatic, increased incidence in atopic patients, ± nail dystrophy

Tests Histopathology: lichenoid infiltrate ± dyskeratotic cells and parakeratosis

Associated systemic disease atopy

Treatment pearls topical corticosteroids if needed

Epidermal nevus

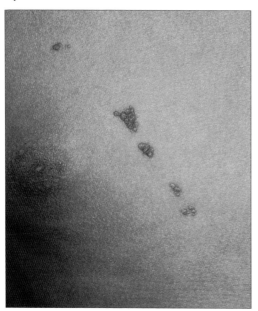

Description pink to brown linear, confluent, verrucous papules

Location linear distribution on scalp, trunk or extremities following lines of Blaschko, usually unilateral but can be bilateral in ichthyosis hystrix

Characteristics appears at birth or shortly after, chronic, asymptomatic, ± wooly hair or alopecia if occurs on scalp, rarely BCC, SCC or KA may develop within nevus after puberty

Tests Histopathology: hyperplasia of epidermis with hyperkeratosis, acanthosis and papillomatosis, ± acantholysis/epidermolysis (no 'nevus' cells)

Associated systemic disease can be associated with epidermal nevus syndrome which includes CNS, skeletal and ocular abnormalities

Treatment pearls no treatment necessary; can try surgical excision, laser therapy or oral retinoids; if extensive, evaluate for systemic associations

Phytophotodermatitis

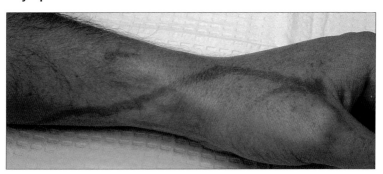

Description linear erythema or hyperpigmentation
Location patchy or linear distribution in areas touched by plant containing psoralens/furocoumarins
Characteristics occurs after exposure to plant and sun in approximately 24 h (lime, celery, parsnip, fig, parsley, lemon, rue)
Tests Histopathology: necrotic keratinocytes in epidermis, lymphocytic infiltrate
Associated systemic disease none
Treatment pearls topical corticosteroids

Linear verruca vulgaris/planae

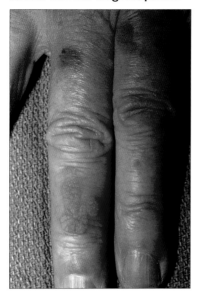

Description skin-colored/pink/brown verrucous papules ± tiny black dots on surface
Location linear distribution on extremities

Characteristics children>adults, may resolve within 2 years vs. chronic, associated with loss of dermatoglyphics if occurs on finger pads, asymptomatic
Tests Histopathology: viral changes in epidermal cells, acanthosis, compact hyperkeratosis, hypergranulosis
Associated systemic disease cryotherapy, topical imiquimod, topical retinoids, laser, oral cimetidine, oral retinoids, intralesional bleomycin, topical DNCB or squaric acid

Linear lichen planus
See page 259, Lichen planus

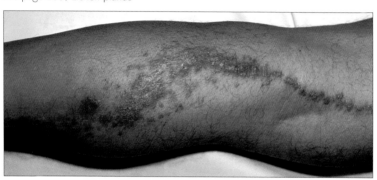

Linear morphea
See page 99, Morphea

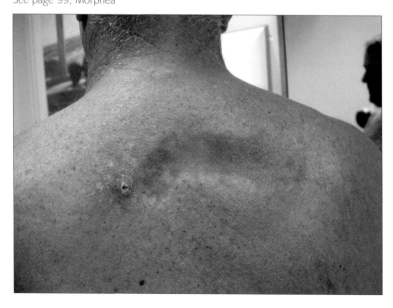

Linear psoriasis
See page 397, Psoriasis

Linear porokeratosis

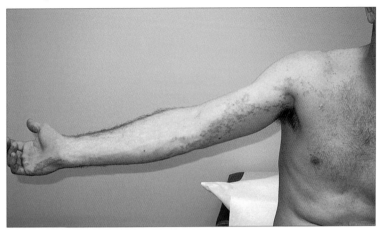

Description erythematous annular plaque with elevated scaly border with groove or 'moat' in between two layers of scale at periphery
Location linear arrangement down an extremity commonly, usually unilateral
Characteristics males>females, adolescent or early adult onset, chronic and progressive
Tests monitor for malignant changes; Histopathology: cornoid lamella correlates with collarette of scale seen clinically, hyperkeratosis, mild perivascular infiltrate
Associated systemic disease none
Treatment pearls difficult to treat: topical 5-FU, cryotherapy, topical or systemic retinoids

Incontinentia pigmenti

Focal dermal hypoplasia (Goltz syndrome)

Pigmentary demarcation lines
See page 269

Pigmentary mosaicism
See page 270

Bleomycin flagellate hyperpigmentation

Linear and whorled nevoid hypermelanosis

Inflammatory linear verrucous epidermal nevus (ILVEN)

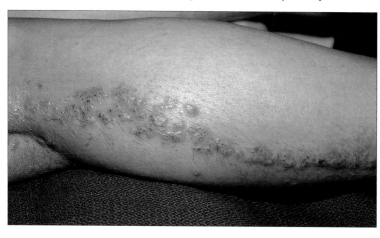

Striae

Thrombophlebitis

Postinflammatory hyperpigmentation

Factitial

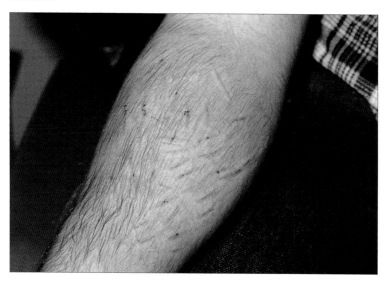

Darier's disease

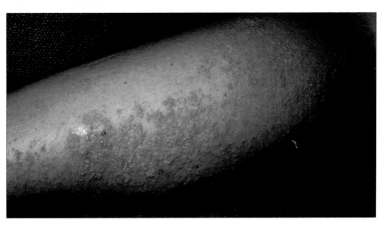

Sporotrichosis

Plant dermatitis (Rhus)

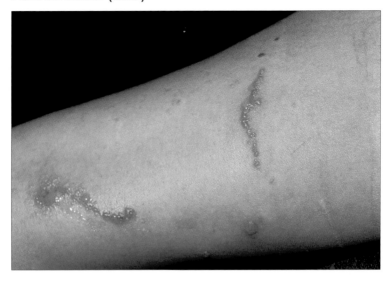

Herpes zoster

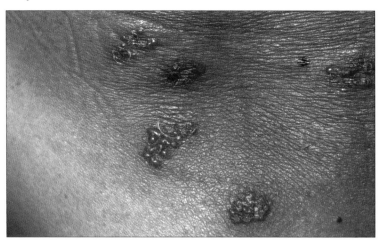

Bites

Electrical burns

Excoriations/trauma

LINEAR LESIONS – FLAT AND HYPERPIGMENTED

Postinflammatory hyperpigmentation
See page 207

Pigmentary demarcation lines

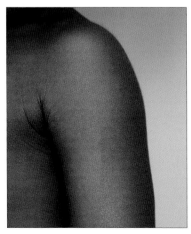

Epidermal nevus (early and evolving)

Phytophotodermatitis

Pigmentary mosaicism

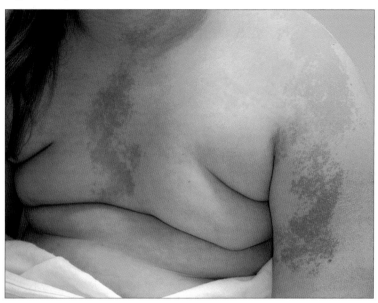

Linear morphea

Post-sclerotherapy

Bleomycin flagellate hyperpigmentation

Lichen striatus (usually hypopigmented)

Incontinentia pigmenti

Linear and whorled nevoid hypermelanosis

LINEAR LESIONS – HYPOPIGMENTED OR DEPIGMENTED

Lichen striatus
See page 262

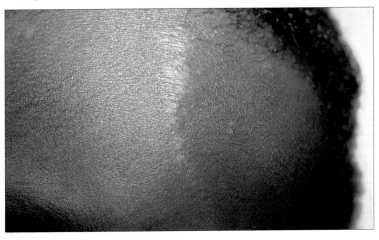

Scar
See page 97

Vitiligo – segmental (depigmented)

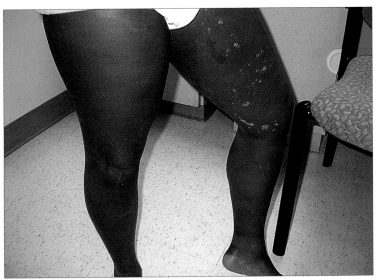

Description depigmented, well-demarcated macules

Location common on extremities or trunk in a linear distribution confined to a segment of the body
Characteristics children>adults, self-limited vs. chronic
Tests Histopathology: absence of melanocytes
Associated systemic disease none
Treatment pearls high-potency topical corticosteroids, sunlight, light therapy, tacrolimus

Corticosteroid-induced hypopigmentation
See page 98, Steroid atrophy

Nevus depigmentosus
See page 231

Hypomelanosis of Ito
See page 232

Ash leaf macule spot (segmental)
See page 233

Incontinentia pigmenti (fourth stage)

Linear morphea

Focal dermal hypoplasia (Goltz syndrome)

Menkes' syndrome carriers

LIP ENLARGEMENT

Acquired
Trauma
Angioedema
Lupus (SLE or DLE)

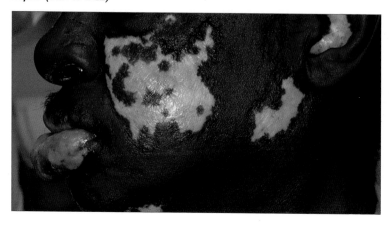

Hemangioma
Neurofibroma
Secondary syphilis
Leishmaniasis
Herpes simplex
Bacterial infection (Staph, anthrax, diphtheria)

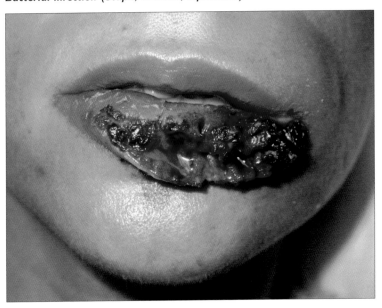

Leprosy
Rhinoscleroma
Melkersson–Rosenthal syndrome

Congenital
Familial (normal variant)
Double lip
Ascher's syndrome
Lymphangioma

Hemangioma

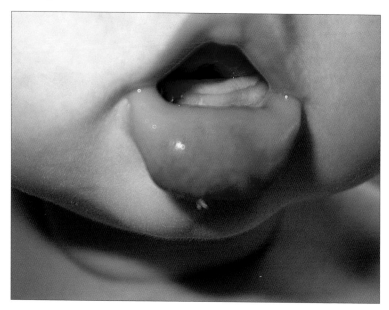

Neurofibroma

Neoplastic
Basal cell carcinoma
Squamous cell carcinoma
Melanoma

LIPS – ECZEMATOUS

Contact dermatitis – lips (toothpaste, nickel, rubber, nail polish, denture paste)

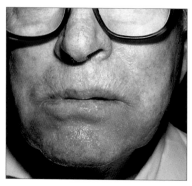

Mechanical (lip lickers, dentures)

Medication effect (oral retinoids, doxycycline)

Photosensitive (systemic lupus erythematosus)

Actinic cheilitis
Description hyperkeratotic, scaly patches and plaques on vermilion lips that progress to ulceration
Location vermilion lips, may extend onto cutaneous lip
Characteristics male>females, light skin>dark skin, >50 years, chronic and progressive, painful, exacerbated by sun
Tests Histopathology: hyperkeratosis ± epidermal dysplasia
Associated systemic disease none
Treatment pearls monitor for malignant changes, topical or oral retinoids, cryotherapy, topical 5-FU, CO_2 laser

Atopic dermatitis

Oral candidiasis (thrush)
See page 258

Nutritional deficiency (B$_1$, B$_2$, B$_6$, iron)

Seborrheic dermatitis

Pemphigus vegetans

Acanthosis nigricans

Secondary syphilis

Irritant dermatitis (spices)

Squamous cell carcinoma

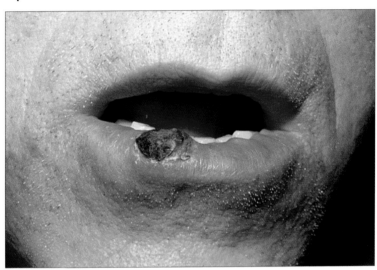

Acrodermatitis enteropathica

Impetigo

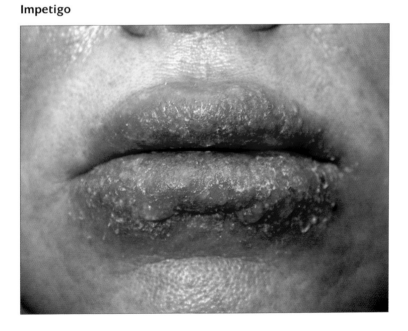

LIPS – HYPERPIGMENTED MACULES

Solar lentigo

Peutz–Jeghers syndrome

Laugier–Hunziker syndrome

Osler–Weber–Rendu syndrome (hereditary hemorrhagic telangiectasia)

Melanoma

LEOPARD syndrome

Labial melanosis

Nevus

LIPS – PERLÈCHE

Oral commisures – 'corners of mouth'.

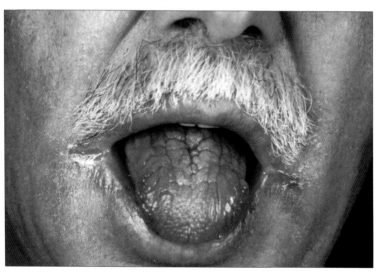

Oral candidiasis

Salivary drooling (secondary to malocclusion)

Infection (especially Strep and Staph)

Vitamin deficiency (B$_1$, B$_2$, B$_6$, iron)

Verruca vulgaris/planae

Acanthosis nigricans

Secondary syphilis (split papules)

Pemphigus vegetans

Oral florid papillomatosis

LIVEDO RETICULARIS
Cutis marmorata

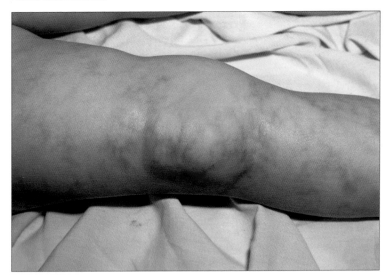

Idiopathic

Connective tissue diseases
Systemic lupus erythematosus (SLE)
Dermatomyositis
Morphea/scleroderma

Arteriosclerosis

Polyarteritis nodosa (PAN)

Rheumatoid arthritis

Rheumatic fever (Strep infection)

Hypercholesterolemia

Secondary syphilis

Tuberculosis

Pancreatitis

Arterial emboli/thrombi

Thrombocytosis

Cryoglobulinemia

Hyperparathyroidism

Erythema ab igne

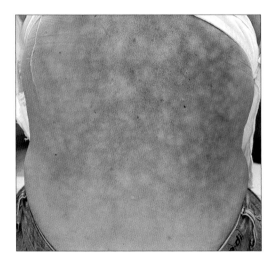

Capillary nevus

Cutis marmorata telangiectatica congenita

MALAR ERYTHEMA

Rosacea
See page 40

Systemic lupus erythematosus (SLE)
See page 425

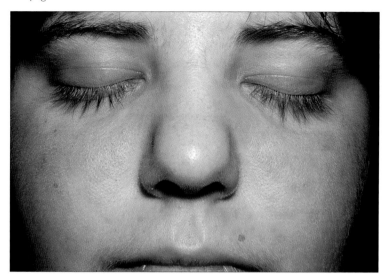

Discoid lupus erythematosus (DLE)
See page 78

Polymorphous light eruption (PMLE)
See page 422

Contact dermatitis
See page 189

Atrophy
See page 8

Seborrheic dermatitis
See page 398

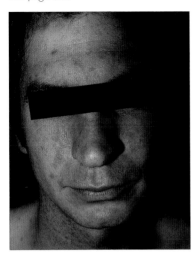

Erysipelas

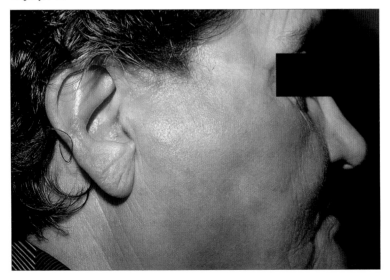

Description erythematous, warm, well-demarcated plaque ± pustules, vesicles, bulla

Location face or lower extremity most common, areas of chronic lymphedema
Characteristics *adults*: female>male, *children*: male>female; painful, associated with fever, malaise and local lymphadenopathy, resolves with treatment
Tests bacterial culture often + for *Streptococcus pyogenes*, elevated CBC, check ASO titer; Histopathology: superficial dermal edema with neutrophils unlike deeper involvement of cellulites, areas of necrosis and dilation of lymphatics
Associated systemic disease none
Treatment pearls oral antibiotics

Cellulitis
See page 154

Dermatomyositis
See page 427

Lymphocytic infiltrate of Jessner

Pemphigus erythematosus

Erythrasma

MALIGNANCY – CUTANEOUS MARKERS

Generalized pruritus

Exfoliative dermatitis/erythroderma

Icterus

Erythema nodosum

Sweet's syndrome

Urticaria

Eczema

Cutaneous metastases

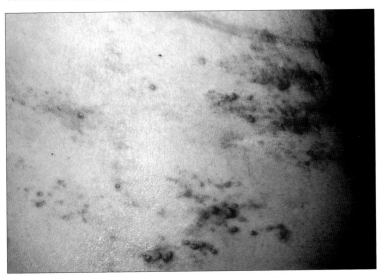

Sister Mary Joseph nodule

Bullae
Bullous pemphigoid
Paraneoplastic pemphigus
Dermatitis herpetiformis
Herpes gestationis
Erythema multiforme
Epidermolysis bullosa acquisita
Linear IgA

Flushing

Purpura

Palmar erythema

Acquired ichthyosis

Infections
Herpes zoster
Herpes simplex
Bacterial infection
Fungal and yeast infection

Clubbing of nails

Seborrheic keratosis – eruptive (Leser–Trélat sign)

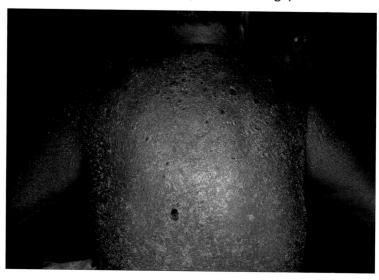

Fibroepitheliomas (excessive skin tags and colon polyps)

Hemochromatosis

Erythema multiforme

Figurate erythema/erythema gyratum repens

Necrolytic migratory erythema

Telangiectasias

Melanosis

Hypertrichosis lanuginosa acquisita

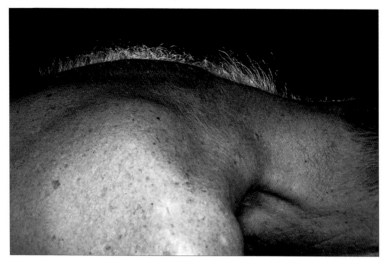

Xanthomas
Acanthosis nigricans

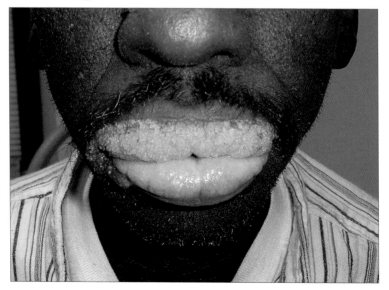

Dermatomyositis
Scleroderma

Palmar hyperkeratosis

Subcutaneous fat necrosis

Pachydermoperiostosis

Primary amyloid

Gardner's syndrome

Superficial phlebitis

Alopecia mucinosa

Paraneoplastic pemphigus

Paraneoplastic acrokeratosis of Bazex

MORBILLIFORM ERUPTION

Drug reaction

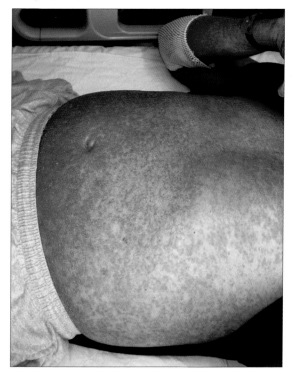

Description erythematous macules and papules (morbilliform, exanthematous), can be urticarial, purpuric, vesicular, pustular or with erythroderma

Location usually starts on trunk and upper extremities and spreads diffusely over body, becoming confluent in some areas

Characteristics associated pruritus, ± fever, history of drug either prescribed or OTC, onset can be immediate or delayed, may persist for 6–8 weeks after discontinuation of drug based on the drug half-life; factors predisposing to drug reactions include female, increased age, number of drugs, immunosuppressed, HIV+ and atopy

Tests ± peripheral eosinophilia; Histopathology: perivascular superficial infiltrate with eosinophils

Associated systemic disease none

Treatment pearls discontinue drug, oral and topical corticosteroids, oral antihistamines

Viral exanthem

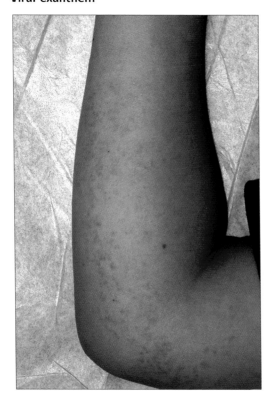

Description blanchable fine erythematous papules and patches

Location diffusely over body especially trunk and extremities, less on face

Characteristics children>adults, self-limited course – usually resolves in 1 week, asymptomatic

Tests clinical diagnosis, ASO titer or other viral serology; Histopathology: non-specific

Associated systemic disease viral infection

Treatment pearls supportive treatment

EXANTHEM – PEDIATRIC

- First disease – measles (rubeola virus)
- Second disease – scarlet fever (Strep)
- Third disease – German measles (rubella virus)
- Fourth disease – Duke's/common viral exanthem (Coxsackie or echovirus)
- Fifth disease – erythema infectiosum (erythrovirus [formerly parvovirus] B19)
- Sixth disease – roseola (exanthem subitum, HHV 6)

Gianotti–Crosti syndrome (papular acrodermatitis of childhood)

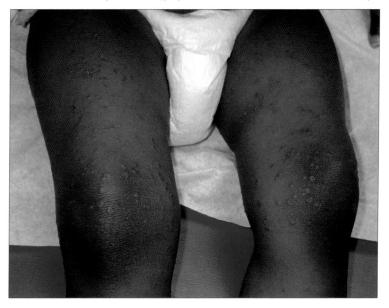

Description erythematous morbilliform eruption of macules and papules, rarely vesicular or purpuric

Location symmetric distribution on extremities, face and buttocks with sparing of trunk

Characteristics children, acute onset after a viral illness in springtime, spontaneously resolve within weeks, asymptomatic but may be associated with fever or lymphadenopathy

Tests Histopathology: acanthosis, hyperkeratosis, perivascular lymphohistiocytic infiltrate

Associated systemic disease viral illness, most commonly EBV or hepatitis B

Treatment pearls no treatment necessary

Meningococcemia

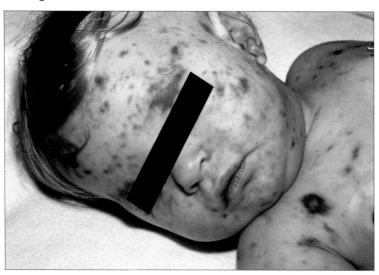

Description petechiae which may progress to purpura and hemorrhagic bulla, less commonly a blanchable morbilliform eruption is seen

Characteristics abrupt onset of rash in young children especially males, associated with fever, chills, arthralgias, hypotension, meningitis, rare chronic form where rash recurs

Location most common on trunk and lower extremities, can affect mucosal surfaces

Tests blood cultures for *Neisseria meningitidis*, CSF analysis; Histopathology: leukocytoclastic vasculitis (LCV), thrombosis and commonly see organisms

Associated systemic disease none

Treatment pearls I.V. antibiotics

Meningococcemia

Graft-versus-host disease

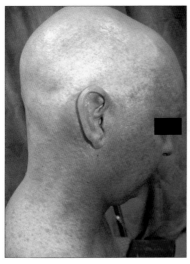 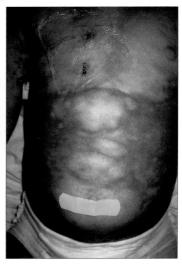

Acute GVHD   *Chronic sclerodermoid GVHD*

Description *acute*: morbilliform erythematous macules, papules and petechiae that can progress to bulla ± erythroderma with desquamation resembling TEN; *chronic* (early lichenoid vs. late sclerodermoid): erythematous/violaceous papules and plaques ± progression to sclerotic, mottled skin

Location *acute* GVHD is often morbilliform and diffuse with accentuation on the head (especially ears), proximal trunk and extremities (especially palms), mucous membrane involvement; *chronic* GVHD often affects dorsal hands, arms and trunk ± mucous membrane involvement

Characteristics can be acute and/or chronic, can be associated with diarrhea, fever and hepatitis

Tests LFTs; Histopathology: *acute* – necrotic keratinocytes ± surrounding lymphocytes (satellite cell necrosis), interface change, perivascular lymphocytic infiltrate, ± epidermal necrosis; *chronic* – hyperkeratosis, necrotic keratinocytes, interface change, lichenoid infiltrate with epidermal atrophy and underlying fibrotic changes in sclerodermoid variant

Associated systemic disease history of bone marrow, stem cell or less commonly solid organ transplant

Treatment pearls oral corticosteroids or other immunosuppressive medications

Rocky Mountain spotted fever (RMSF)

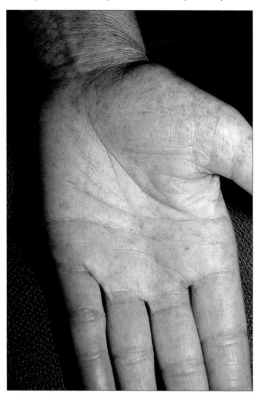

Description erythematous macules and papules with central petechiae and purpura
Location starts on extremities, spreads centripetally, palm and sole involvement, spares the face
Characteristics children>adults, resolves with treatment, associated with fever and headache, increased incidence in summer
Tests serology; Histopathology: vasculitis, extravasated erythrocytes
Associated systemic disease none
Treatment pearls doxycycline

Secondary syphilis (lues)
See page 401

Pityriasis rosea
See page 400

Primary HIV (initial high viral load)

Leptospirosis

Q fever

Scarlet fever

Toxoplasmosis

Typhus

Systemic lupus erythematosus (SLE)

Vasculitis

Juvenile rheumatoid arthritis

Hodgkin's lymphoma

NAILS – ANONYCHIA (PARTIAL OR COMPLETE ABSENCE OF NAIL)

Acquired

Nail–patella syndrome

Aplastic anonychia

Acitretin/isotretinoin/etretinate

NAILS – ATROPHIC (ALL NAILS INVOLVED)

Idiopathic

Dyskeratosis congenita

NAILS – BEAU'S LINES

Transverse depressions secondary to damage in proximal matrix.

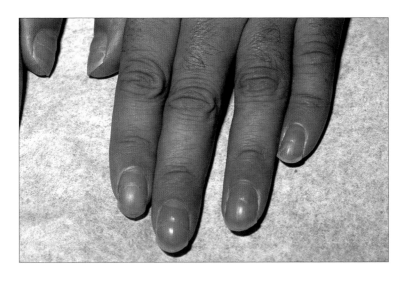

Febrile systemic illness

Emotional stress – severe episode

Zinc deficiency

Carpal tunnel syndrome

Paronychia (chronic)

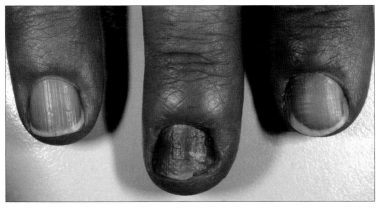

Cryosurgery/trauma

NAILS – BRITTLE

Hand dermatitis

Wetting and drying (chronic)

Trauma

Chemicals

Thyroid disease/myxedema

Psoriasis

Alopecia areata

Lichen planus

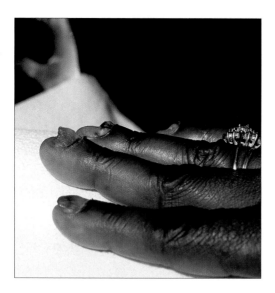

Severe/chronic Illness

Iron deficiency

Vitamin deficiency (A, C, B$_6$)

Arsenic poisoning

NAILS – CLUBBING

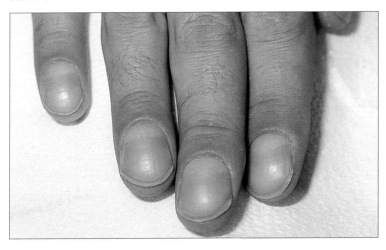

Pulmonary disorders with hypoxia
Bronchiectasis
Lung cancer
Congestive heart failure
Sarcoidosis
Cystic fibrosis
Tuberculosis

Liver/GI disease
Chronic active hepatitis
Cirrhosis

Mediastinal tumors

Idiopathic

Familial variety (autosomal dominant)

Vascular malformation (particularly unilateral/single digit clubbing)

Aortic aneurysm

Congestive heart failure

Bacterial endocarditis

Hyperthyroidism

HIV infection

Pachydermoperiostosis

NAILS – DYSTROPHIC

Fungus

Psoriasis

External (trauma, chemical)

Habit tick

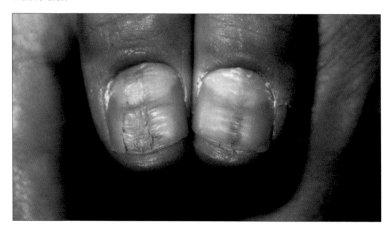

Lichen planus with pterygium

Alopecia areata

NAILS – HALF AND HALF

Distal red/pink/brown discoloration, proximal half is white, most distinct on fingers

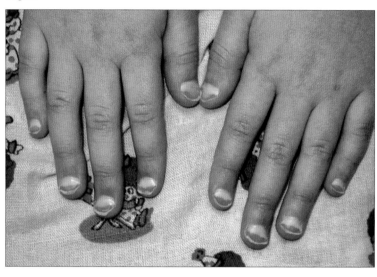

Renal disease

NAILS – HAPALONYCHIA (SOFT NAILS)

Chronic arthritis

Cachexia

Chemicals

Peripheral neuritis

Myxedema

Leprosy

NAILS – HYPERPIGMENTATION

Nevus

Longitudinal melanonychia (normal variant)

Melanoma

Hematoma

NAILS – HYPERTROPHY

Idiopathic

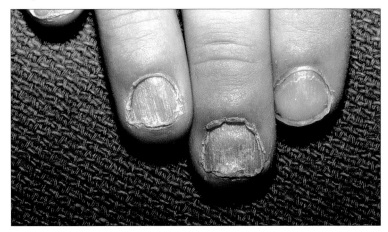

Lichen planus

Alopecia areata

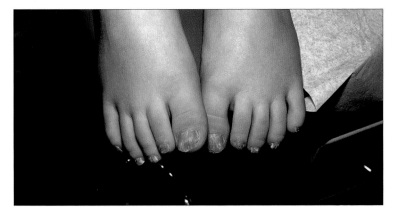

Psoriasis

Pachyonychia congenita

Mucocutaneous candidiasis

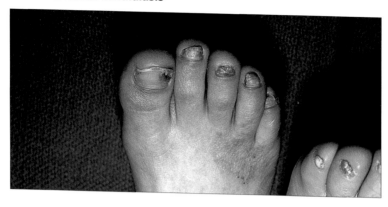

Eczema

Advanced age

Pityriasis rubra pilaris (PRP)

Fungal infections

NAILS – KOILONYCHIA (SPOON NAILS)

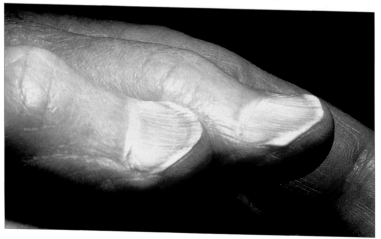

Normal children

Iron deficiency anemia

Occupational (trauma)

Hemochromatosis

Lichen striatus

Familial variety

Plummer–Vinson syndrome

NAILS – LEUKONYCHIA (APPARENT)

Apparent leukonychia – nail plate is normal, color change in nail bed

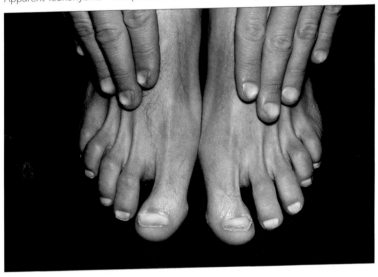

Drugs

Terry's nails

NAILS – LEUKONYCHIA (TRUE)

True leukonychia is due to parakeratosis in nail plate/distal nail matrix changes

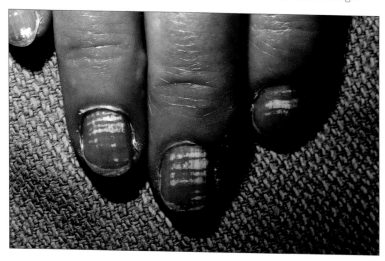

Trauma

Psoriasis

Familial (associated with keratoderma)

NAILS – LONGITUDINAL GROOVES

Old age

Lichen planus

Rheumatoid arthritis

Darier's disease

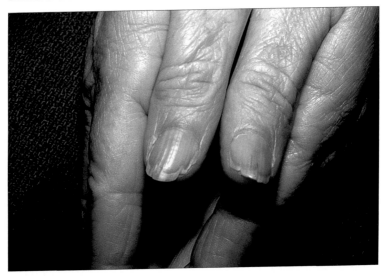

Inherited

Persistent trauma (median nail dystrophy)

Tumors near matrix

NAILS – MEE'S LINES

Transverse white bands, nail plate changes which do grow out with nail

Heavy metals (e.g. arsenic) deposited in nail plate

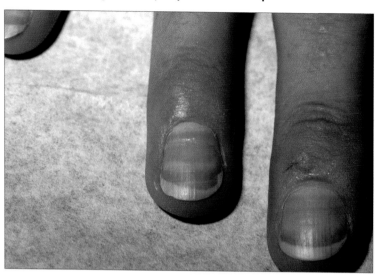

Acute rejection of renal transplant

Breast cancer

Poisoning
Carbon monoxide
Lead
Thallium

Cardiac failure

Chemotherapeutic agents

Hodgkin's lymphoma

Immunohemolytic anemia

Malaria

Parasitic infection

Pneumonia

Psoriasis

Renal failure

Myocardial infarction

Leprosy

Sickle cell anemia

Systemic lupus erythematosus (SLE)

NAILS – MUEHRCKE'S LINES

Parallel transverse white bands, can blanch; nail bed changes which do not grow out with nail

Hypoalbuminemia (nephritic syndrome)

NAILS – ONYCHAUXIS (PACHYONYCHIA)

Nail thickening with subungual hyperkeratosis

Onychomycosis

Psoriasis

Eczema

NAILS – ONYCHOLYSIS

Separation of nail plate and bed at distal and lateral margin

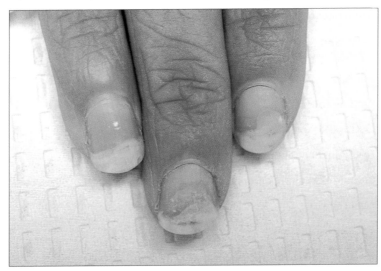

Systemic
Hyper- or hypothyroid
Iron deficiency
Decreased peripheral blood supply
Blistering diseases
> Porphyria cutanea tarda
> Epidermolysis bullosa acquisita
> Bullous pemphigoid
> Pemphigus

Pregnancy
Secondary syphilis

Yellow nail syndrome
Description yellow/green, thick, convex nails with onycholysis and loss of surrounding cuticle
Location all nails affected
Characteristics asymptomatic, associated with very slow growth of the nail
Tests clinical diagnosis
Associated systemic disease respiratory tract disease, lymphedema, AIDS, nephrotic syndrome, hypothyroidism or penicillamine use
Treatment pearls oral vitamin E, pulse itraconazole

Hyperhidrosis

Cutaneous diseases
Contact dermatitis
Nail products: formaldehydes in nail polishes, monoacrylates, cyanoacrylates
Psoriasis (nails)

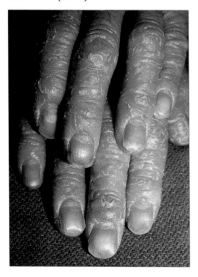

Description irregular, deep pits, round yellow/brown discoloration (oil spots), onycholysis with surrounding erythema, subungual hyperkeratosis of toenails
Location most nails affected

Characteristics chronic, asymptomatic, can be associated with hand arthritis
Tests Histopathology: parakeratosis, regular acanthosis, small neutrophilic abscesses within epidermis
Associated systemic disease none, may be only manifestation of psoriasis
Treatment pearls topical or intralesional corticosteroids

Lichen planus (nails)

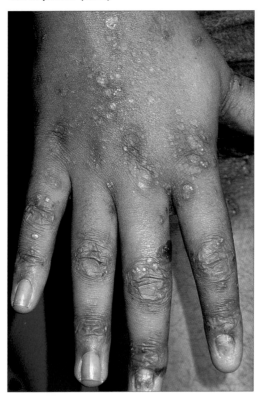

Description thin dystrophic nails with ridging, onycholysis, ± pterygium
Location several nails affected
Characteristics chronic
Tests Histopathology: wedge-shaped hypergranulosis, saw-toothed rete ridges, lichenoid lymphocytic infiltrate with vacuolar basal layer changes and Civatte bodies
Associated systemic disease none
Treatment pearls oral, topical or intralesional corticosteroids

Eczema/atopic dermatitis
Congenital ectodermal defect
Alopecia areata
Lichen striatus

Local
Mechanical trauma
Foreign body

Infections
Bacterial infection
Description onycholysis, erythema and swelling; green discoloration of the nail if Pseudomonas infection
Location nails and surrounding tissue
Characteristics resolves with treatment, painful
Tests bacterial culture
Associated systemic disease none
Treatment pearls oral and topical antibiotics ± incision and drainage of the area

Onychomycosis (dermatophytosis)

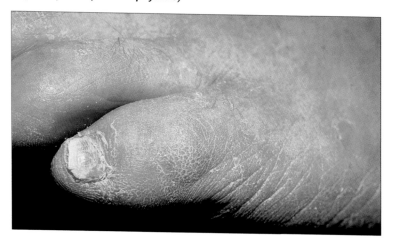

Description thick, yellow, dystrophic nails, ± onycholysis
Location one to all nails affected
Characteristics chronic unless treated, asymptomatic
Tests KOH+, fungal elements seen within nail plate on biopsy, +fungal culture
Associated systemic disease none
Treatment pearls oral antifungals, topical antifungals

Candida
Viral infection

Drugs
Tetracyclines
Nail hardener with formaldehyde
Gasoline/paint remover
Phenothiazine
Chloramphenicol

Fluoroquinolones
Psoralens
NSAIDs
Retinoids
Quinine
Thiazides

Neoplastic
Melanoma
Fibroma
Glomus tumor
Myxoid cyst

NAILS – ONYCHORRHEXIS

Thinning of nail with fine longitudinal ridging and fissuring

Old age (mild disease)

Lichen planus

Impaired vascular supply

Trauma

Tumors compressing nail matrix

NAILS – ONYCHOSCHIZIA

Splitting of nail layers, lamellar dystrophy

Water (repeated soaking)

Lichen planus

Retinoids

Hereditary onychoschizia

Polycythemia vera

NAILS – PIGMENTED (BLACK)

Nevus

Subungual hematoma

Melanoma

Fungus

Peutz–Jeghers syndrome

Vitamin B$_{12}$ deficiency

Pinta

Cyclophosphamide

Ammoniated mercuric sulfide

Postradiation

Photographic developer (brown–black)

Pseudomonas infection (green–black)

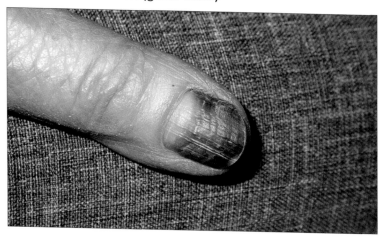

Longitudinal melanonychia (normal variant)

Laugier–Hunziker syndrome

NAILS – PIGMENTED (BLUE/BLUE–BROWN)

Minocycline

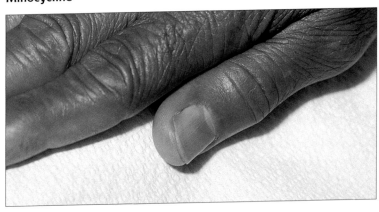

Quinacrine

Chloroquine

Wilson's disease

NAILS – PIGMENTED (BROWN)

Striate melonychia (normal variant)

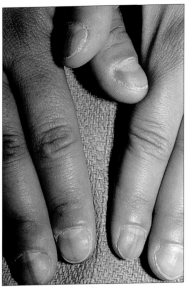

Resorcin/nail lacquer (red–brown)

Zidovudine (AZT)

Doxorubicin (brown–blue)

Bleomycin

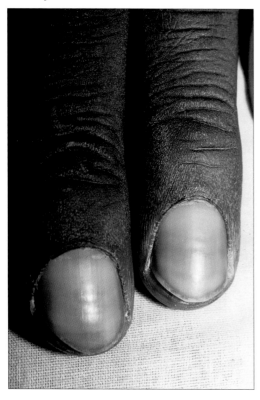

Melphalan

Photographic developer (brown–black)

NAILS – PIGMENTED (GRAY)

Argyria (slate gray)

Phenolphthalein

Melanoma (systemic/metastatic)

Mercuric chloride

NAILS – PIGMENTED (GREEN)

Pseudomonas infection

See image of Pseudomonas infection (green–black), page 309

NAILS – PIGMENTED (ORANGE)

Secondary to nail polish (discoloration can be removed by scraping nail)

Pyridium overdose

Atabrine

Carotenemia

Azo dyes

Tetracyclines (including doxycycline) plus sun-exposure to nails

Cigarette stain

NAILS – PIGMENTED (WHITE, TERRY'S NAILS)

Diffuse, milky, ground glass appearance involving all but distal 1–2 mm of nail – obliterates lunula

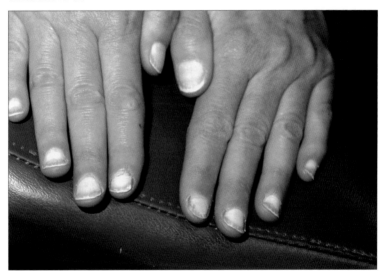

Hepatic cirrhosis

Hypoalbuminemia

Idiopathic

NAILS – PITTING

Parakeratotic cells in foci on dorsum of nail fall out leaving pits

Psoriasis (irregular, deep)

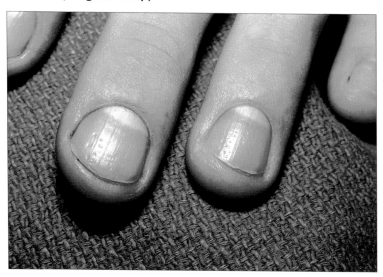

Alopecia areata (fine, symmetrical)

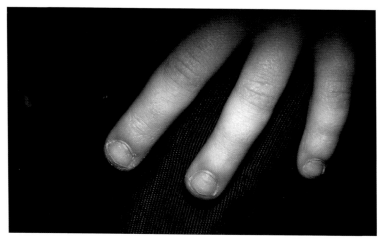

Eczematous dermatitis/hand dermatitis (coarse, irregular pits)

Paronychia, chronic

Fungus

Lichen planus

Trauma

Normal nail (a few pits can be normal)

Pityriasis rosea

Secondary syphilis

Hereditary

NAILS – PTERYGIUM

Cuticle becomes fused to nail bed

Lichen planus

Ischemia

Bullous dermatosis

Trauma

Congenital

NAILS – SPLINTER HEMORRHAGE

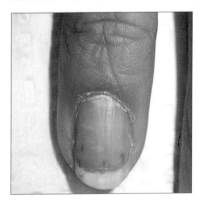

Thin longitudinal dark-red subungual lines secondary to damage to longitudinally oriented capillaries of nail bed

Trauma

Psoriasis

Endocarditis

Vasculitis

Cirrhosis

Mountain sickness (altitude)

Antiphospholipid syndrome

Trichinosis

Mitral stenosis

Chronic glomerulonephritis

Scurvy

Onychomycosis

Normal variant

NAILS – SUBUNGUAL HYPERKERATOSIS

Psoriasis

Verruca vulgaris

Onychomycosis

Chronic eczema

Lichen planus

Darier's disease

Norwegian scabies

Pityriasis rubra pilaris (PRP)

Reiter's syndrome

NAILS – TRACHYONYCHIA (ROUGH NAIL)

Rough nail surface, brittleness, splitting of free edge, gray opacity, may have longitudinal ridging

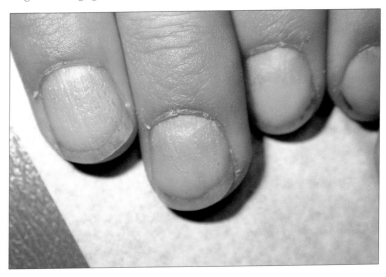

20 nail dystrophy

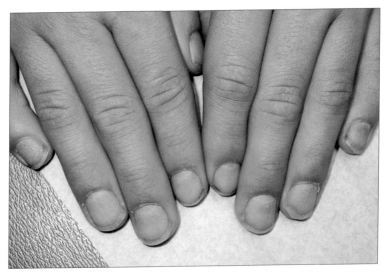

Psoriasis

Eczema

Alopecia areata

Lichen planus

Chemicals

Idiopathic

Ichthyosis vulgaris

Ectodermal dysplasia

NAILS – TUMORS

Verruca vulgaris

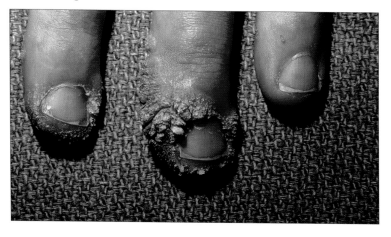

Pyogenic granuloma

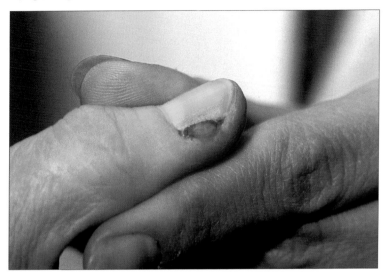

Fibroma

Myxoid cysts

Subungual exostosis

Glomus tumor

Nevus

Melanoma

Keratoacanthoma

Squamous cell carcinoma

Verrucous carcinoma

Bowen's disease

Onychomatricoma

NECROSIS

Trauma

Pressure ulcer

Injections
Sclerotherapy
Epinephrine

Electrical injury

Radiation injury

Septic emboli

Fat or cholesterol emboli

Cryoglobulinemia

Vascular disease
Arteriosclerosis obliterans
Thromboangiitis obliterans

Frostbite/chilblains

Connective tissue disease

Raynaud's phenomenon

Viral
Herpes simplex virus
Herpes zoster virus
Varicella
Vaccinia
Orf

Bacterial
Necrotizing fasciitis
Anthrax
Diphtheria
Group A/B Streptococcus

Atypical mycobacteria
Leprosy
Tuberculosis

Deep fungal infections

Rickettsial infections
Rocky Mountain spotted fever
Typhus

Syphilis (primary, secondary and tertiary)

Yaws/bejel

Coagulopathies

Spider bite

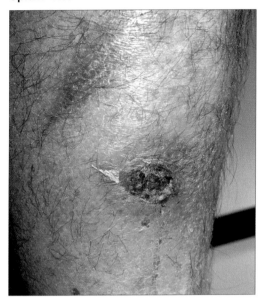

Snake bite

Marine life (jellyfish, others)

Metastatic disease

Leukemia/lymphoma

NIPPLE LESIONS – HYPERKERATOTIC

Florid papillomatosis of nipples

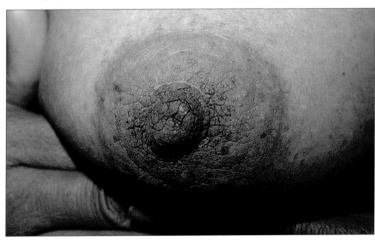

Eczema/atopic dermatitis

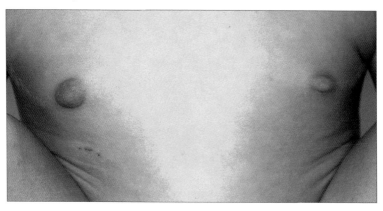

Lichen simplex chronicus

Psoriasis

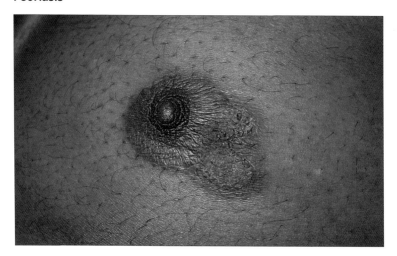

Paget's disease

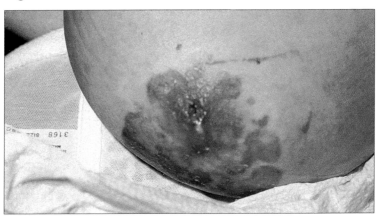

Description erythematous, well-demarcated scaly patches ± scale and erosions
Location breast, usually in nipple area, or extramammary in genital region especially vulva
Characteristics light skin>dark skin, female>male, elderly, pruritus and burning vs. asymptomatic
Tests Histopathology: large, plump clear cells grouped in the epidermis
Associated systemic disease underlying ductal adenocarcinoma of the breast in Paget's; extramammary Paget's is associated with underlying malignancy in 25% of patients (usually GU cancer: bladder, rectum, etc.)
Treatment pearls Mohs excision, CO_2 laser, radiation

Acanthosis nigricans

Bowen's disease

Verruca vulgaris/planae

Contact dermatitis

Estrogens (endogenous in pregnancy or exogenous)

Prostate cancer

Chronic friction (joggers)

Ichthyosis

Epidermal nevus

NODULES – RED

See page 366, Papules and nodules – red

NODULES – SKIN-COLORED/BROWN

See page 379, Papules and nodules – skin-colored/brown

NODULES – YELLOW/BROWN/RED

See page 392, Papules and nodules – yellow/brown/red

NUMMULAR PATCH

See page 498, Scaly red patch

ORAL LESIONS – COBBLESTONING

Darier's disease

Cowden's syndrome

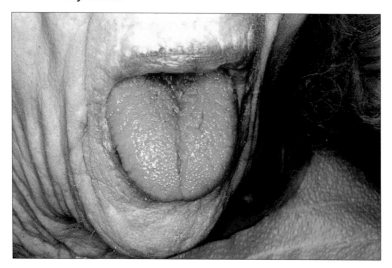

Crohn's disease

Lipoid proteinosis

ORAL LESIONS – HYPERTROPHIC

Contact dermatitis (oral)
Description eroded or white hyperkeratotic areas of mucosa ± erythema
Location oral mucosa including gingiva
Characteristics self-limited but recurs with re-exposure to offending agent, painful
Tests Histopathology: hyperkeratosis, perivascular or lichenoid lymphocytic infiltrate ± exocytosis, ± erosion
Associated systemic disease none
Treatment pearls topical corticosteroids, avoid offending agent (if amalgam, may need removal)

Fordyce granules

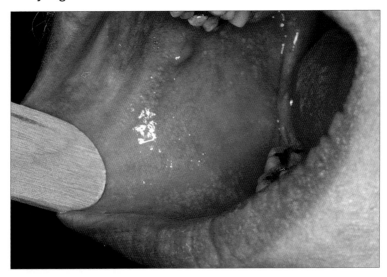

Darier's disease
See page 196

White sponge nevus
See page 256

Florid oral papillomatosis
Description white 'cauliflower-like' mass
Location oral mucosa: tongue, buccal, palate or laryngeal
Characteristics chronic, ± progression to squamous cell carcinoma
Tests Histopathology: acanthosis, papillomatosis, ± keratinocyte dysplasia
Associated systemic disease none
Treatment pearls excision, CO_2 laser, interferon, monitor for progression to malignancy

Verruciform xanthoma
Description solitary 1–2 cm pink/yellow verrucous or flat patch or plaque
Location oral mucosa or genital mucosa or skin
Characteristics asymptomatic, persists for years
Tests Histopathology: hyperkeratosis, acanthosis, papillomatosis, few to many foamy cells in submucosa and superficial dermis
Associated systemic disease normal lipids
Treatment pearls excision

Pemphigus vegetans

Dyskeratosis congenita

Pachyonychia congenita

ORAL ULCERS
Aphthous ulcers

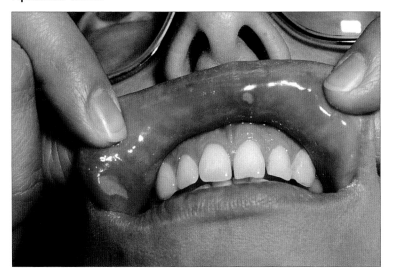

Description round, white eroded area of mucosa with surrounding halo of erythema
Location oral mucosa
Characteristics female>male, young adults, self-limited, painful
Tests Histopathology: mucosal erosion with perivascular infiltrate
Associated systemic disease Behçet's, Crohn's, SLE, HIV, cyclic neutropenia, vitamin deficiency
Treatment pearls topical anesthetics, topical corticosteroids, colchicine, dapsone, thalidomide

Herpes simplex virus (HSV)
See page 116

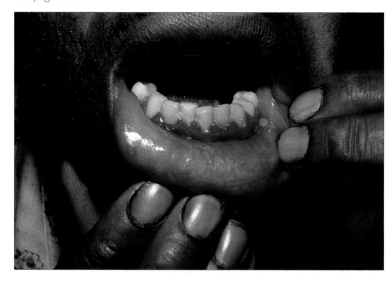

Lichen planus (mucosal)
See page 257

Contact dermatitis (oral)
See page 324

Trauma/burn (thermal or chemical)
Description eroded areas with overlying white or yellow membrane ± white hyperkeratosis
Location oropharynx
Characteristics self-limited, painful
Tests Histopathology: epithelial necrosis ± underlying inflammation
Associated systemic disease none
Treatment pearls drink plenty of water when taking aspirin and other pills, topical anesthetic

Stevens–Johnson syndrome (SJS, erythema multiforme major)
See page 64

Erythema multiforme
See page 484

Systemic lupus erythematosus (SLE-oral)
Description small erosions and ulcerations
Location oral mucosa
Characteristics female predominance, young adult onset, chronic, can be drug induced (HCTZ, NSAIDs, ACE-I)

Tests ANA+; Histopathology: epithelial erosion, interface change, superficial and deep perivascular lymphocytic infiltrate
Associated systemic disease lupus is a systemic disease
Treatment pearls antimalarials, topical, intralesional or systemic corticosteroids, thalidomide

Syphilis – oral

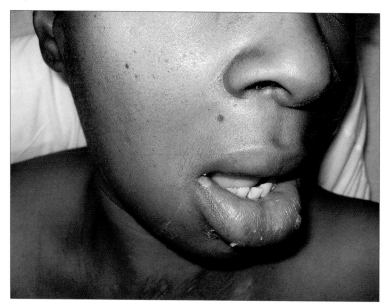

Description *primary syphilis chancre*: ulcerated mucosal nodule; *secondary syphilis*: small 'aphthous-like' ulcers
Location *primary*: genital or less likely oral mucosa; *secondary*: oral and genital mucosa
Characteristics *primary*: resolves spontaneously in 1–4 months or faster with antibiotic treatment, painless, local lymphadenopathy; *secondary*: resolves spontaneously in weeks to months but can recur, ± pain, local lymphadenopathy
Tests serology: RPR/VDRL and confirmatory MHA-TP/FTA-ABS; Histopathology: *primary*: ulcer surrounded by lymphocytic and plasma cell infiltrate, endothelial swelling, can stain for spirochetes in primary lesions with Warthin–Starry stain *secondary*: lymphocytic and plasma cell perivascular infiltrate with normal epidermis or psoriasiform and lichenoid changes, ± granulomas, Warthin–Starry stain for spirochetes + 30% in secondary lesions
Associated systemic disease syphilis is a multisystem infection which can affect the kidneys, brain, GI tract, eyes and joints
Treatment pearls I.M. penicillin G, azithromycin or PCN desensitization if PCN allergic

Cicatricial pemphigoid
See page 128

Behçet's syndrome

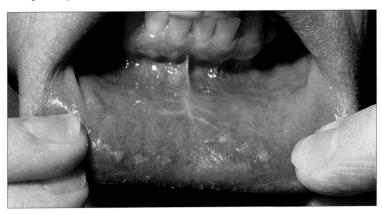

Description multiple, small, round erosions with surrounding erythema
Location oral and genital mucosa
Characteristics male>female, young adults, resolves in 1–3 weeks but
recurrent with chronic course, increased incidence if from the Middle East
(especially Turkey and Japan), painful, ± associated CNS and GI symptoms,
± thrombophlebitis
Tests +pathergy, >three episodes of oral ulcers in 1 year plus two of the
following: genital ulcers, eye findings, acne-like lesions or erythema nodosum-
like lesions; Histopathology: erosion of epidermis with leukocytoclastic vasculitis,
perivascular lymphocytic infiltrate and endothelial changes ± thrombosis
Associated systemic disease Behçet's is a multisystem disease of unknown
etiology which can include ocular abnormalities (uveitis, conjunctivitis, retinal
vasculitis), recurrent oral and genital ulcers, arthritis/synovitis, nervous system
abnormalities (neuropathies, meningoencephalitis), cutaneous findings (papules,
pustules, erythema nodosum) and thrombophlebitis of any vessel
Treatment pearls topical anesthetics, NSAIDs, colchicine, dapsone,
thalidomide, oral prednisone, methotrexate; avoid trauma to mucosa

Pemphigus vulgaris/vegetans (oral)

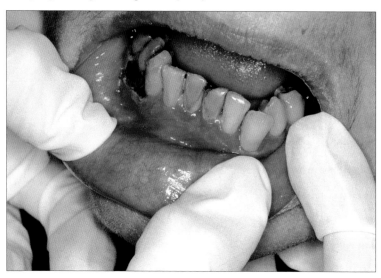

Description few to diffuse erosions with irregular borders that heal without scarring, cerebriform changes of the tongue in pemphigus vegetans
Location buccal and palate mucosa most commonly but can extend into esophagus and onto vermilion lip; conjuctiva and genital mucosa also involved
Characteristics peak onset 50–60 years, chronic, painful
Tests +Nikolsky sign (bulla forms with gentle rubbing on skin of active patients) and +Asboe–Hansen sign (bulla extends laterally when placing pressure on top of bulla); Histopathology: suprabasilar cleft ('tombstone'), perivascular infiltrate, intraepidermal bulla with acantholysis; DIF: +intercellular IgG with or without C3; autoantibody titers can be used to follow disease course
Associated systemic disease underlying malignancy can be associated with paraneoplastic pemphigus (skin disease can precede malignancy in up to 30%)
Treatment pearls oral corticosteroids or other systemic immunosuppressants, plasmapheresis

Viral (Coxsackie: hand, foot and mouth disease)

Drug reaction

Oral candidiasis (thrush)

Reiter's syndrome

Fungal (histoplasmosis)

Dermatomyositis (rare, mild)

Tuberculosis

Gonococcemia

EBV

Diphtheria

PALATE OR NASAL SEPTUM PERFORATION

Trauma (often pediatric)

Squamous cell carcinoma

Wegner's granulomatosis

Tertiary syphilis

Yaws

Leprosy

Leishmaniasis (new world mucocutaneous)

Salivary gland neoplasm

Nasal NK/T-cell lymphoma (lethal midline granuloma)

Lymphoma

Melanoma

Tuberculosis

Actinomycosis

Paracoccidioidomycosis

Histoplasmosis

Rhinoscleroma

Mucormycosis

Arsenic (chronic)

PALMAR PITS

Verruca palmaris and plantaris

Basal cell nevus syndrome

Darier's disease

Cowden's syndrome

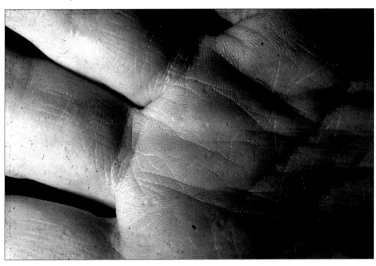

Sarcoid

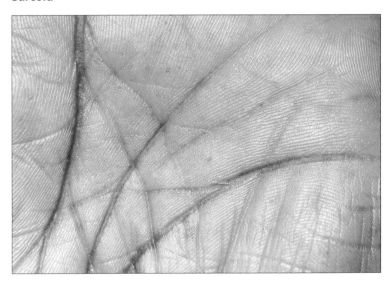

Arsenic poisoning

PAPILLOMATOSIS – RETICULATED

Acanthosis nigricans
See page 111

Confluent and reticulated papillomatosis of Gougerot and Carteaud (CARP)

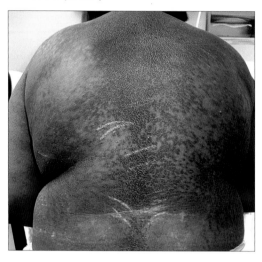

Description hyperpigmented, hyperkeratotic verrucous papules and plaques
Location seborrheic/dermatitis distribution on anterior chest and upper back with confluent plaques in central areas and more reticulated pattern laterally
Characteristics dark skin>light skin, female>male, young adults, onset during puberty, asymptomatic
Tests Histopathology: hyperkeratosis, acanthosis, papillomatosis, increased pigmentation of basal layer, sparse infiltrate
Associated systemic disease none
Treatment pearls minocycline, topical and oral retinoids

Pseudoatrophoderma colli

Darier's disease

Epidermodysplasia verruciformis

Verruca planae (flat warts)

PAPULES – GENERALIZED

Acne vulgaris
See page 39

Folliculitis

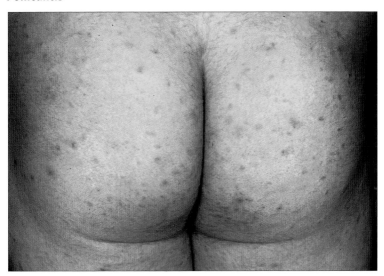

Description erythematous follicular papules and pustules ± collarette of scale
Location areas with terminal hairs especially head and neck, buttocks and trunk
Characteristics all ages, pain, pruritus
Tests bacterial culture; Histopathology: lymphocytic and neutrophilic inflammation surrounding a follicle with neutrophils within follicle, ± rupture of follicle with a granulomatous reaction
Associated systemic disease none
Treatment pearls topical and oral antibiotics, benzoyl peroxide

Pityrosporum folliculitis

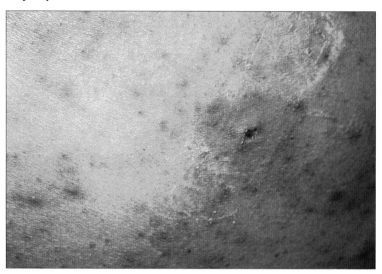

Description erythematous follicular papules and pustules
Location upper trunk most commonly
Characteristics female>male, young adults, very pruritic, resistant to typical acne treatments
Tests Histopathology: dilated follicles packed with Pityrosporum and surrounded by inflammation
Associated systemic disease may be associated with systemic immunosuppression
Treatment pearls topical or oral antifungals, selenium sulfide shampoo

Eosinophilic folliculitis

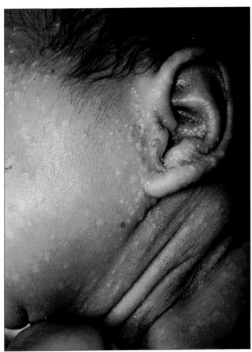

Description erythematous follicular papules and pustules, some edematous papules, ± annular patches with pustules at edge; HIV variant has more papules with fewer pustules
Location face, trunk and proximal extremities; scalp and brows in infants
Characteristics male>female, typically young adults, rarely infants, increased incidence in Japan, intensely pruritic, abrupt onset, resolves in about 1 week then reoccurs in crops several weeks later; infant variant is self-limited, the HIV variant does not spontaneously resolve
Tests ± peripheral eosinophilia; Histopathology: follicular spongiosis with neutrophils and eosinophils within the follicular epithelium and within the follicle
Associated systemic disease increased incidence in HIV+ with CD4 counts <300
Treatment pearls indomethacin, dapsone, antihistamines, topical or oral corticosteroids, light therapy, oral antibiotics, colchicine, topical antipruritics

'Hot tub' folliculitis
Description edematous follicular papules and pustules
Location trunk in bathing suit distribution
Characteristics young adults, onset within 2 days of exposure to hot tub, resolves in 1–2 weeks, may be associated with inguinal and axillary lymphadenopathy, fever, sore throat, malaise or abdominal pain

Tests bacterial cx.+ for Pseudomonas; Histopathology: mixed inflammatory infiltrate surrounds follicle ± ruptured follicle with granulomatous inflammation

Associated systemic disease none

Treatment pearls no treatment necessary, can use oral antibiotics with pseudomonal coverage (fluoroquinolone)

Keratosis pilaris
See page 171

Viral exanthem
See page 287

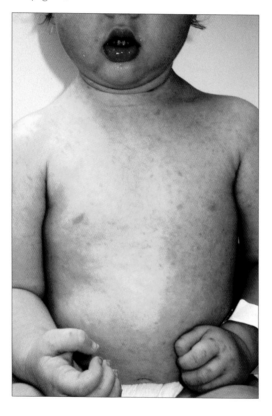

Bites
See page 120

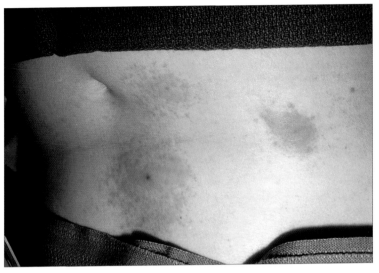

Miliaria rubra (MR) and miliaria profunda (MP)

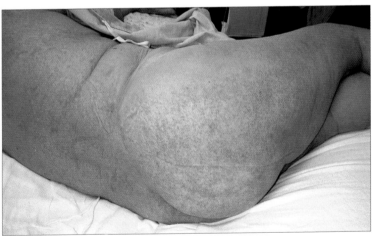

Description *MR*: pinpoint erythematous papules/vesicles/pustules on an erythematous base ± maceration; *MP*: skin-colored to white deep papules
Location *MR*: upper trunk, flexor and intertriginous surfaces; *MP*: trunk and extremities

Scabies

Characteristics infants to elderly, *MR*: pruritic ± burning sensation; *MP*: asymptomatic, resolves spontaneously (MP within 1–2 hours), exacerbated by heat and occlusion, worse in humid environments

Tests Histopathology: *MR*: intraepidermal spongiotic vesicle with neutrophils surrounding the occluded eccrine duct, + perivascular dermal inflammation, *MP*: epidermal/dermal junction occlusion of eccrine duct with spongiosis and perivascular inflammation in dermis

Associated systemic disease none

Treatment pearls avoid occlusion and heat of area, powder to absorb moisture

Scabies
See page 52

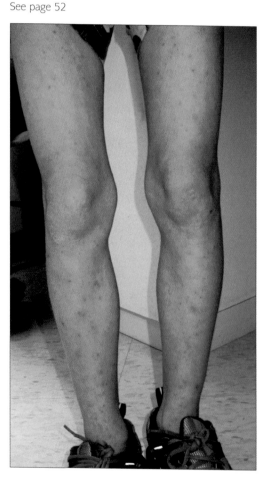

Steatocystoma multiplex

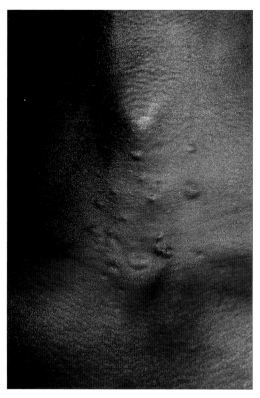

Steatocystoma multiplex

Description multiple, small, mobile skin-colored to yellow nodules
Location upper trunk (especially anterior chest) and proximal extremities
Characteristics chronic, asymptomatic, may be AD inherited
Tests Histopathology: flattened cysts in dermis lined by an interior pink cuticle and cuboidal epithelium with flattened sebaceous glands along the edge
Associated systemic disease rarely associated with type II pachyonychia congenita
Treatment pearls no treatment necessary; excision

Eruptive vellus hair cysts

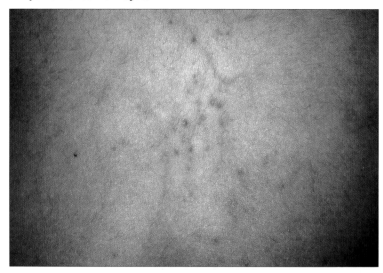

Description tiny skin-colored or red/hyperpigmented papules
Location trunk (especially anterior chest) and lateral thighs most common
Characteristics female>male, young adults, may be AD inherited, chronic, asymptomatic
Tests Histopathology: small cysts in the dermis lined by stratified squamous epithelium with numerous vellus hairs and loose keratin within cyst
Associated systemic disease rarely associated with type II pachyonychia congenita
Treatment pearls no treatment necessary; laser, topical retinoids, keratolytics

Drug reaction
See page 286

Nevus
See page 379

Hemangioma
See page 370

Neurofibroma
See page 107

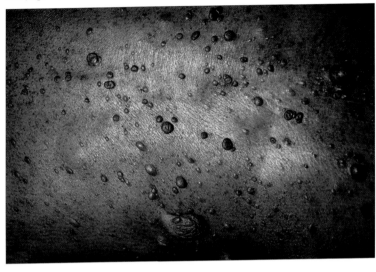

Epidermal cyst
See page 136

Reactive perforating collagenosis

Perforating folliculitis

Kyrle's disease

Elastosis perforans serpiginosa

Eruptive xanthomas

Xanthoma disseminatum

Generalized eruptive histiocytosis

Pityriasis lichenoides et varioliformis acuta (PLEVA)

Lymphomatoid papulosis

Candidiasis

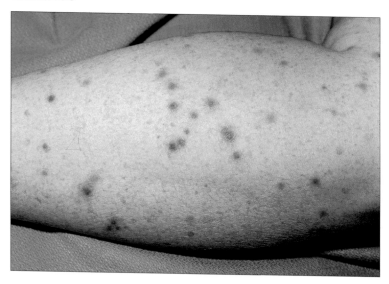

Disseminated granuloma annulare

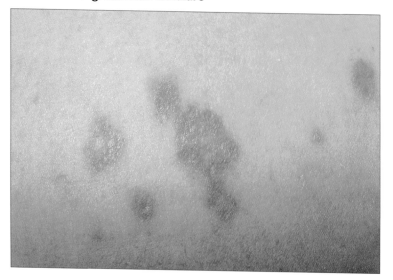

Basal cell carcinoma

Melanoma (metastatic)

PAPULES – HYPERKERATOTIC

See page 196, Hyperkeratotic papules

PAPULES – NON-PIGMENTED PERIORBITAL AND NASOLABIAL

Dermal nevus
See page 379, Nevus

Fibrous papule
See page 373, Angiofibroma

Sebaceous hyperplasia

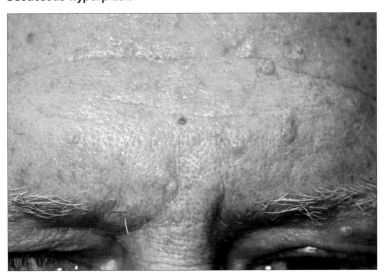

Description multiple, small, yellow lobular, umbilicated papules
Location face
Characteristics males>females, >40 years, asymptomatic, chronic, increased incidence with cyclosporine use
Tests Histopathology: hyperplasia of sebaceous glands in dermis
Associated systemic disease none
Treatment pearls no treatment necessary, electrocautery, liquid nitrogen, laser

Syringoma

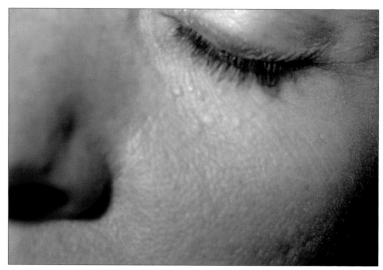

Description skin-colored/yellow small 1–3 mm flat, firm papules

Location periorbital most commonly but may occur anywhere including acral, axillary and genital

Characteristics females>males, occurs at any age but rarely before puberty, can be familial

Tests Histopathology: pale pink nested cells in dermis, some forming ducts with a 'tadpole' or 'comma' shape, thought to be either eccrine or apocrine in origin

Associated systemic disease common in females with Down's syndrome

Treatment pearls reassurance as lesions are benign, cryotherapy, electrodessication, laser ablation or chemical peels for cosmetic improvement

Hidrocystoma
See page 167

Xanthelasma
See page 167

Trichoepithelioma

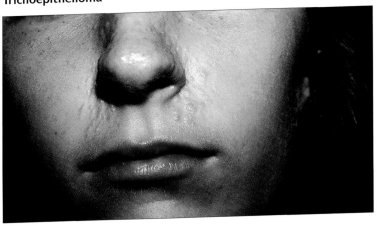

Description solitary or multiple grouped skin-colored to red, shiny, firm papules or cysts
Location symmetric on face especially periorbital, periorificial and nasolabial
Characteristics female>male, children or adults, chronic
Tests Histopathology: solid and cystic small groups of basaloid cells without surrounding retraction
Associated systemic disease none
Treatment pearls no treatment necessary, excision, curettage, electrocautery, laser

Trichilemmoma
Description single or multiple skin-colored wart-like verrucous papules
Location face especially periorbital and around nose, or genital
Characteristics chronic, asymptomatic
Tests Histopathology: nodular acanthosis of pale cells commonly with squamous eddies and with overlying hypergranulosis, papillomatosis and hyperkeratosis
Associated systemic disease if multiple, may be associated with Cowden's syndrome (± adenocarcinoma of the breast, thyroid, or GI tract)
Treatment pearls no treatment necessary, electrocautery, excision

Basal cell carcinoma
See page 366

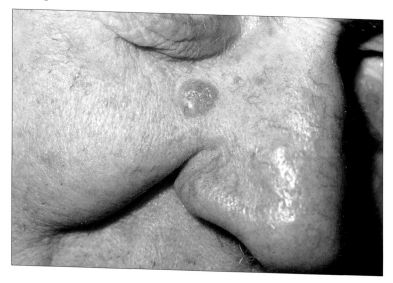

Sarcoid
See page 443

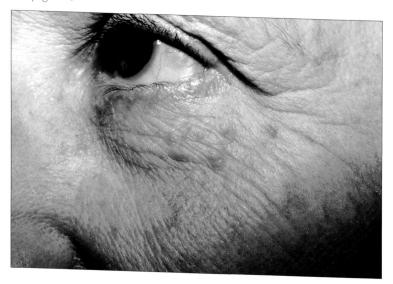

Dermoid cyst
See page 138

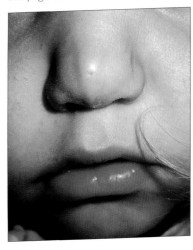

Epidermal cysts – multiple
See page 136

Adenoma sebaceum
See page 589 – Tuberous sclerosis

Steatocystoma multiplex (usually trunk)
See page 339

Trichofolliculoma

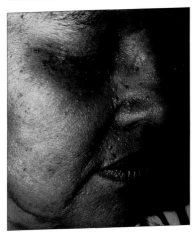

Cylindroma

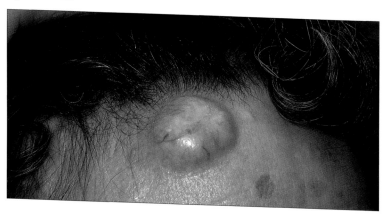

PAPULES – PEARLY

Basal cell carcinoma
See page 366

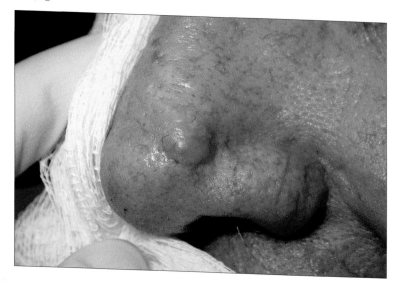

Molluscum contagiosum
See page 355

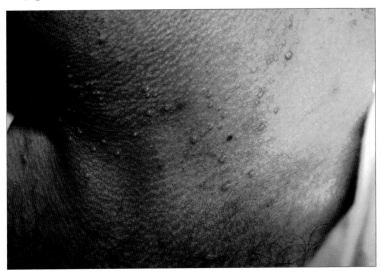

Milia
See page 42

Trichoepithelioma
See page 345

Hidrocystoma
See page 167

Sarcoid
See page 443

Granuloma annulare
See page 87

Sebaceous hyperplasia
See page 343

Trichilemmoma
See page 345

Palisaded and encapsulated neuroma

Malignant fibrous histiocytoma/atypical fibroxanthoma

Cryptococcosis

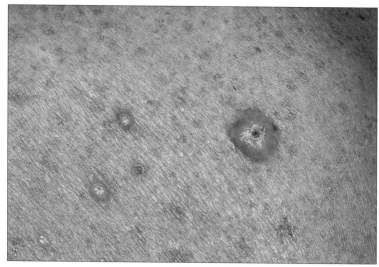

Dermatofibroma

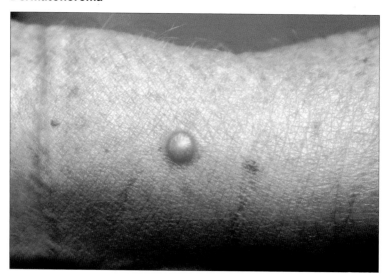

PAPULES – RED, ACRAL

See page 52, Acral papules and plaques

PAPULES – SCALY (ANGIOKERATOMA-LIKE)

Angiokeratoma

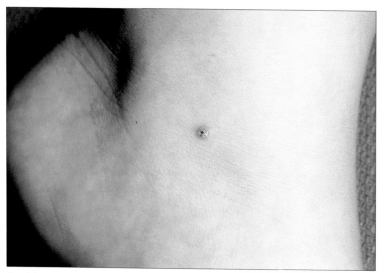

Angiokeratoma

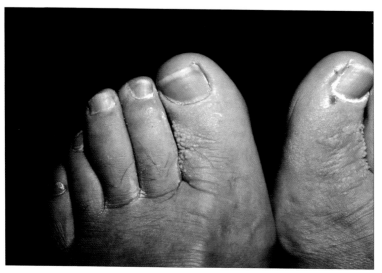

Angiokeratoma of Mibelli

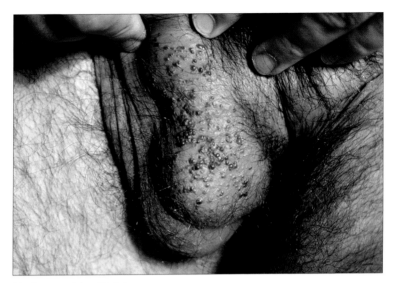

Fordyce angiokeratoma

Description red/brown/violaceous/black discrete papule with scaly surface
Location usually on extremities and may appear black (solitary type); multiple and discrete on scrotum with underlying erythema in elderly men, less commonly on vulva of elderly women (Fordyce type); diffuse especially in 'bathing trunk' distribution (Fabry's angiokeratoma corporis diffusum); dorsal hands and feet and extensor surfaces (angiokeratoma of Mibelli); grouped and confluent papules on trunk or extremities (angiokeratoma circumscriptum)
Characteristics asymptomatic, solitary type may occur after trauma in young adults, Fordyce type presents in elderly men, Fabry's usually present at birth, angiokeratoma of Mibelli presents in young children (especially females) prior to puberty, angiokeratoma circumscriptum is rare variant in young females>males
Tests Histopathology: dilated capillaries in the papillary dermis with overlying hyperkeratosis
Associated systemic disease no systemic association with solitary or scrotal angiokeratomas; Fabry's is an inherited systemic glycolipid storage disease with manifestations in many organ systems; angiokeratoma of Mibelli is associated with chilblains
Treatment pearls if diffuse, evaluate for Fabry's; otherwise no treatment necessary (can try cryotherapy, laser therapy or electrocautery)

Lymphangioma circumscriptum (superficial lymphatic malformation)

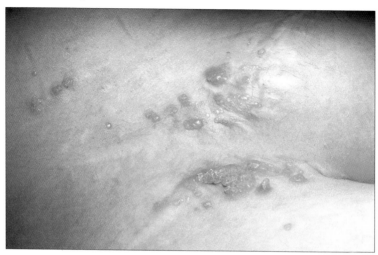

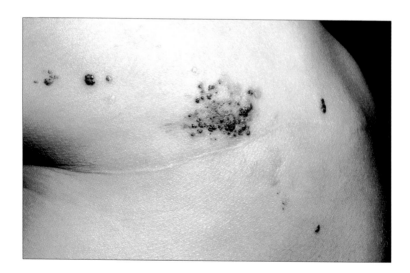

Description clear/yellow to deep red, grouped deep-seated vesicles and papules that look like 'frog spawn'
Location localized; usually on tongue, abdomen, axillae, or scrotum
Characteristics congenital; when pierced, clear fluid is released
Tests Histopathology: dilated lymphatic vessels

Associated systemic disease none
Treatment pearls excision, electrocautery, laser therapy only if malformation does not extend deep

Lichen planus
See page 259

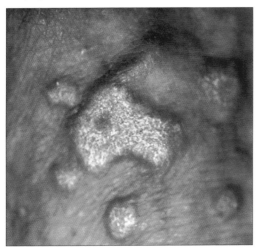

Acral pseudolymphomatous angiokeratoma (APACHE)
Description red/brown/violaceous discrete papules
Location unilateral, dorsal hands
Characteristics sporadic in children, no associated cold intolerance
Tests Histopathology: dense lymphohistiocytic infiltrate with multinucleated giant cells, eosinophils and plasma cells; no vascular changes appreciated
Associated systemic disease none
Treatment pearls no treatment necessary, but can try laser or cryotherapy

Angiolymphoid hyperplasia with eosinophils

Kimura's disease

PAPULES – SUBCUTANEOUS
See page 512, Subcutaneous papules and nodules

PAPULES – UMBILICATED (MOLLUSCUM CONTAGIOSUM-LIKE)

Molluscum contagiosum

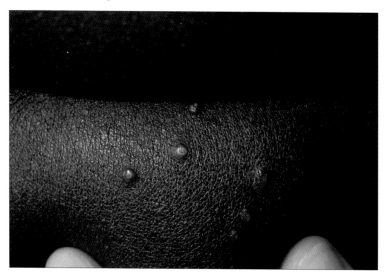

Description multiple, skin-colored to pink, firm, umbilicated papules that vary in size from 2 to 6 mm

Location most common on hands and face, or genital in young adults and HIV+

Characteristics young children, sexually active young adults and immunosuppressed, usually resolves spontaneously within 2 years, can be spread by contact

Tests Histopathology: rounded acanthosis with magenta epidermal cell inclusions (Henderson–Paterson bodies)

Associated systemic disease may be associated with immunosuppression (HIV)

Treatment pearls curettage, cantharone, cryotherapy, laser, imiquimod, topical retinoid, topical 5-FU, podophyllin

Cryptococcosis

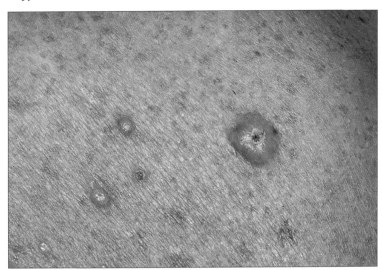

Description umbilicated yellow to red papules and pustules with areas of ulceration
Location head and neck as well as diffuse over body
Characteristics adults most common, resolves with treatment, more common in HIV+
Tests tissue culture, serology for Cryptococcus antigen; Histopathology: pseudoepitheliomatous hyperplasia with areas of necrosis and areas of suppurative granulomas, cryptococcal organisms of varying sizes noted with India ink, PAS or mucin stains
Associated systemic disease often disseminated in HIV/AIDS involving lungs, CNS and bone
Treatment pearls I.V. antifungals, HAART therapy

Sebaceous hyperplasia
See page 343

Lichen nitidus

Perforating granuloma annulare

Vaccinia

Elastosis perforans serpiginosa

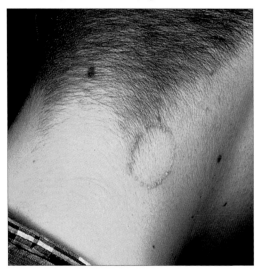

Kyrle's disease

Perforating folliculitis

Reactive perforating collagenosis

Keratoacanthoma

Basal cell carcinoma

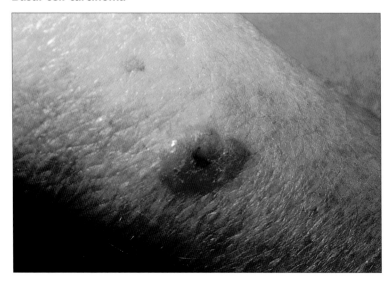

Atypical mycobacteria

Histoplasmosis

***Penicillium marneffei* lesions**

***Pneumocystis carinii* (now termed *P. jiroveci*) (disseminated in HIV+ patients)**

PAPULES AND NODULES – BLUE

Blue nevus

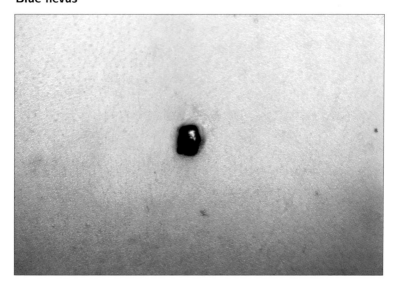

Description well-demarcated blue/black macule or papule
Location common on dorsal hands and feet, scalp and buttocks/sacrum
Characteristics female>male, chronic, asymptomatic
Tests Histopathology: loose collection of pigmented spindle-shaped melanocytes in the dermis
Associated systemic disease none
Treatment pearls no treatment necessary

Glomus tumor

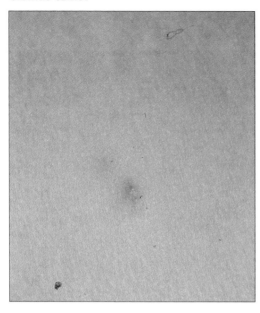

Description solitary blue/red small, firm nodule or subungual blue/red patch
Location extremities especially periungual and subungual
Characteristics young adults, painful
Tests pain with changes in pressure and temperature; Histopathology: plump, clear glomus cells, with increased surrounding small blood vessels
Associated systemic disease none
Treatment pearls excision, electrocautery, sclerotherapy

Kaposi's sarcoma
See page 364

Melanoma

Blueberry muffin baby
Toxoplasmosis
Rubella
Cytomegalovirus (CMV)
Herpes virus

Congenital neuroblastoma metastases

PAPULES AND NODULES – CENTRAL ULCERATION

Basal cell carcinoma (BCC)
See page 366

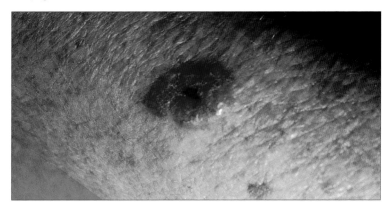

Molluscum contagiosum
See page 355

Keratoacanthoma
See page 368

Pyoderma gangrenosum
See page 487

Trauma

Foreign body

Leishmaniasis

Atypical mycobacteria

Sporotrichosis

Cat scratch fever

Sarcoid

Lymphocytic infiltrate of Jessner

Granuloma annulare (rarely)

Cutaneous anthrax

Malignant fibrous histiocytoma/atypical fibroxanthoma

Pityriasis lichenoides et varioliformis acuta (PLEVA)

Hydroa vacciniforme

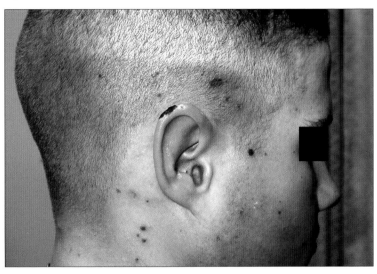

Kyrle's disease

Anthrax

PAPULES AND NODULES – PAINFUL, DERMAL ('ANGEL' ACRONYM)

Angiolipoma
Description multiple, soft, skin-colored subcutaneous nodules usually <2 cm
Location forearms followed by trunk and upper arms
Characteristics onset at puberty, mildly painful
Tests Histopathology: well-demarcated mature adipose cells with small blood vessels and some mast cells, ± fibrin thrombi, ± fibrosis
Associated systemic disease none
Treatment pearls excision

Neurilemmoma (schwannoma)
Description single pale-pink, soft or firm, dermal or subcutaneous nodule
Location follows nerves of extremities (especially flexor arms and legs), head and neck

Characteristics female>male, mid-adult onset, mildly painful
Tests Histopathology: spindle cells encapsulated, ± nuclear palisading (Verocay bodies), no axons, +mast cells, ± degenerative changes
Associated systemic disease if multiple, may be associated with neurofibromatosis
Treatment pearls excision

Glomus tumor
See page 359

Eccrine spiradenoma

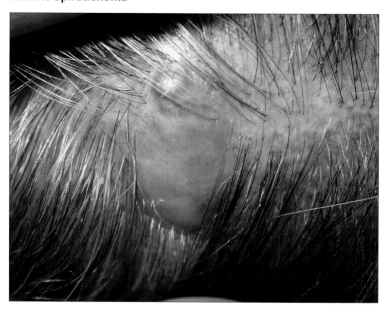

Description solitary, skin-colored, blue or pink deep nodule
Location usually on ventral surface of upper body
Characteristics young adults (15–35 years), severe paroxysmal pain
Tests Histopathology: basaloid cells with pale cells intermixed in multilobular well-circumscribed arrangement, 'blue balls in the dermis'
Associated systemic disease if multiple and occurs with other adnexal tumors, consider Brooke–Spiegler syndrome
Treatment pearls excision

Leiomyoma
Description solitary or multiple in clusters, firm, smooth, mobile red/violaceous/pink/brown nodules
Location grouped in linear or dermatomal arrangement on trunk, extremities or tongue
Characteristics child to early adult onset, mildly painful especially in cool weather

Tests pain can be elicited by rubbing lesion with ice cube; Histopathology: fascicles of long muscle cells with 'cigar-shaped' nuclei
Associated systemic disease none
Treatment pearls excision, CO_2 laser

Piezogenic pedal papule

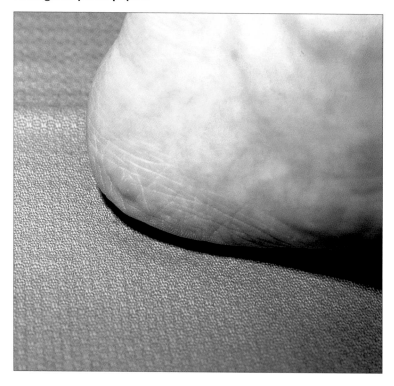

Description large, 1 cm transitory, soft, subcutaneous nodules
Location lateral sides of feet
Characteristics female>male, >40 years, painful
Tests lesions and pain disappear when supine and not weight bearing
Associated systemic disease none
Treatment pearls no treatment

Traumatic neuroma

Cutaneous endometriosis

Chondrodermatitis nodularis helicis

Erythema nodosum

PAPULES AND NODULES – PURPLE

Cherry angioma
See page 371

Hemangioma
See page 370

Lichen planus
See page 259

Leukocytoclastic vasculitis
See page 479

Sweet's syndrome
See page 447

Kaposi's sarcoma

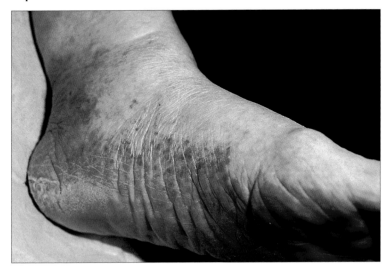

Description violaceous to black macule that may progress to papule/tumor
Location lower legs in Middle-Eastern men and immunosuppressed patients; symmetric and often diffuse especially on face, trunk, oral and genital mucosa of HIV+ males; lower extremities of African men or diffusely in children with the most aggressive African type
Characteristics elderly Middle-Eastern men (classic type), iatrogenically immunosuppressed patients, HIV+ homosexual males, or African endemic variant which is aggressive with lymphadenopathy, lymphedema and systemic involvement often leading to death in children
Tests Histopathology: increase in dermal, abnormal, dilated vessels with thin walls which dissect through collagen bundles, extravasation of RBCs, sparse

infiltrate including lymphocytes, mast cells and plasma cells; Slide can be stained for HHV 8

Associated systemic disease HIV, all types can be associated with systemic involvement including the GI tract, lymph nodes, heart, liver and bone

Treatment pearls topical retinoid (alitretinoin) for solitary lesion, surgery, aggressive cryosurgery, laser, irradiation and chemotherapy for more extensive lesions, intralesional vinblastine, interferon-α and treatment of underlying HIV with HAART treatment

Blue nevus
See page 358

Acroangiodermatitis

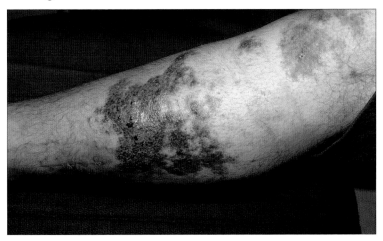

'Blood blister' secondary to trauma

Erythema elevatum diutinum

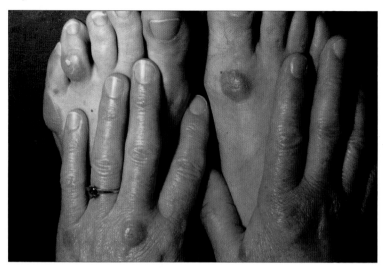

Lichenoid drug reaction

PAPULES AND NODULES – RED

Neoplastic
Basal cell carcinoma (BCC)

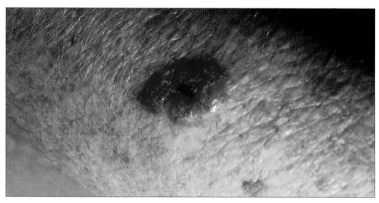

Description translucent pearly pink papule with overlying telangiectasias and rolled border ± central ulceration, can also present as a dark brown nodule or a pink/white sclerotic, atrophic plaque

Location sun-exposed areas especially the head and neck
Characteristics adults, light skin >dark skin, progresses without treatment, may bleed spontaneously
Tests Histopathology: basaloid cells in groups with palisading of cells at border of group surrounded by an area of retraction, distinctive stroma surrounds groups as well
Associated systemic disease none
Treatment pearls surgical excision, ED&C, topical 5-FU, topical imiquimod, photodynamic therapy

Squamous cell carcinoma (SCC)

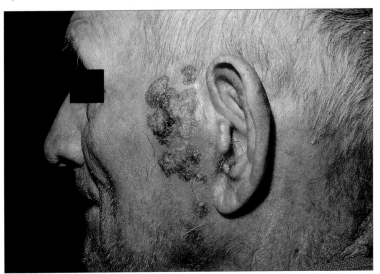

Description pink to erythematous scaly papule or plaque ± ulceration
Location most common in sun-exposed areas especially dorsal hands, may arise within a scar (Marjolin's ulcer)
Characteristics older age, progressive without treatment and may metastasize internally, may spontaneously bleed
Tests Histopathology: atypical epithelial cells in irregular arrangement invading the dermis typically with surrounding inflammation, +cytokeratin staining
Associated systemic disease none
Treatment pearls surgical excision, topical 5-FU oral retinoids, photodynamic therapy

Keratoacanthoma

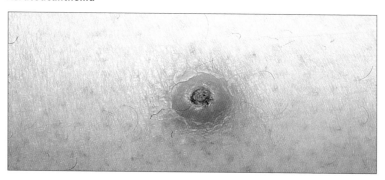

Description rapidly growing erythematous papule with depressed central cavity usually with ulceration and crust .

Location sun-exposed areas most common

Characteristics male>female, older adults, may resolve without treatment but have been known to metastasize, painful

Tests Histopathology: acanthosis with atypical epithelial cells 'cupping' area of central depression which is filled with eosinophilic keratin, +inflammatory infiltrate

Associated systemic disease multiple KAs can be associated with internal malignancy

Treatment pearls treatment is recommended given reports of metastasis: surgical excision, ED&C, intralesional 5-FU, oral retinoids

Spitz nevus

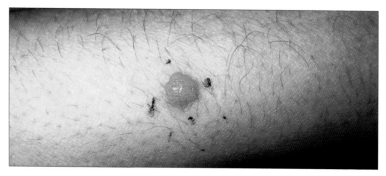

Description single, well-demarcated pink to brown to black papule appearing abruptly

Location common on face and neck, can occur anywhere in groups

Characteristics children>adults, asymptomatic

Tests Histopathology: well-demarcated lesion with large, atypical-appearing melanocytes and spindle cells in a 'school of fish' or 'raining down' pattern

Associated systemic disease none
Treatment pearls excision with clear margins is recommended

Melanoma
See page 380
Cutaneous T-cell lymphoma (CTCL)
See page 402

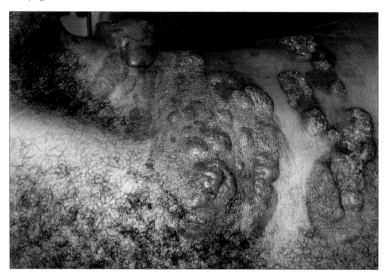

Glomus tumor
See page 359
Kaposi's sarcoma
See page 364
Nevus
See page 379
Blue nevus
See page 358
Leukemia/lymphoma cutis
See page 445
Lymphomatoid papulosis

Metastatic lesion

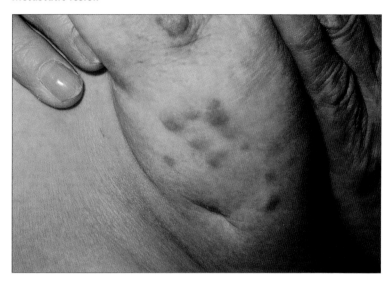

Trichoepithelioma
Eccrine poroma
Malignant fibrous histiocytoma/atypical fibroxanthoma
Dermatofibrosarcoma protuberans (DFSP)
Merkel cell carcinoma

Vascular
Hemangioma (infantile)

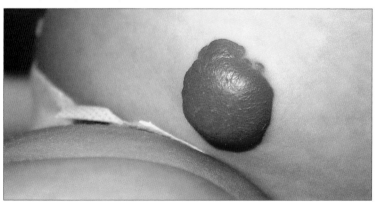

Description blue/erythematous/violaceous patch or papule ± ulceration, firm in early stage to soft in later stages
Location head and neck common, can occur anywhere

Characteristics female>male, increased in premature infants, appears shortly after birth, resolves spontaneously in years

Tests Histopathology: mass of numerous endothelial cells which may extend to deep dermis, ± increase in mast cells in early stage

Associated systemic disease if >6 hemangiomas, MRI to rule out internal hemangiomas, high output congestive heart failure in larger hemangiomas, ± underlying congenital abnormalities in face, neck hemangiomas (especially beard distribution) and over spinal area

Treatment pearls no treatment necessary unless organ or functional abnormality; oral or intralesional corticosteroids, laser, excision, interferon

Cherry angioma

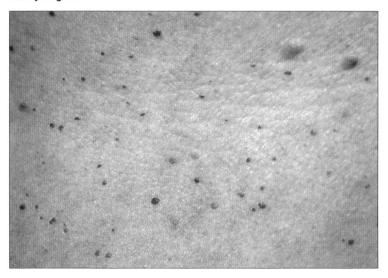

Description bright erythematous/violaceous papule

Location trunk and proximal extremities most common

Characteristics onset in third decade, number increases with age, chronic, asymptomatic

Tests Histopathology: increased blood vessels in papillary dermis with flattening of overlying rete ridges

Associated systemic disease none

Treatment pearls no treatment necessary, electrocautery, excision, laser

Vascular

Pyogenic granuloma

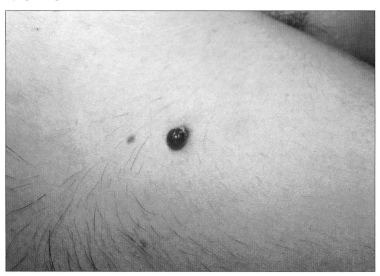

Description solitary, erythematous, friable papule usually with a collarette of skin ± central ulceration

Location can occur anywhere; most common on digits, oral mucosa and at sights of trauma

Characteristics any age but common in children, young adults and during pregnancy, frequently recur after removal, rapid growth is characteristic, asymptomatic vs. painful

Tests Histopathology: collarette of acanthosis surrounding a nodular proliferation of capillaries.

Associated systemic disease none

Treatment pearls shave ED&C, laser

Vascular

Angiofibroma (pearly penile papules, adenoma sebaceum, fibrous papule of the nose)

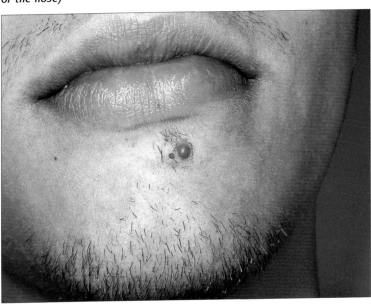

Description small, skin-colored to pink, dome-shaped papules
Location around nose, corona of glans penis and periungual in tuberous sclerosis patients
Characteristics adults or children in tuberous sclerosis, chronic, asymptomatic
Tests Histopathology: groups of fibroblasts in the dermis intermixed with stroma and an increase in number of small, dilated blood vessels, S100–, Factor XIIIa+
Associated systemic disease tuberous sclerosis if multiple
Treatment pearls excision

Angiokeratoma
See page 351
Leukocytoclastic vasculitis
Cutaneous polyarteritis nodosa (PAN)
Angiosarcoma

Infectious
Molluscum contagiosum
See page 355

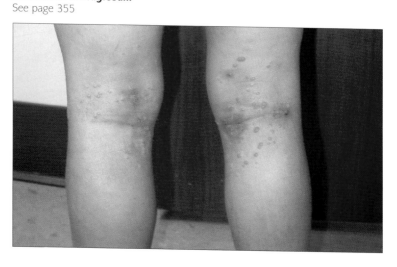

Deep fungal infection

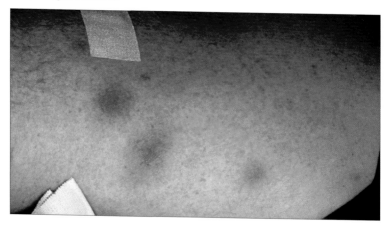

Atypical mycobacteria infection
Furuncle/carbuncle

Infectious • Other

Scabies

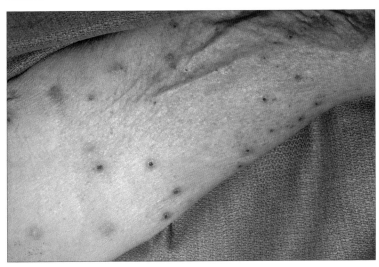

Sporotrichosis
Orf
Leprosy
Leishmaniasis

Other
Sarcoid
See page 443

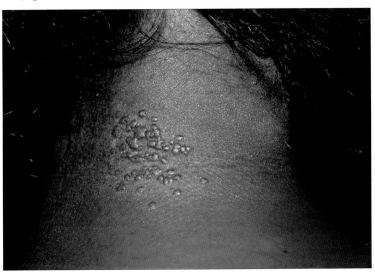

Other

Granuloma annulare
See page 87

Sweet's syndrome
See page 447

Keloid

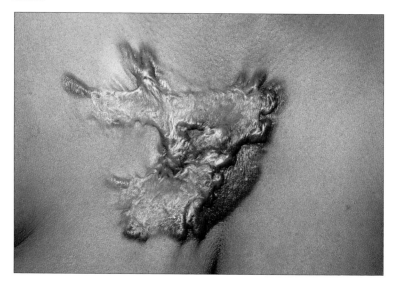

Description pink/violaceous/red/brown firm nodule which surpasses wound margins

Location occurs in areas of previous trauma especially earlobes, upper chest and back

Characteristics adults>children and elderly, dark skin>light skin, chronic, ± pain and pruritus

Tests Histopathology: thickened collagen bundles in parallel arrangement and in clumps and swirls with loss of adnexal structures and increased blood vessels

Associated systemic disease none

Treatment pearls can try excision, however often recurs; intralesional corticosteroids, laser, radiation

Dermatofibroma
See page 381

Giant cell reticulohistiocytoma (GCR)/multicentric reticulohistiocytoma (MR)

Description solitary (*GCR*) or multiple (*MR*) red/brown papules and nodules; 'coral beads'

Location over joints of hands, head, elbows, 50% with mucous membrane involvement

Characteristics light skin>dark skin, *GCR*: young adults, asymptomatic, resolves spontaneously; *MR*: adult females, painful, resolves spontaneously in 5–10 years, can be associated with mutilating arthritis, hyperlipidemia, malignancy, +PPD, vasculitis or autoimmune diseases

Other

Tests if multiple lesions, evaluate patient for systemic involvement which can affect any organ: check ESR, CBC, lipid panel, PPD; Histopathology: giant cells and histiocytes with 'ground glass', purple cytoplasm within granulomatous nodule, CD68+, HAM56+
Associated systemic disease if multiple, can be associated with solid organ involvement
Treatment pearls excision; if systemic involvement, difficult to treat, but can try NSAIDs or immunosuppressives (oral corticosteroids, methotrexate, cytoxan, imuran)

Clear cell acanthoma
Description pink/red blanchable, firm papule ± scale around edge of papule
Location lower legs most commonly
Characteristics adults >50 years, chronic, asymptomatic
Tests Histopathology: symmetric clearly defined area of acanthosis with clear/pale pink PAS+ keratinocytes, parakeratosis, decreased granular layer, prominent blood vessels in the papillary dermis, sparse infiltrate
Associated systemic disease none
Treatment pearls excision

Erythema elevatum diutinum (EED)
Nodular amyloidosis
Bite (tick bite, spider bite or other)

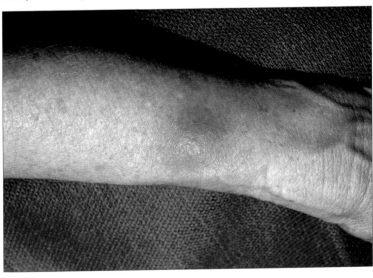

Folliculitis
Granuloma faciale
Epithelioid cell histiocytoma

Other

Subcutaneous fat necrosis of the newborn

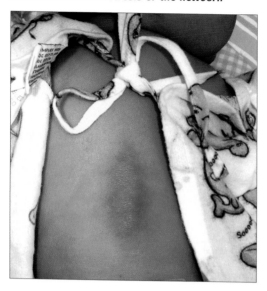

Mastocytosis (urticaria pigmentosa)
See page 385
Foreign body
Xanthoma
Juvenile xanthogranuloma
Rheumatoid nodule
Gout tophus
Cutaneous polyarteritis nodosa (PAN)
Erythema nodosum
Lupus profundus
Panniculitis
Verruca vulgaris

PAPULES AND NODULES – SKIN-COLORED/BROWN
Nevus

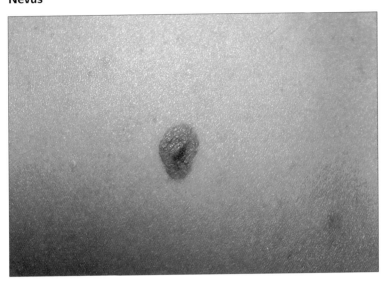

Description well-demarcated, round or oval, pink or brown, macule or papule
Location can occur anywhere
Characteristics female>male, light skin>dark skin, asymptomatic, may continue to arise in early childhood, number usually stabilizes as a young adult and decreases as person ages
Tests Histopathology: nests of melanocytes in epidermis and/or dermis
Associated systemic disease none
Treatment pearls no treatment necessary

Melanoma

Melanoma

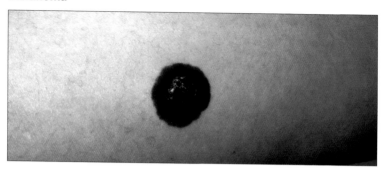

Description dark brown, black or pink/red macule or papule often with irregular borders and asymmetrical in size and color

Location can occur anywhere on skin, even plantar surface of foot and perineal area; can also occur in eye or brain

Characteristics any age, light skin>dark skin, can metastasize, asymptomatic, may spontaneously bleed

Tests Histopathology: large abnormal melanocytes with prominent nucleoli that extend into upper layers of the epidermis as well as into the dermis, +mitotic figures

Associated systemic disease none

Treatment pearls surgical excision; if depth >1 mm, sentinel lymph node biopsy may be recommended to guide in choosing possible adjunct treatments including I.V. interferon.

Seborrheic keratosis

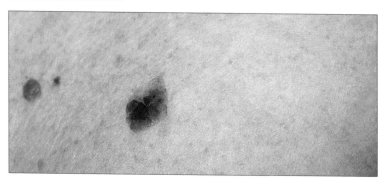

Description brown, verrucous, well-demarcated, 'stuck-on' papule
Location common on trunk, but can occur anywhere
Characteristics older adults, chronic, benign, asymptomatic or pruritic
Tests Histopathology: hyperkeratosis, acanthosis with horn pseudocysts
Associated systemic disease Leser–Trélat syndrome; abrupt eruption of many pruritic seborrheic keratoses may be associated with internal malignancy (especially gastric adenocarcinoma)
Treatment pearls no treatment necessary, LN2 or ED&C

Milia
See page 42

Epidermal cyst
See page 136

Dermatofibroma

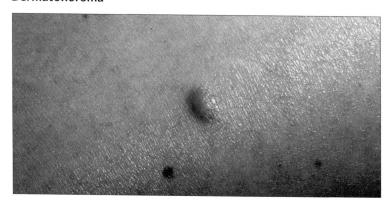

Description skin-colored to brown, firm nodule
Location in areas of trauma (especially extremities)
Characteristics adults, chronic course, may resolve in years, asymptomatic vs. rarely tender

Lipoma

Tests +'dimple sign' (dimple in center of lesion when pinching it);
Histopathology: nodule of dense swirls of plump fibroblasts with entrapped
'keloidal' collagen at edges of nodule, ± hyperpigmented and hyperplastic
overlying epidermis, Factor XIIIa+, S100– and CD34–
Associated systemic disease none
Treatment pearls no treatment necessary

Lipoma

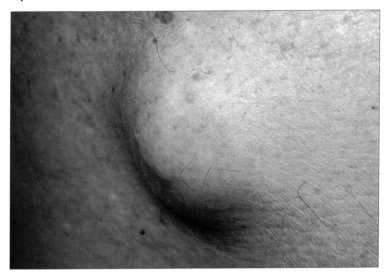

Description soft, round, mobile subcutaneous skin-colored nodule ranging in
size from 5 mm to >10 cm
Location neck, trunk, arms, buttocks and upper legs most common
Characteristics adults>children, chronic, asymptomatic
Tests Histopathology: proliferation of mature adipocytes
Associated systemic disease may be associated with Gardner's,
Bannayan–Riley–Ruvalcaba and Proteus syndromes
Treatment pearls no treatment necessary, excision

Neurofibroma
See page 107

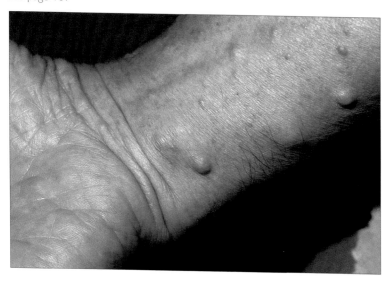

Verruca planae (flat warts)
See page 60, Wart

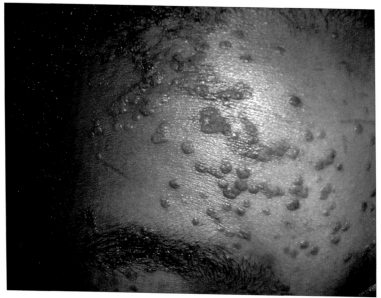

Molluscum contagiosum
See page 355

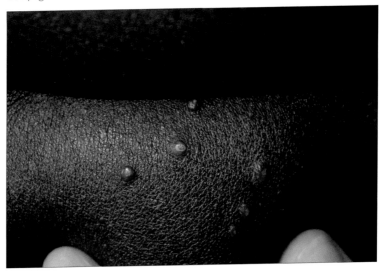

Mastocytoma

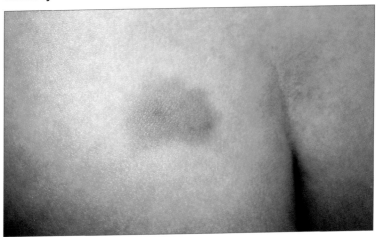

Description solitary yellow/brown papule, patch or plaque that 'urticates' and becomes red upon stroking (Darier's sign) with possible progression to bulla
Location distal extremities most common, but can occur anywhere
Characteristics most present prior to 2 years, most resolve spontaneously over years (may be persistent if presents in an adult), asymptomatic vs. pruritic

Tests +Darier's sign; Histopathology: increase in mast cells seen by Leder stain
Associated systemic disease if multiple, can be a sign of urticaria pigmentosa
(diffuse mastocytosis)
Treatment pearls avoidance of manipulation, antihistamines, excision

Mastocytosis (urticaria pigmentosa)

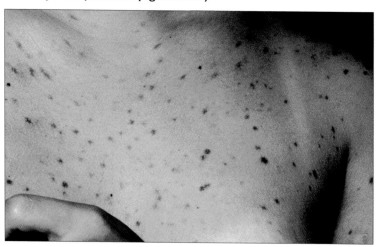

Description multiple yellow/brown/red macules and papules that may urticate
with stroking (Darier's sign) to produce a bulla; telangiectasia macularis eruptiva
perstans (TMEP) variant with red/brown patches and papules with telangiectasias
Location distal extremities and trunk common in children, proximal extremities
and trunk common in adults, typically spares the face
Characteristics bimodal with largest incidence in children <2 years followed by
adults 30–40 years; childhood form often resolves, adult form typically chronic;
asymptomatic usually but may have pruritus, flushing, diarrhea, syncope,
abdominal pain, dizziness, fever and/or malaise; exacerbated by stroking,
exercise, temperature increase or alcohol
Tests +Darier's sign; Histopathology: infiltrate of mast cells in dermis seen with
Leder stain, ± subepidermal bulla
Associated systemic disease adult types more likely to have associated
internal organ involvement and/or association with hematologic disease such as
polycythemia rubra vera, hypereosinophilic syndrome, CML, CLL and Hodgkin's
lymphoma
Treatment pearls antihistamines (H_1 and H_2 blockers), cromolyn sodium (mast
cell stabilizer), oral, intralesional and/or topical corticosteroids, PUVA to relieve
pruritus or interferon if severe; also avoid manipulation of lesions, NSAIDs,
alcohol and other mast cell degranulators

Lichen nitidus

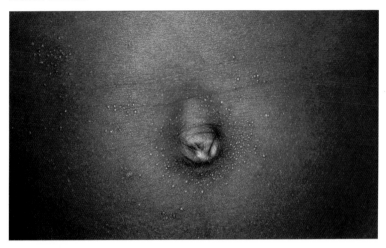

Description multiple, firm, tiny 1–2 mm skin-colored papules
Location grouped on flexor surface of wrists and dorsal arms, trunk and genitalia
Characteristics young children, spontaneous resolution after months to years, asymptomatic vs. pruritic
Tests +Koebner phenomenon; Histopathology: atrophic epidermis 'cups' lichenoid lymphohistiocytic infiltrate ('ball and claw'), ± granulomas
Associated systemic disease none
Treatment pearls topical corticosteroids, oral antihistamines

Calcinosis cutis
See page 453

Pseudoxanthoma elasticum (PXE)

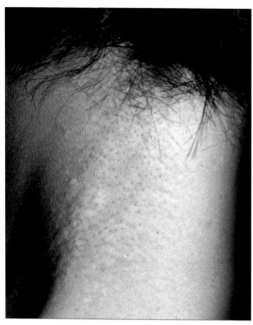

Description skin-colored to yellow 'cobblestoned' papules and plaques which give the appearance of 'plucked chicken skin' superimposed on lax skin, ± yellow mucosal papules

Location lateral neck and flexor surfaces most common, ± oral mucosal involvement

Characteristics AR inheritance (ABCC6 gene), females>males, onset during childhood, chronic, associated with ocular angioid streaks (decreased visual acuity) and vascular calcification in many organs (especially cardiovascular)

Tests Histopathology: purple, calcified, oblong elastic fibers in dermis on H&E

Associated systemic disease PXE is a multisystem disease

Treatment pearls no treatment required in skin lesions, ophthalmology and cardiology to follow other signs

Xanthoma
See page 392

Juvenile xanthogranuloma
See page 393

Angiofibroma
See page 373

Pseudoxanthoma elasticum • Xanthoma • Juvenile xanthogranuloma • Angiofibroma

Sarcoid
See page 443

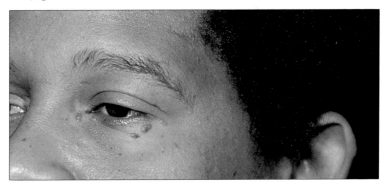

Mucous cyst
See page 60

Dermoid cyst
See page 138

Rheumatoid nodule
See page 183

Gout tophus
See page 182

Granuloma faciale
See page 213

Leiomyoma
See page 362

Angiolipoma
See page 361

Neurilemmoma
See page 361

Lymphangioma
See page 353

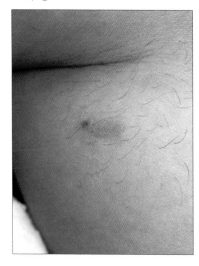

Eccrine spiradenoma
See page 362

Connective tissue nevus

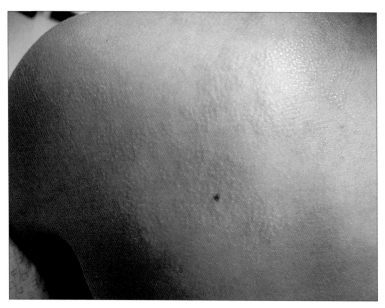

Thyroglossal cyst (bow cleft)

Scleromyxedema

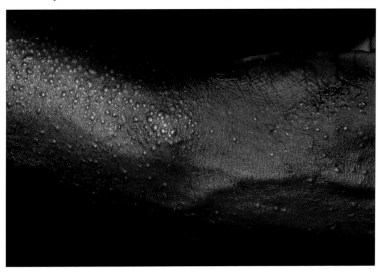

Papular mucinosis (lichen myxedematosus)

Follicular mucinosis

Steatocystoma multiplex

Cylindroma

Fox–Fordyce disease

Spitz nevus

Dermatofibrosarcoma protuberans (DFSP)

Desmoid tumor

Nodular fasciitis

Morphea (early nodules)

Trichoepithelioma

Trichilemmoma (face)

Ganglion cyst

Hemangiopericytoma

Cystic hygroma

Osteoma cutis

Lymph node

Perforating folliculitis

Reactive perforating collagenoses

Gardner's syndrome

PAPULES AND NODULES – WITHIN SCARS

Hematoma

Foreign body reaction (suture, starch, talc)

Epidermal inclusion cyst

Hypertrophic granulation tissue

Hypertrophic scar

Keloid

Traumatic nodule

Locally recurrent neoplasm

Metastatic neoplasm

Infectious granuloma

Psoriasis

Sarcoid

Desmoid tumor

Prurigo nodularis

Squamous cell carcinoma (Marjolin's ulcer)

Endometriosis

Cystic hygroma • Osteoma cutis • Lymph node • Perforating folliculitis • Reactive perforating collagenoses • Gardner's syndrome

PAPULES AND NODULES – YELLOW/BROWN/RED

Xanthoma: eruptive (ER), tuberous (Tub), tendinous (Ten), plane (including xanthelasma)

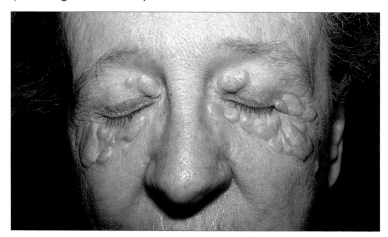

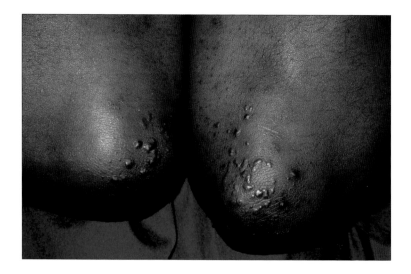

Description firm yellow/brown/orange/red patches, papules, plaques or nodules
Location *ER, Tub, Ten:* extensor surfaces, hands, buttocks; *plane:* often periorbital and intertriginous (in finger web spaces is pathognomonic for homozygous familial hypercholesterolemia, in palmar creases is pathognomonic for dysbetaproteinemia)

Characteristics most resolve with correction of underlying lipid abnormality (xanthelasmas are chronic); ± pain and pruritus, may be exacerbated by obesity, alcoholism or oral retinoid use

Tests Histopathology: variable amounts of foam cells in the dermis (Tub and Ten>Er>plane), ± cholesterol clefts, ± mixed inflammatory infiltrate (xanthelasmas are non-inflammatory)

Associated systemic disease ± hyperlipidemia, cholestasis, monoclonal gammopathy or increased estrogen states (only 50% of patients with xanthelasmas have abnormal lipids)

Treatment pearls treat underlying lipid abnormalities, low fat diet, excision, electrocautery, laser; avoid alcohol

Juvenile xanthogranuloma

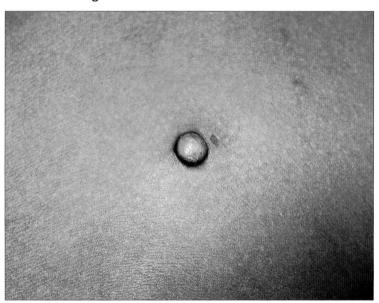

Description yellow/brown small, firm papule

Location head and neck most common followed by trunk and proximal extremities

Characteristics male>female, infants/children>adults, light skin>dark skin, resolves in years, asymptomatic, ocular lesions can lead to blindness, rare systemic lesions

Tests Histopathology: dense groups of histiocytes with Touton giant cells (large histiocyte with a wreath of nuclei at edge), HAM56+, CD68+, CD1a–, Factor XIIIa+, S100 usually +

Associated systemic disease multiple JXGs may be associated with neurofibromatosis or CML

Treatment pearls no treatment necessary, excision

Dermatofibroma
See page 381

Mastocytoma
See page 384

Keloid
See page 376

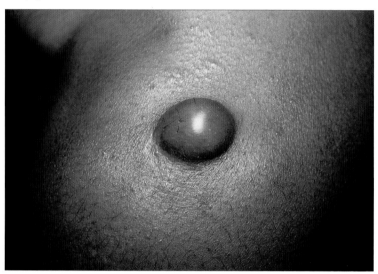

Neurofibroma
See page 107

Nevus
See page 379

Epidermal cyst
See page 136

Benign cephalic histiocytosis

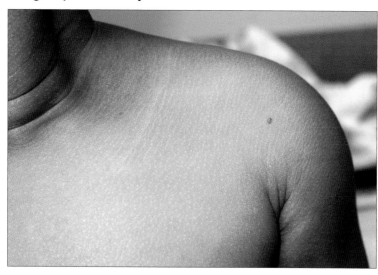

Giant cell reticulohistiocytoma (GCR)/multicentric reticulohistiocytoma (MR)
See page 376

Malignant fibrous histiocytoma/atypical fibroxanthoma

Sarcoid

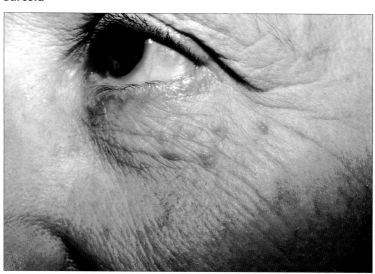

Syringoma

Trichoepithelioma

Pilomatrixoma

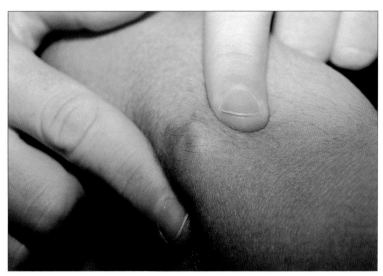

Hidradenoma/acrospiroma

Trichilemmoma

Hidrocystoma

PAPULOSQUAMOUS
Psoriasis

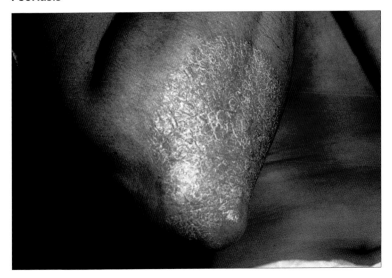

Description erythematous well-demarcated patches and plaques of varying size with thick, silvery scale, large plaques and treated plaques can be annular; pustular lesions are possible; oil spots, pits and/or onycholysis in nails

Location symmetric on extensor surfaces, scalp, sacrum, or diffusely; inverse psoriasis is intertriginous; pustular psoriasis often involves palms and soles

Characteristics any age, chronic, asymptomatic, +Koebner phenomenon, drugs can exacerbate (beta-blockers, lithium, antimalarials, terbinafine, calcium channel blockers, lipid lowering drugs, captopril, glyburide, interferon)

Tests +Auspitz sign (pinpoint areas of bleeding if scale removed); Histopathology: parakeratosis, regular acanthosis, small neutrophilic abscesses within epidermis

Associated systemic disease ~25% have psoriatic arthritis (asymmetric oligoarthritis especially of DIP joints), guttate psoriasis can occur abruptly after upper respiratory infection (usually Strep)

Treatment pearls topical corticosteroids (*avoid* systemic corticosteroids), topical calcipotriene, tar, light therapy, methotrexate, cyclosporine, topical or systemic retinoids, biologics (etanercept, alefacept, efaluzimab, adalimumab, infliximab)

Seborrheic dermatitis • Atopic dermatitis

Atopic dermatitis
See page 141

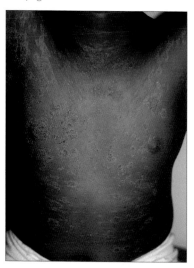

Seborrheic dermatitis

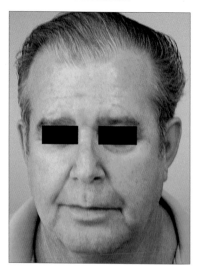

Description poorly demarcated greasy, erythematous, scaly patches; can appear as hyper- or hypopigmented scaly patches

Location scalp, eyebrows, nasolabial folds, central chest and intertriginous areas

Characteristics infants and elderly men>women, asymptomatic or pruritic
Tests Histopathology: spongiosis, perivascular and perifollicular lymphocytic infiltrate, ± acanthosis and parakeratosis
Associated systemic disease none; however, severe seborrheic dermatitis can be seen in the HIV and Parkinson's population
Treatment pearls topical azoles, zinc pyrithione, emollients, tacrolimus or pimecrolimus, mild topical corticosteroids if severe

Tinea versicolor
See page 225

Drug reaction
See page 286

Tinea corporis (dermatophytosis)
See page 86

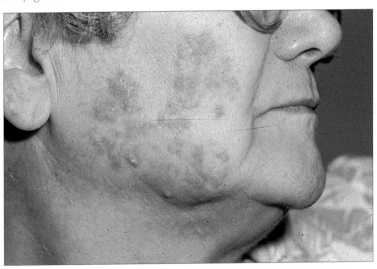

Pityriasis rosea

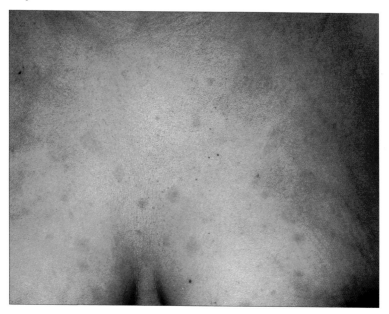

Description annular, erythematous patches with collarette of scale, may appear gray and more papular in dark skin

Location starts as a larger herald patch which appears days to weeks prior to eruption on trunk and proximal extremities (usually spares the face), follows skin cleavage lines ('Christmas tree' pattern); can be atypical: inverse/intertriginous (more common in young children), vesicular, pustular or purpuric

Characteristics ± pruritus, young adults, slight female predominance, resolves spontaneously in 6 weeks, increased incidence in spring and fall, possible viral etiology

Tests Histopathology: mounds of parakeratosis, extravasation of RBCs, mild spongiosis, perivascular infiltrate

Associated systemic disease may be associated with HHV 6 and 7

Treatment pearls no treatment necessary, topical corticosteroids for pruritus

Lichen planus
See page 259

Lichen simplex chronicus
See page 201

Scabies
See page 52

Systemic lupus erythematosus (SLE)
See page 425

Dermatomyositis
See page 427

Id reaction
See page 142

Secondary syphilis

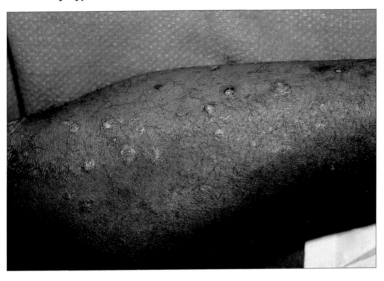

Description erythematous macules, papules, erosions or targetoid/annular lesions with slight scale
Location genital and oral mucosa, oral commissures, palms and soles and/or symmetrically distributed diffusely over body
Characteristics any age, local lymphadenopathy, resolves spontaneously in weeks to months but can recur
Tests serology: RPR/VDRL and confirmatory MHA-TP/FTA-ABS; Histopathology: lymphocytic and plasma cell perivascular infiltrate with normal epidermis or psoriasiform and lichenoid changes, ± granulomas, Warthin–Starry stain for spirochetes + 30% in secondary lesions
Associated systemic disease syphilis is a multisystem infection which can affect the kidneys, brain, GI tract, eyes and joints
Treatment pearls I.M. penicillin G, azithromycin or PCN desensitization if PCN allergic

Sarcoid
See page 443

Pityriasis rubra pilaris
See page 159

Lichen striatus
See page 262

Cutaneous T-cell lymphoma (CTCL)

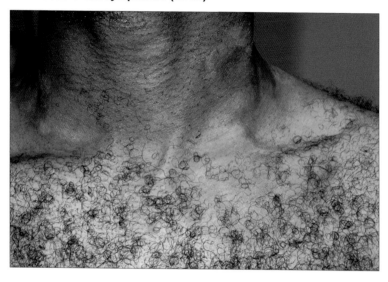

Description erythematous patches and papules, ± overlying atrophy, telangiectasias or hypopigmentation, may be annular, may progress to plaques and tumors ± ulceration

Location trunk, buttocks and proximal extremities (covered sites) most common

Characteristics male>female, increased incidence with age, chronic course ± remissions and relapses, patches and plaques typically asymptomatic, tumors may be painful

Tests +T-cell gene rearrangement; Histopathology: lymphocyte epidermotropism in a linear array or in clumps (Pautrier's microabscesses), lichenoid infiltrate with atypical lymphocytes with cerebriform nuclei

Associated systemic disease CTCL is a systemic disease that may progress to lymph node and organ involvement

Treatment pearls topical corticosteroids, nitrogen mustard, topical or oral bexarotene, light therapy (PUVA or UVB), interferon, electron beam radiation, extracorporeal photophoresis

Pityriasis lichenoides chronica (PLC)
See page 411

Leprosy
See page 186

Prurigo nodularis
See page 198

Gianotti–Crosti syndrome (papular acrodermatitis of childhood)
See page 288

Contact dermatitis

Intertrigo

Lichen nitidus
See page 386

Chronic mucocutaneous candidiasis

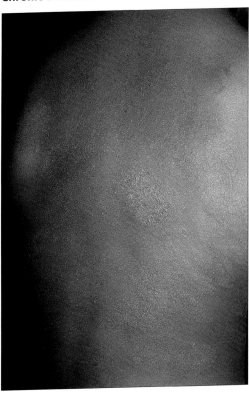

PAPULOSQUAMOUS – FACE AND CHEST (SEBORRHEIC–DERMATITIS-LIKE)

Seborrheic dermatitis
See page 398

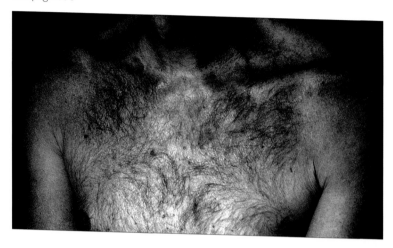

Psoriasis
See page 397

Contact dermatitis
See page 189

Pityriasis rosea
See page 400

Tinea versicolor
See page 225

Darier's disease (keratosis follicularis)

Tinea barbae (dermatophytosis)

Pemphigus erythematosus

Perioral dermatitis

Histiocytosis X

Systemic lupus erythematosus (SLE)

PAPULOSQUAMOUS – INFANTS

Seborrheic dermatitis (cradle cap)
See page 398

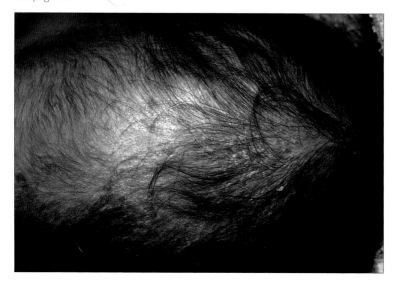

Atopic dermatitis
See page 141

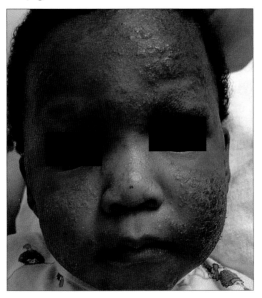

Psoriasis
See page 397

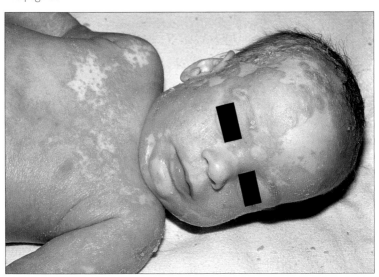

Contact dermatitis
See page 189

Viral exanthem
See page 287

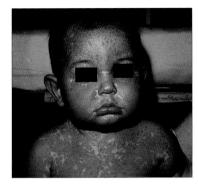

Tinea corporis (dermatophytosis)
See page 86

Candidiasis
See page 145

Intertrigo
See page 145

Scabies
See page 52

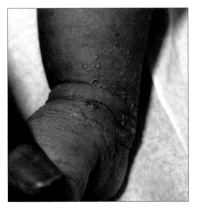

Acrodermatitis enteropathica

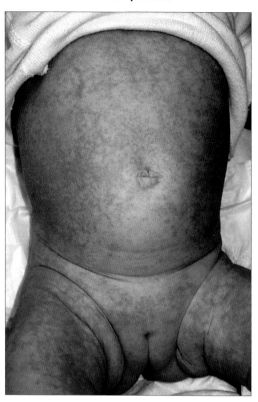

Histiocytosis X

Syndromes
Wiskott–Aldrich syndrome
Leiner's syndrome
Bruton's agammaglobulinemia
Job's syndrome
Hartnup's syndrome
Phenylketonuria
Ataxia telangiectasia
Chronic granulomatous disease
Netherton's syndrome

PAPULOSQUAMOUS – SCALP

See page 497, Scalp – scaly

PARAPSORIASIS ('PSORIASIS-LIKE')
Parapsoriasis

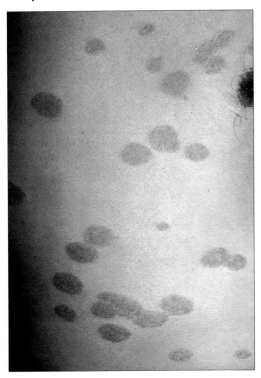

Description erythematous round patches with fine scale (<5 cm in small plaque, >5 cm in large plaque)

Location symmetric and diffuse distribution sometimes accentuated in sun-protected areas; digitate variant of small plaque with long, oval patches like fingers on bilateral flanks; retiform variant of large plaque with diffuse lacy/striped pattern

Characteristics male>female, adults, chronic course, some spontaneously resolve, large plaque form (especially retiform variant) may progress to cutaneous T-cell lymphoma (CTCL), asymptomatic

Tests Histopathology: spongiosis, parakeratosis, perivascular or lichenoid ، infiltrate

Associated systemic disease large plaque parapsoriasis may be associated with CTCL

Treatment pearls topical corticosteroids, light therapy, topical tar

Pityriasis lichenoides et varioliformis acuta (PLEVA)

(PLEVA = Mucha–Habermann syndrome – more acute on spectrum of PLC entities)

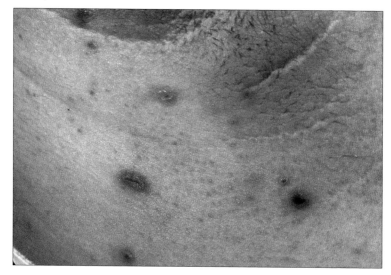

Description erythematous papules with central hemorrhagic crust, vesicles or pustules

Location diffusely over body

Characteristics male>female, spontaneously resolves within weeks but recurs in crops, asymptomatic to pruritic

Tests Histopathology: lichenoid infiltrate, crust, parakeratosis, necrotic keratinocytes ± areas of epidermal necrosis, extravasated RBCs

Associated systemic disease none

Treatment pearls light therapy, tetracycline, erythromycin, topical corticosteroids, topical tar, low dose methotrexate, antihistamines

Pityriasis lichenoides chronica (PLC)

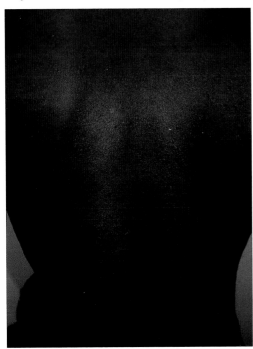

Description scaly guttate erythematous to brown patches
Location diffusely over body
Characteristics male>female, spontaneously resolves within months but can be chronic and typically recurs in crops, asymptomatic to pruritic
Tests Histopathology: lichenoid infiltrate, areas of parakeratosis, few necrotic keratinocytes, mild extravasation of RBCs
Associated systemic disease none
Treatment pearls PUVA

Pityriasis rosea
See page 400

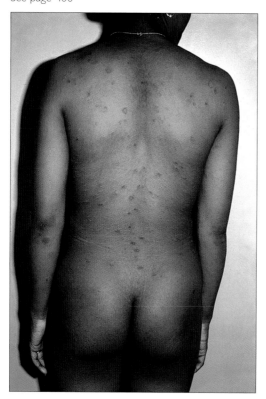

Cutaneous T-cell lymphoma (CTCL)
See page 402

Poikiloderma vasculare atrophicans (atrophic parapsoriasis en plaque)

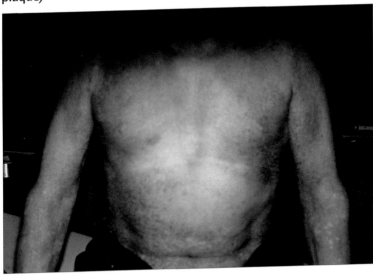

PENIS – ULCERS

See page 524, Ulcers – genital

PENIS AND SCROTUM – PAPULES AND PLAQUES

Scabies
See page 52

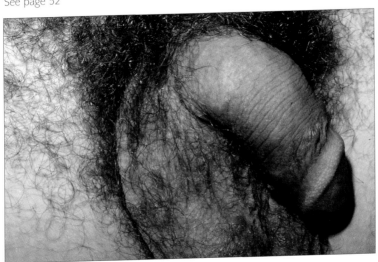

Pearly penile papules
See page 373, Angiofibroma

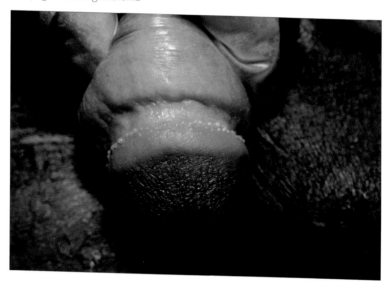

Lichen nitidus
See page 386

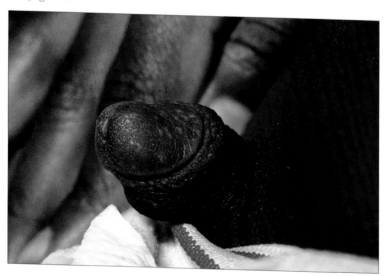

Bowenoid papulosis

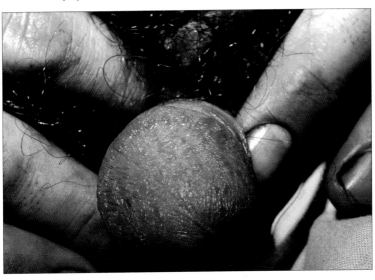

Lichen planus

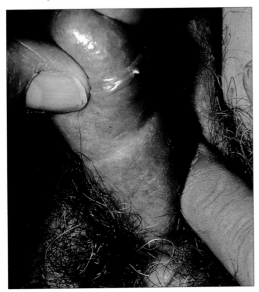

Fixed drug reaction

Erosive balanitis

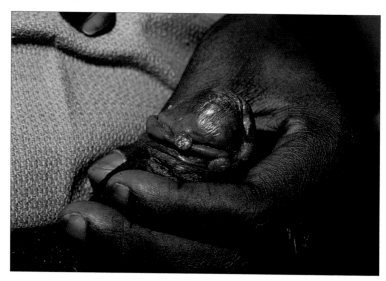

Herpes simplex virus

Angiokeratoma of the scrotum (Fordyce)

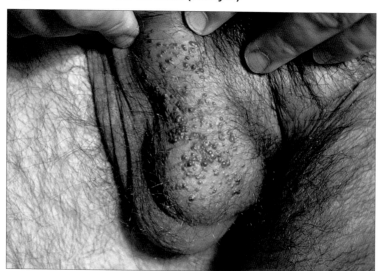

Psoriasis

Molluscum contagiosum

Condyloma accuminata

Seborrheic keratosis

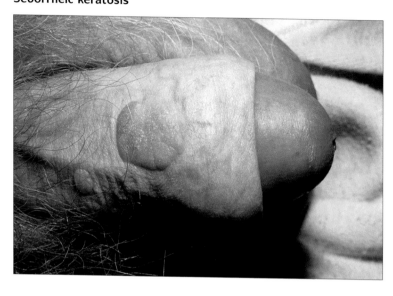

Accessory urethra

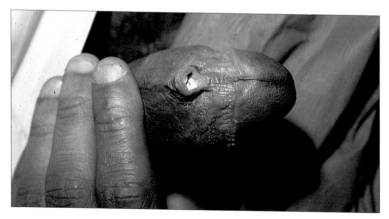

PERIANAL STENOSIS

Cicatricial pemphigoid

Pemphigus vegetans

Eosinophilic granuloma

Lymphogranuloma venereum (LGV)

Crohn's disease

Amebiasis

Blastomycosis

Cryptococcosis

Sporotrichosis

Tuberculosis

Actinomycosis

Nocardia

PERIORBITAL EDEMA

Acute contact dermatitis

Angioedema

Infection
Dental abscess
Mononucleosis
Sinusitis
Mucormycosis
Erysipelas
Herpes

Obstructive
Postinfection
Cavernous sinus thrombosis
Superior vena cava syndrome

Infiltrative
Leukemia/lymphoma
Tumor
Sarcoid

Metabolic
Myxedema
Nephritic syndrome

Connective tissue diseases
SLE
Dermatomyositis

Trichinosis

Allergic gastric enteropathy

Melkersson–Rosenthal syndrome

Acne

PETECHIAE
Pigmented purpuric eruption

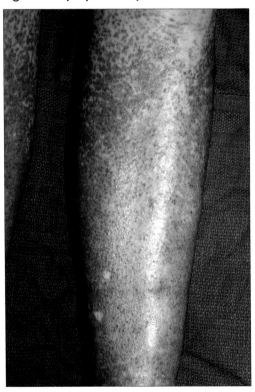

Schamberg's

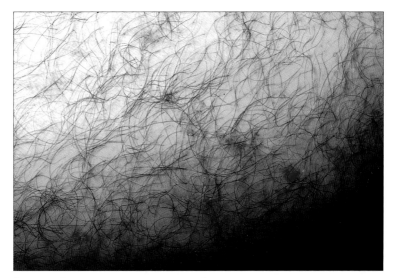

Pigmented purpuric eruption, non-specific

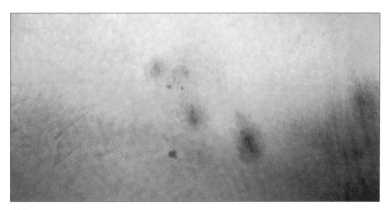

Lichen aureus

Description petechiae and purpura on light yellow/red/brown macules
Location lower extremities most common
Characteristics asymptomatic; Schamberg's variety resembles 'cayenne pepper' and occurs at any age but most often in older men where it is chronic; Majocchi's variety is more annular with telangiectasias, appears in young women and usually resolves spontaneously; Gougerot and Blum variety appears more lichenoid in older men; Doucas and Kapetanakis variety appears scaly and eczematous; lichen aureus variety is usually solitary and rust-colored and appears in adults
Tests Histopathology: RBC extravasation, endothelial cell swelling, perivascular lymphocytic infiltrate and hemosiderin macrophages (lichen aureus and Gougerot

and Blum varieties have a lichenoid infiltrate, Doucas and Kapetanakis variety has spongiosis)
Associated systemic disease none
Treatment pearls topical corticosteroids, compression hose if element of stasis

Thrombocytopenia

Drug reaction

Valsalva maneuvers – vomiting, childbirth, coughing

Hemolytic anemia

Bacterial endocarditis

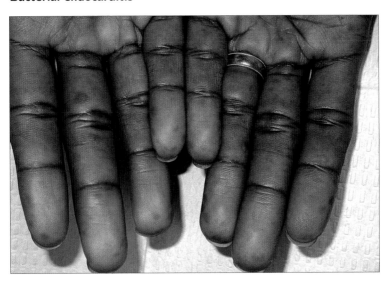

Infectious mononucleosis

Coxsackie virus

Echovirus

Meningococcemia

Rubella

Rocky Mountain spotted fever

Leptospirosis

Wiskott–Aldrich syndrome

PHOTOSENSITIVE DERMATOSES
Polymorphous light eruption (PMLE)

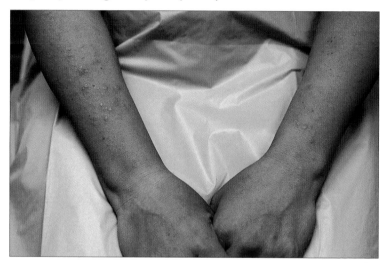

Description erythematous scaly patches, papules, vesicles and plaques
Location sun-exposed areas, rarely sun-protected sites are involved
Characteristics females>males, adults, pruritic and burning, usually occurs minutes to 4 days after increased exposure to sunlight, duration of days to weeks, may recur each spring, usually improves as summer progresses and improves with age, more common in temperate climates
Tests Histopathology: papillary dermal edema, superficial and deep lymphocytic perivascular infiltrate
Associated systemic disease none
Treatment pearls sunscreen, PUVA or narrowband UVB each spring, topical or oral corticosteroids, antihistamines, hydroxychloroquine (Plaquenil), thalidomide, azathioprine, cyclosporine

Photoallergic reaction

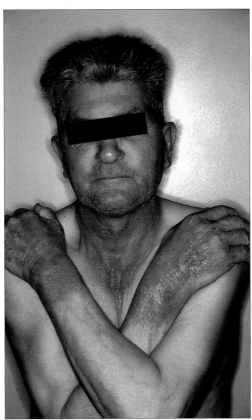

Description erythematous, scaly papules and plaques ± crust
Location usually starts in sun-exposed areas but can spread diffusely over body with even sun-protected areas becoming confluent
Characteristics associated pruritus, ± fever, +history of drug (oral or topical) either prescribed or OTC (*see box*), onset can be immediate or delayed but typically occurs within 24–48 h after sun exposure in previously sensitized individuals (UVA 320–425 nm), may persist for 6–8 weeks or become chronic after discontinuation of drug; requires a state of acquired altered reactivity involving an antigen–antibody reaction
Tests ± peripheral eosinophilia; Histopathology: spongiotic dermatitis with perivascular superficial infiltrate with eosinophils
Associated systemic disease none
Treatment pearls discontinue drug, oral and topical corticosteroids, oral antihistamines

PHOTOALLERGIC DRUGS AND CHEMICALS

- Sunscreens (PABA, benzophenones, digalloyl trioleate)
- Antibacterial cleansers (chlorhexidine, hexachlorophene, bithionol)
- Sulfa drugs
- Quinidine
- Quinine
- Tricyclic antidepressants
- NSAIDs
- Thiazide diuretics

- Antimalarials
- Phenothiazines (chlorpromazine, promethazine)
- Griseofulvin
- Carbonilide
- Fragrances (musk ambrette, sandalwood oil, 6-methylcoumarin)
- Antifungal agents (fentichlor, jadit, multifungin)
- Gold
- Silver

Phototoxic reaction

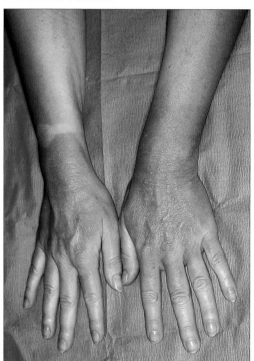

Description confluent erythema and edema ± vesicles like a severe sunburn
Location sun-exposed distribution
Characteristics occurs within hours after exposure to sunlight (285–450 nm), resolves within weeks; burning, stinging, painful; may be associated with onycholysis, hyperpigmentation or lichenoid papules; eruption occurs by a non-immunologic mechanism (*see box*)

Tests Histopathology: necrotic keratinocytes high within the epidermis, edema, perivascular lymphocytic infiltrate ± neutrophils
Associated systemic disease none
Treatment pearls discontinue drug, oral and topical corticosteroids, antihistamines

---

PHOTOTOXIC DRUGS AND CHEMICALS MORE COMMON THAN PHOTOALLERGIC

- Phenothiazines (Compazine, Stelazine, Thorazine, Temaril, Phenergan, chlorpromazine, promethazine)
- Sulfonamides
- Sulfonylureas (orinase, diabenase)
- Furocoumarins (psoralens, 8-MOP, TMP)
- Tetracyclines (especially demeclocycline, doxycycline)
- Thiazides (especially HCTZ)
- Coal tars (acridine, anthracene, pyridine)
- Furosemide (frusemide)
- Amiodarone
- NSAIDs (especially naproxen, piroxicam)
- Artificial sweeteners (saccharin)
- Dyes (anthraquinone, eosin, Rose Bengal)
- Quinolone (nalidixic acid, ciprofloxacin)

Systemic lupus erythematosus (SLE)

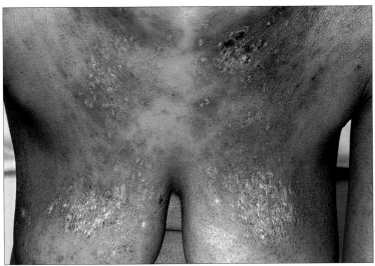

Description erythematous patches and plaques ± scale, ± central clearing; erythematous macules in malar distribution
Location face and sun-exposed areas
Characteristics female predominance, young adult onset, chronic, UV light exacerbates, SLE can be drug induced (*see box*)

Tests ANA, dsDNA, anti-Smith, Ro (SS-A) and La (SS-B) antibodies; Histopathology: interface change ± scale/crust, superficial and deep perivascular and periadnexal lymphocytic infiltrate with follicular plugging; urinalysis to rule out proteinuria

Associated systemic disease SLE is a systemic disease with manifestations in the lungs, liver, kidneys and other internal organs

Treatment pearls daily sunscreen, antimalarials, corticosteroids (oral and topical), thalidomide

---

COMMON DRUGS THAT CAUSE DRUG-INDUCED SLE

- 5-Aminosalicylic acid (pentasa, mesalamine, asacol)
- Chlorpromazine*
- Chlorprothixene
- Chlorthalidone
- Estrogens (including OCPs)
- Ethosuximide
- Furosemide
- Griseofulvin
- Hydralazine*
- Hydrochlorothiazide (HCTZ)
- Isoniazid (INH)*
- Methyldopa*
- Methylthiouracil
- NSAIDs (including ibuprofen, naproxen)
- Penicillamine*
- Penicillin
- Phenytoin
- Phenylbutazone
- Phenothiazines
- Phenytoin
- Procainamide*
- Propylthiouracil*
- Psoralen*
- Quinidine
- Streptomycin
- Sulfa drugs
- Tetracyclines (including doxycycline and minocycline)*
- Thiazides*

Positive antihistone antibodies often, antibodies to ssDNA in many cases, ds-DNA negative, ± Ro (SS-A) antibodies.
* Indicates the most common.

Dermatomyositis

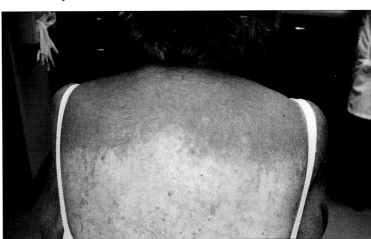

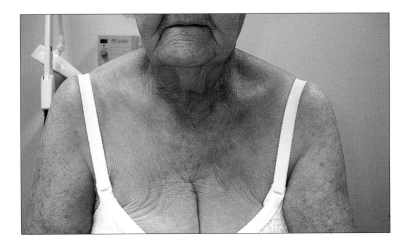

Description poikilodermatous, red, scaly patches and papules
Location erythematous patches occur in sun-exposed areas and in a 'shawl' distribution on upper back and shoulders, periorbital 'heliotrope' violaceous patches, Gottron's papules over joints and extensor surfaces especially dorsal hand joints; proximal nailfold telangiectasias and 'ragged' cuticles
Characteristics female>male; bimodal: children and adults, chronic course may include exacerbations and remissions, rash is exacerbated by sunlight and may be associated with proximal muscle weakness that typically presents after skin lesions and pulmonary interstitial fibrosis; childhood cases may be associated with calcinosis cutis

Tests +SS-A, ± ANA, elevated muscle enzymes (aldolase and CK); muscle biopsy; Histopathology: interface change, perivascular lymphocytic infiltrate with increased dermal mucin

Associated systemic disease 25% of adult cases are associated with malignancy that can develop up to 2 years after cutaneous lesions

Treatment pearls sunscreen, oral corticosteroids, methotrexate, azathioprine, hydroxychloroquine (Plaquenil), oral retinoids, dapsone, thalidomide, mycophenolate mofetil

Porphyria (porphyria cutanea tarda, erythropoietic protoporphyria)

See page 46, Porphyria cutanea tarda

Chronic actinic dermatitis (actinic reticuloid, severe variant)

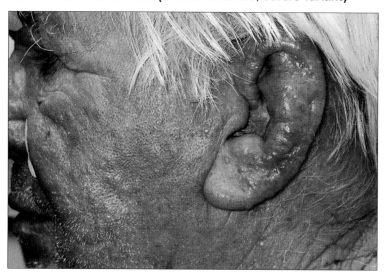

Description erythematous, edematous, scaly patches and plaques ± lichenification

Location sun-exposed areas (face, neck, arms, hands)

Characteristics male>female, older adults, chronic course but may slowly resolve after years, worse in summer, pruritic, may occur in conjunction with contact dermatitis

Tests Histopathology: psoriasiform dermatitis with mild inflammatory infiltrate

Associated systemic disease none

Treatment pearls avoidance of sun and allergens, sunscreens, topical corticosteroids and emollients, low dose PUVA with an immunosuppressive such as an oral corticosteroid, mycophenolate mofetil, azathioprine or cyclosporine

Phytophotodermatitis
See page 264

Pseudoporphyria
See page 47

Hydroa vacciniforme

Solar urticaria

Summertime actinic lichenoid eruption

Actinic prurigo

Xeroderma pigmentosum

Erythema multiforme
See page 484

Herpes simplex
See page 116

Atopic dermatitis
See page 141

Lichen planus
See page 259

Pityriasis rubra pilaris
See page 159

Darier's disease
See page 196

Hypopituitary disease

Chronic photosensitive dermatitis

Persistent light reaction

Actinic granuloma
See page 92

Syndromes with an element of photosensitivity
Rothmund–Thomson syndrome

Cockayne syndrome
Trichothiodystrophy
Kindler–Weary syndrome
Albinism
Piebaldism
Bloom's syndrome
Hartnup's syndrome

PIGMENTATION – RETICULATED

Livedo reticularis

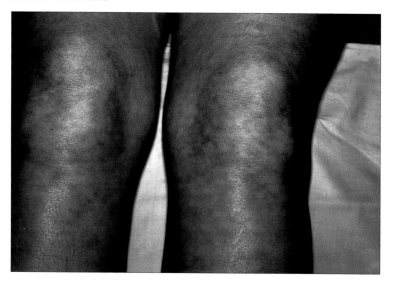

Description violaceous pigmentation in a lacy/reticular pattern
Location lower legs most common, can occur anywhere
Characteristics female>male, middle-aged adults, chronic, asymptomatic vs.
tingling and numbness, exacerbated by cool temperature
Tests Histopathology: non-specific
Associated systemic disease may be associated with micro-occlusive disease,
lymphoproliferative disorders, autoimmune disease or medications
Treatment pearls treat any underlying condition, avoid cold temperature

Erythema ab igne

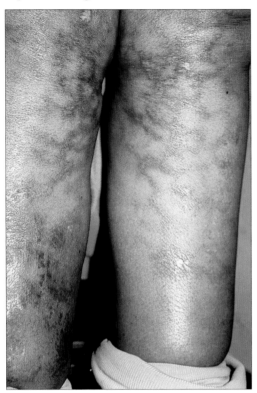

Description erythema in a lacy/reticular pattern
Location anywhere exposed to chronic heat most commonly back, sacrum and shins
Characteristics female>male, adults, chronic, asymptomatic, may rarely progress to SCC
Tests Histopathology: epidermal atrophy with atypical keratinocytes, interface dermatitis, hemosiderin macrophages, dilated capillaries
Associated systemic disease none
Treatment pearls avoid heat source

Cutis marmorata

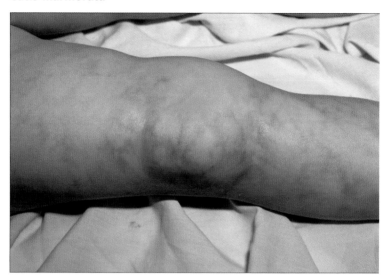

Dowling–Degos disease

Atopic dermatitis
See page 141

Post-inflammatory hyperpigmentation
See page 207

Confluent and reticulated papillomatosis of Gougerot and Carteaud
See page 332

Parvovirus B19 (erythrovirus) (erythema infectiosum)

Cryoglobulinemia

Disseminated intravascular coagulation (DIC)

Waldenström's macroglobulinemia

Scleroderma (often follows course of vein)

Reticulated erythematous mucinosis (REM)

X-linked reticulate pigmentary disorder

Naegeli–Franceschetti–Jadassohn syndrome

Prurigo pigmentosa

Epidermolysis bullosa herpetiformis (Dowling–Mera variant)

Dyskeratosis congenita

Mendes da Costa syndrome

Fanconi's anemia

Dermatopathia pigmentosa reticularis

Reticulate acropigmentation of Kitamura

CREST syndrome

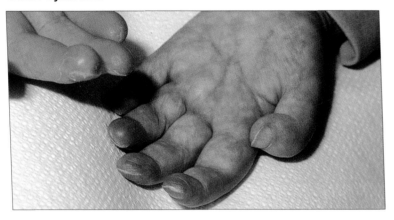

Polyarteritis nodosa (PAN)

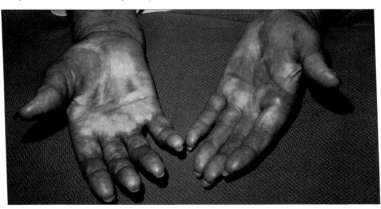

Calciphylaxis

PIGMENTED SKIN – BLUE

Blue nevus
See page 358

Nevus of Ota/Ito

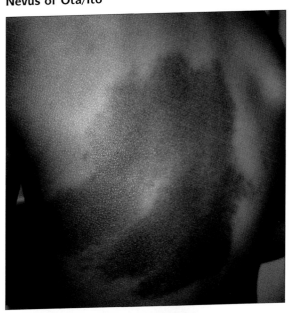

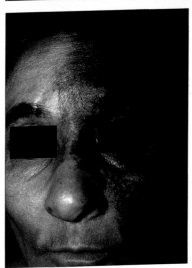

Description poorly demarcated hyperpigmented/bluish unilateral mottled patch

Location usually within distribution of V1 or V2 on head especially periorbital in Ota, across shoulder in Ito
Characteristics female>male, darker skin>lighter skin, present at birth or shortly thereafter or arises at puberty, asymptomatic
Tests Histopathology: dendritic melanocytes in the dermis, normal epidermis
Associated systemic disease none
Treatment pearls no treatment necessary, laser

Mongolian spot

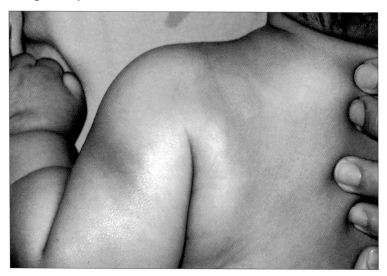

Description hyperpigmented bluish patch
Location lower back common, can occur anywhere
Characteristics darker skin>lighter skin, present at birth or shortly thereafter, resolves in years vs. rarely chronic, asymptomatic
Tests Histopathology: few dendritic melanocytes in the dermis, normal epidermis
Associated systemic disease none
Treatment pearls no treatment necessary, laser

Drugs – minocycline, amiodarone, antimalarials, clofazimine, chlorpromazine

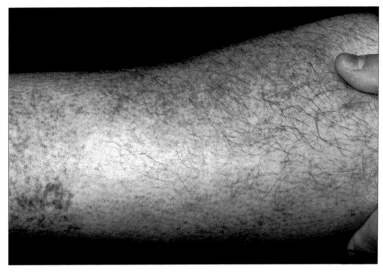

Maculae cerulae *(after spider bite)*

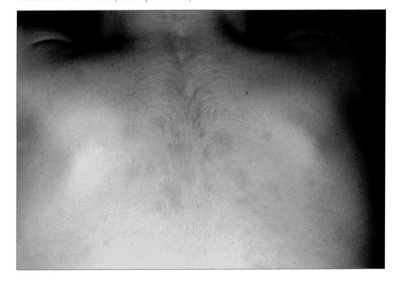

Melanoma
See page 380

Blue rubber bleb nevus syndrome

Argyria

Cyanosis (methemoglobinemia)

Ochronosis

PIGMENTED SKIN – GREEN

Tattoo

Pseudomonas infection

Chloroma

PIGMENTED SKIN – GREY

Argyria

Antimalarials

Amiodarone
Biopsy shows yellow/brown granules within dermal macrophages

Mongolian spot

Nevus of Ota/Ito

Erythema dyschromicum perstans

Carbon residue (coalminers – linear marks on forearms)

Heavy metal toxicity (gold, bismuth)

Degos' disease

PIGMENTED SKIN – WHITE/PORCELAIN

Degos' disease

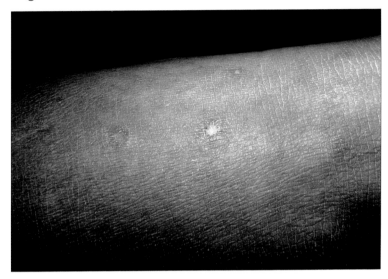

Description erythematous papules that resolve with a centrally depressed white porcelain scar surrounded by telangiectasias

Location can occur anywhere but common on lower legs

Characteristics onset 20–40 years, occur in crops and resolve over weeks to months with scarring, poor prognosis

Tests Histopathology: atrophic epidermis with underlying focal area of perivascular lymphocytic infiltrate, sclerosis, mucin and edema ± a deep thrombosed vessel

Associated systemic disease associated with vaso-occlusion in GI tract and CNS

Treatment pearls aspirin, pentoxifylline

Atrophie blanche (livedo vasculopathy)

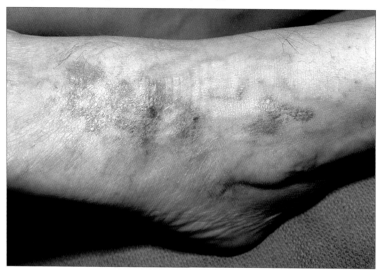

Description round, deep ulcers and stellate white scars surrounded by lacy violaceous pigmentation and telangiectasias
Location lower legs especially around ankles
Characteristics female>male, adults, chronic, painful
Tests check antiphospholipid, anticardiolipin, antinuclear antibodies and factor V Leiden; Histopathology: perivascular lymphocytic infiltrate with extravasated RBCs and fibrin thrombi within vessels
Associated systemic disease can be associated with venous stasis, varicose veins and hypercoagulable states
Treatment pearls anticoagulants, aspirin, danazol, stanozolol, PUVA

Scar
See page 97

PIGMENTED SKIN – YELLOW

Jaundice

Hepatitis
Can occur as hives in prodrome/anicteric phase of hepatitis

Solar elastosis

Carotenemia

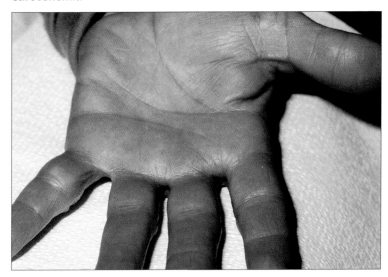

Quinacrine

Pseudoxanthoma elasticum (PXE)

Lycopenemia
Excess of lycopene often from excessive intake of tomatoes or papaya

PIGMENTED TUMORS

Nevus
See page 379

Seborrheic keratosis
See page 381

Dermatofibroma
See page 381

Basal cell carcinoma
See page 366

Hemangioma
See page 370

Spitz nevus
See page 368

Melanoma
See page 380

Blue nevus
See page 358

Pyogenic granuloma
See page 372

Thrombosed verruca

Hematoma

PLANTS – CONTACT URTICARIA

Fruits
Apricot
Plum
Peach
Pear
Banana
Apple
Mango
Kiwi
Pineapple
Lemon
Grapefruit
Sweet orange
Fig

Vegetables
Endive
Celery
Onion
Cabbage
Cauliflower
Potato
Corn
Cucumber
Carrot
Lettuce

Spices
Chili pepper (capsaicin)
Garlic
Chicory
Dill
Parsley

Other
Great nettle *(stinging hairs contain histamine, acetylcholine, 5-hydroxytryptamine)*
Cowhage *(itch powder – mucanain)*
Tulip
Chrysanthemum
Castor oil
Thistle

PLANTS – IRRITANT CONTACT DERMATITIS

Prickly pear

May apple

Buttercup

Juniper

Croton

Pencil tree

Dumb cane

Black mustard

Ivy

Fig

Thistle

Grass

PLAQUES – AXILLARY

See page 111, Axillary – plaques

PLAQUES – GRANULOMATOUS

Sarcoid

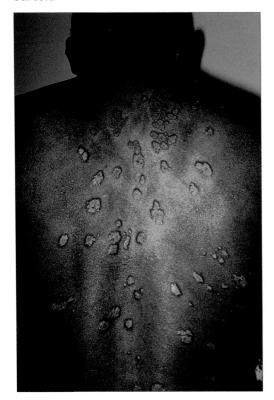

Description erythematous/violaceous, skin-colored, yellow/brown, hypopigmented or hyperpigmented firm, flat papules and plaques; may also be annular, ulcerative or ichthyosiform

Location common on face (periorificial), neck, upper extremities, often in areas of previous trauma, may also affect the nails and oral mucosa and may cause a scarring alopecia

Characteristics bimodal with peaks between 25–35 years and 45–65 years, Dark>fair in the US, chronic waxing and waning course, skin lesions are asymptomatic

Tests elevated serum ACE and ESR, anemia, lymphopenia, thrombocytopenia and eosinophilia, 10% with hypercalcemia, some with +ANA and rheumatoid factor (RF); CXR with hilar lymphadenopathy, hand and feet x-ray with cystic cavities seen in the bones of the digits; Histopathology: dermal non-caseating epithelioid granulomas with minimal to no surrounding inflammation ('naked granulomas'). (Historically: Kveim–Siltzbach test: intradermal injection of Kveim antigen from sarcoidal tissue elicits a sarcoidal granulomatous response noted on biopsy of injection site in 6 weeks; no longer done because of universal precautions.)

Associated systemic disease sarcoidosis is a systemic disease (90% have pulmonary manifestations, although almost any organ can be involved); *Löfgren syndrome*: sarcoidosis with hilar lymphadenopathy, fever, polyarthritis, iritis and erythema nodosum; *Heerfordt syndrome*: sarcoidosis with uveitis, parotid swelling, fever and seventh nerve palsy; *Darier–Roussy syndrome*: subcutaneous sarcoidosis without epidermal involvement; *lupus pernio*: sarcoidosis in 'beaded appearance' on face that scars and has a high association with lung involvement; *Mikulicz's disease*: sarcoidosis with swelling of the parotid, submandibular and lacrimal glands

Treatment pearls corticosteroids (oral, intralesional and topical), hydroxychloroquine (Plaquenil), methotrexate, thalidomide, oral retinoids, minocycline, allopurinol

Granuloma annulare
See page 87

Necrobiosis lipoidica diabeticorum (NLD)
See page 91

Actinic granuloma
See page 92

Granuloma faciale
See page 213

Granuloma gluteale infantum

PLAQUES – HYPERKERATOTIC

See page 201, Hyperkeratotic plaques

PLAQUES – INDURATED (RED/BROWN)

Foreign body
See page 61

Basal cell carcinoma
See page 366

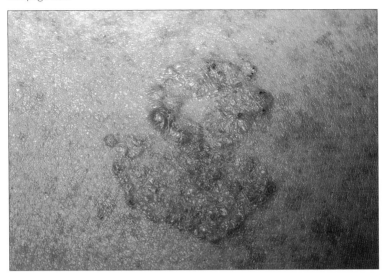

Squamous cell carcinoma
See page 367

Leukemia/lymphoma cutis

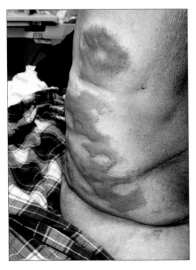

Description erythematous to violaceous firm papules, nodules or plaques ± ulceration, ± purpura
Location head and neck and trunk most common; also within scars
Characteristics adults, chronic, painless
Tests Histopathology: dense dermal infiltrate of atypical lymphocytes or myeloid cells
Associated systemic disease underlying malignancy
Treatment pearls chemotherapy, radiation

Metastatic (breast, renal, ovary, adenocarcinoma, thyroid)

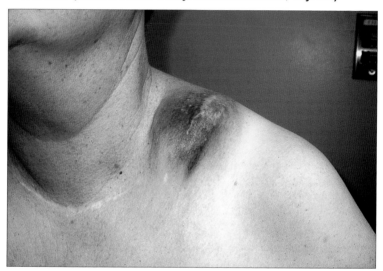

Description erythematous firm papule, nodule or plaque ± peau d'orange appearance
Location can occur anywhere but usually close to the underlying tumor
Characteristics adults, chronic, painless
Tests Histopathology: resembles that of underlying tumor
Associated systemic disease underlying malignancy
Treatment pearls chemotherapy, radiation, excision

Nodular amyloidosis
Description red/brown indurated, waxy plaque with 'apple jelly' appearance, usually solitary
Location face, acral, legs or trunk
Characteristics asymptomatic
Tests Histopathology: dense amorphous pink material (AL amyloid) in dermis, subcutaneous tissue and within blood vessel walls, +plasma cells, ± Russell bodies (plasma cells packed with immunoglobulins), ± lymphohistiocytic infiltrate, +apple-green birefringence
Associated systemic disease usually no systemic involvement but rare cases do progress
Treatment pearls laser, excision

Sweet's syndrome

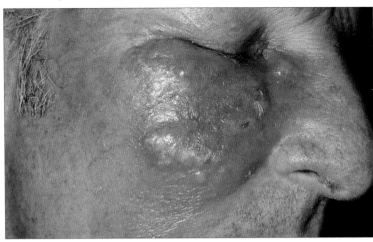

Description solitary to multiple edematous erythematous, violaceous papules and plaques with pustules or vesicles

Location dorsal hands common, can occur anywhere

Characteristics female>male, adults, can occur after a respiratory or GI infection with fever, arthritis, headache, abdominal pain, conjunctivitis and malaise; can occur after drug (GM-CSF, all-trans retinoic acid, bactrim, minocycline, hydralazine, furosemide [frusemide]), resolves in weeks to months but some have recurrences

Tests leukocytosis, elevated ESR; Histopathology: papillary dermal edema, sheets of neutrophils in the dermis

Associated systemic disease Crohn's, ulcerative colitis, myeloproliferative disorders (AML, CML, lymphoma), autoimmune diseases, pregnancy, infection

Treatment pearls dapsone, oral corticosteroids, potassium iodide

Alopecia mucinosa

Papular mucinosis (lichen myxedematosus)

Cutaneous T-cell lymphoma (CTCL)

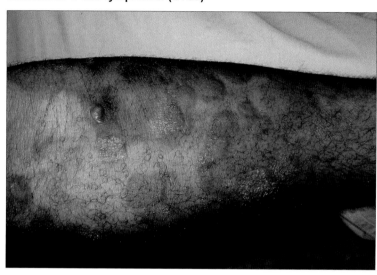

Pseudolymphoma

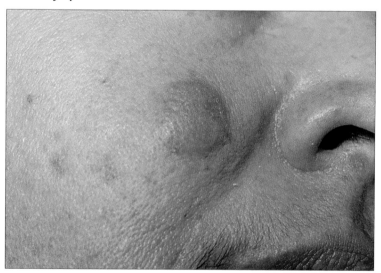

Lymphocytoma cutis (Spiegler–Fendt sarcoid)

Fungal infection
Tinea (dermatophytosis)
Deep fungal infection

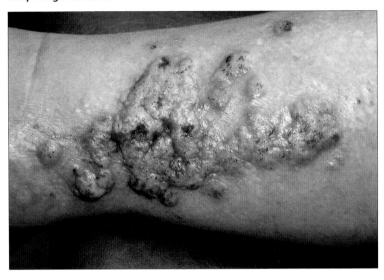

Atypical mycobacteria infection
Leprosy
Tuberculosis
Mycobacterium marinum

Bacterial infection
Cellulitis
Erysipelas
Furuncle

Other infection
Secondary syphilis
Leishmaniasis

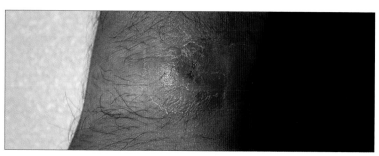

Sarcoid

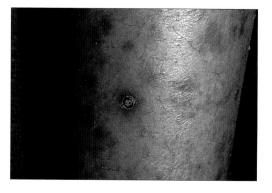

Subcutaneous fat necrosis of the newborn

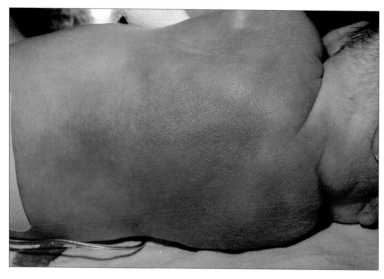

Discoid lupus erythematosus (DLE)

Systemic lupus erythematosus (SLE)

Rheumatoid arthritis

Dermatomyositis

Wegener's granulomatosis

Erythema multiforme

Lymphocytic infiltrate of Jessner

Polymorphous light eruption (PMLE)

Erythema elevatum diutinum (EED)

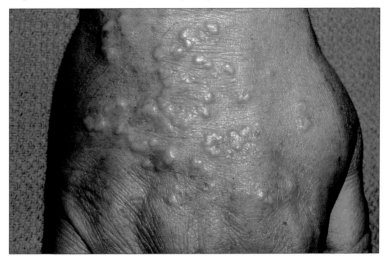

Granuloma faciale

Granuloma annulare

Morphea

Kaposi's sarcoma

Calciphylaxis

Panniculitis

Dermatofibrosarcoma protuberans (DFSP)

Metastatic nodule

Nodular fasciitis

Nephrogenic fibrosing dermopathy

PLAQUES – INDURATED (SKIN-COLORED)

Gout tophi
See page 182

Calcinosis cutis

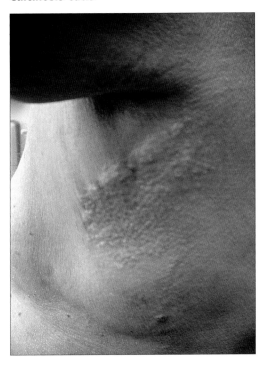

Description skin-colored, white or red, hard, round nodules ± ulceration
Location can occur anywhere
Characteristics chronic, asymptomatic vs. painful,
Tests ± hypercalcemia, hyperphosphatemia, increased PTH or vitamin D3;
Histopathology: calcification seen in dermis
Associated systemic disease malignancy, dermatomyositis,
CREST/scleroderma, renal disease, hyperparathyroidism, Albright's hereditary
osteodystrophy
Treatment pearls excision

Papular mucinosis (lichen myxedematosus)

Colloid milium

Silica, zirconium

Alopecia mucinosa

Lipoid proteinosis

Sarcoid

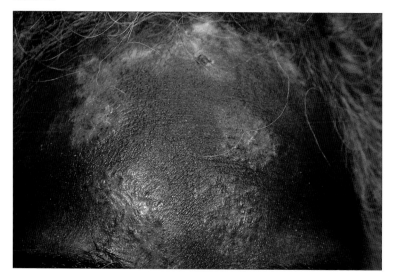

Nephrogenic fibrosing dermopathy

Morphea

Deep granuloma annulare

PLAQUES – INDURATED (YELLOW/BROWN)

Necrobiosis lipoidica diabeticorum

Mastocytosis (urticaria pigmentosa, multiple)

Mastocytoma (solitary)

Histiocytosis X

Sarcoid

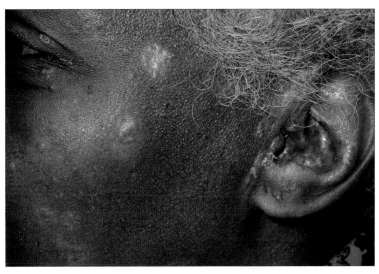

Pseudoxanthoma elasticum (PXE)

Colloid milium

Lipoid proteinosis

PLAQUES – PAPULOSQUAMOUS

Psoriasis
See page 397

Lichen planus
See page 259

Cutaneous T-cell lymphoma (CTCL)
See page 402

Lichen simplex chronicus
See page 201

Parapsoriasis
See page 409

PLAQUES – RED ON FACE

Contact dermatitis

Rosacea

Seborrheic dermatitis

Systemic lupus erythematosus (SLE)

Discoid lupus erythematosus (DLE)

Sarcoid

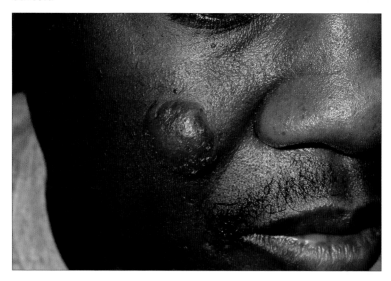

Fixed drug reaction

Polymorphous light eruption (PMLE)

Granuloma faciale

Cellulitis/erysipelas

Lupus vulgaris

Leprosy

Relapsing polychondritis

Microcystic adnexal carcinoma

Angiosarcoma

Sweet's syndrome

PLAQUES – THIN RED/BROWN

Psoriasis
See page 397

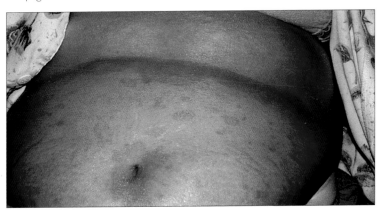

Hypertrophic actinic keratosis
See page 501

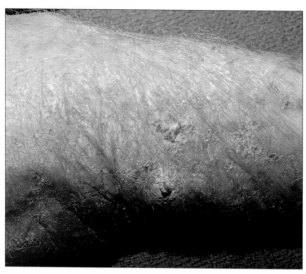

Verruca vulgaris
See page 60

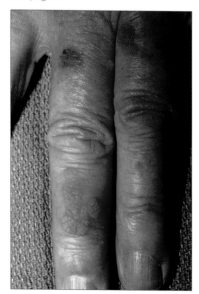

Lichen simplex chronicus
See page 201

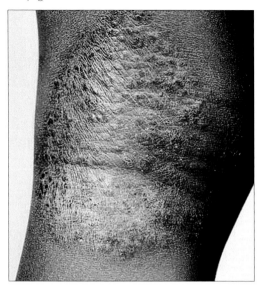

Cutaneous T-cell lymphoma
See page 402

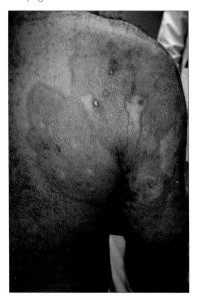

Morpheaform BCC
See page 366

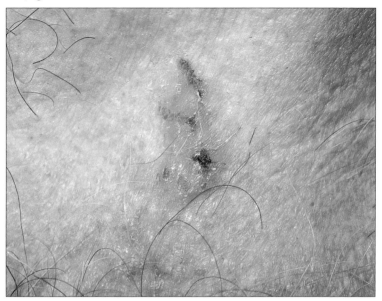

Contact dermatitis
See page 189

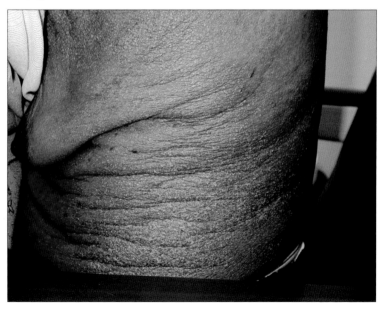

Nummular eczema
See page 498

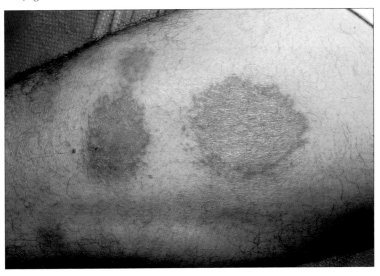

Bowen's disease
See page 499

Sarcoid
See page 443

Tinea corporis (dermatophytosis)
See page 86

Pityriasis rosea
See page 400

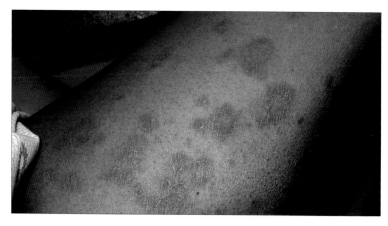

Pityriasis lichenoides chronica (PLC)
See page 411

Granuloma faciale
See page 213

POIKILODERMA

Poikiloderma of Civatte

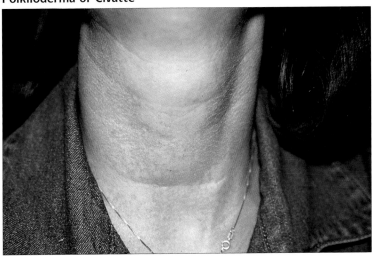

Description hyper- and hypopigmented, mottled atrophic macules
± telangiectasias
Location sun-exposed areas on neck and anterior chest most commonly
Characteristics light skin, older adults, chronic, asymptomatic, worsens with
further sun exposure
Tests Histopathology: dermal atrophy, telangiectasias, irregular pigmentation of
basal layer
Associated systemic disease none
Treatment pearls no treatment necessary, laser

Radiation dermatitis
See page 102

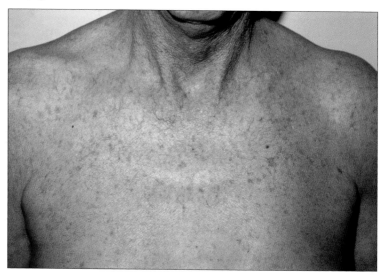

Systemic lupus erythematosus (SLE)
See page 425

Dermatomyositis
See page 427

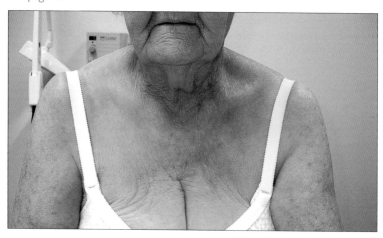

Cutaneous T-cell lymphoma (CTCL)
See page 402

Graft-versus-host disease
See page 290

Corticosteroid overuse

Arsenic toxicity

Parapsoriasis

Hodgkin's lymphoma

Polycyclic hydrocarbon toxicity

Syndromes
Xeroderma pigmentosum
Rothmund–Thompson syndrome
Bloom's syndrome
Dyskeratosis congenita
Goltz syndrome
Cockayne syndrome
Kindler–Weary syndrome (hereditary acrokeratotic poikiloderma)

PREGNANCY – CHANGES

Melasma
See page 208

Cherry angioma
See page 371

Striae

See page 103

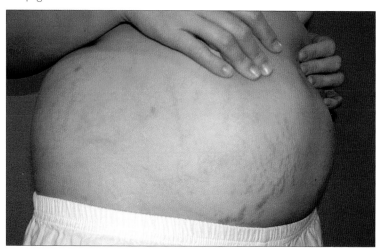

Melanosis (linea nigra, genital, areolae)

Palmar erythema

Edema (face and extremities)

Telogen effluvium

Gingivitis

Hypertrichosis

Erythema multiforme

Urticaria

PRURIGO OF PREGNANCY
Pruritic urticarial papules and plaques of pregnancy (PUPPP)

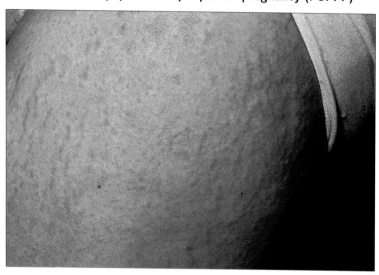

Description erythematous, urticarial patches and plaques
Location starts within striae with periumbilical sparing and spreads diffusely
Characteristics most common in first pregnancy, occurs in third trimester or immediately postpartum and resolves in the early postpartum period; does not recur with subsequent pregnancies, intensely pruritic, more common if excessive weight gain during pregnancy
Tests Histopathology: spongiosis, parakeratosis, with a lymphocytic infiltrate with few eosinophils; DIF is negative
Associated systemic disease none
Treatment pearls topical and oral corticosteroids, antihistamines

Prurigo gravidarum (cholestasis of pregnancy)
Description excoriations common but no primary lesion, patient may appear jaundiced
Location pruritus diffuse without primary skin lesion especially trunk, palms and soles
Characteristics uncommon in women with darker skin, occurs in third trimester often with a UTI, resolves within 1–2 days after delivery, may recur in future pregnancies >60% and with OCP use, intense pruritus, may be associated with meconium and fetal stress and vitamin K malabsorption leading to bleeding abnormalities
Tests abnormal LFTs including direct bilirubin and AST
Associated systemic disease cholestasis
Treatment pearls oral corticosteroids, cholestyramine, phenobarbital, light therapy, low fat diet, ursodeoxycholic acid, oral guar gum

Prurigo of pregnancy

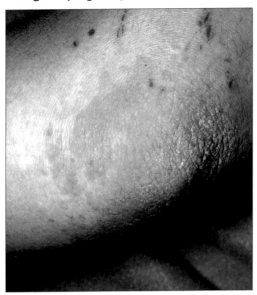

Description erythematous papules and pustules, some follicular, most excoriated
Location can occur anywhere but extensor surfaces and trunk common
Characteristics occurs in second trimester, resolves postpartum, may recur with future pregnancies
Tests LFTs are normal; Histopathology: non-specific inflammatory response ± follicular, DIF is negative
Associated systemic disease none
Treatment pearls topical corticosteroids, light therapy

Impetigo herpetiformis (pustular psoriasis in pregnancy)
Description erythematous patches and plaques with overlying pustules
Location intertriginous areas, neck, palms and soles common, but can occur anywhere
Characteristics occurs during pregnancy, may resolve after pregnancy but can be chronic and will recur with future pregnancies; may be exacerbated by hypocalcemia, associated with fever, associated with fetal death
Tests check for leukocytosis and hypocalcemia; Histopathology: neutrophilic abscesses within stratum corneum and epidermis, psoriasiform hyperplasia, perivascular lymphocytic infiltrate
Associated systemic disease none
Treatment pearls oral and topical corticosteroids

Gestational pemphigoid/herpes gestationis

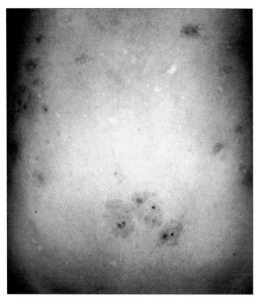

Description erythematous papules and vesicles some urticarial, some annular or polycyclic

Location starts near umbilicus and spreads diffusely including palms and soles but sparing face

Characteristics occurs in second or third trimester or early postpartum period, may flare near delivery, resolves in weeks to months after birth; recurs with subsequent pregnancies, OCPs, or menstruation; can rarely affect the newborn, intensely pruritic, can be associated with prematurity and low birth weight

Tests Histopathology: subepidermal bulla with eosinophilic infiltrate; DIF: C3 along the DEJ

Associated systemic disease none

Treatment pearls oral and topical corticosteroids, dapsone, cyclosporine

PRURITUS ANI

Candidiasis
See page 145

Intertrigo
See page 145

Atopic dermatitis
See page 141

Contact dermatitis
See page 189

Lichen simplex chronicus
See page 201

Seborrheic dermatitis
See page 398

Fungal infection

Pinworms

Scabies

Condyloma accuminata

Gonococcal proctitis

Hemorrhoids, anal fissures, cryptitis, abscess, fistulas

Carcinoma

Extramammary Paget's disease

Idiopathic

Psychogenic

Oral antibiotics (direct irritation, altered bowel flora)

Frequent bowel movements

Excessive moisture

Poor hygiene

PRURITUS – GENERALIZED

Xerosis

Diabetes mellitus

Hepatic/biliary disease

Iron deficiency

Urticaria

Drugs
Opiates
Estrogens

Omeprazole
Erythromycin

Psychogenic

Renal disease/uremia

Underlying malignancy (especially lymphoma/leukemia)

Hyperthyroidism/hypothyroidism

Polycythemia vera

Dermatitis herpetiformis

Hookworm

Onchocerciasis

PSORIATIC ARTHRITIS

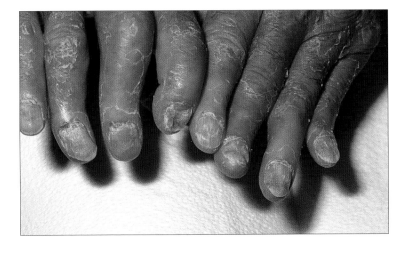

Mono- and asymmetrical oligoarthritis

Arthritis of the distal interphalangeal joints

Rheumatoid arthritis-like presentation

Arthritis mutilans

Spondylitis and sacroiliitis

Raynaud's phenomenon

PURPLE DIGITS
Raynaud's phenomenon

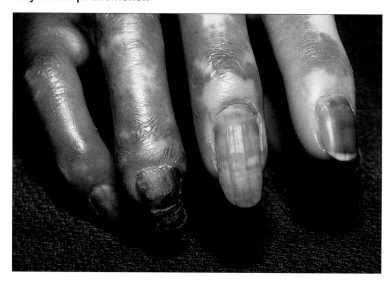

Description symmetrical white to purple poorly demarcated patches
Location distal digits
Characteristics 4:1 female>male, 15–40 years, painful, exacerbated by cold temperature
Tests often resolves with warming
Associated systemic disease can be primary idiopathic or secondary to connective tissue diseases especially scleroderma and others (*see box*)
Treatment pearls calcium channel blockers, alpha-blockers, avoid smoking, avoid cold exposure, I.V. prostaglandin E_1 for refractory cases

CAUSES OF SECONDARY RAYNAUD'S PHENOMENON

- Connective tissue disease (scleroderma, MCTD, SLE, dermatomyositis, Sjögren's syndrome, eosinophilic fasciitis)
- Trauma (vibration, typing, pressure)
- Trauma (surgical)
- Cryoglobulinemia
- Paroxysmal hemoglobinuria
- Drugs (beta-adrenergic blockers, ergotamines, OCPs, bleomycin, vincristine, methysergide, clonidine, cyclosporine, bromocriptine, amphetamines, vinyl chloride)
- Obstructive arterial disease (atherosclerosis, thromboangiitis obliterans, thoracic outlet syndrome)
- Hypothyroidism
- Hyperviscosity (cryoproteins, cold agglutinins, polycythemia, macroglobulins, thrombocytosis)
- Neurological (carpal tunnel syndrome, polio, multiple sclerosis, hemiplegia)
- Paraproteinemia

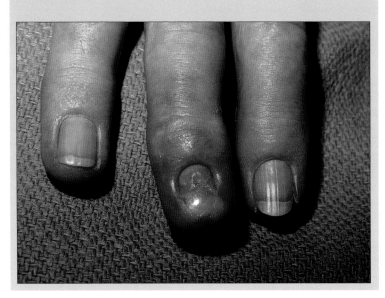

Mixed connective tissue disease

Livedo reticularis
See page 430

Cold digits/frostbite

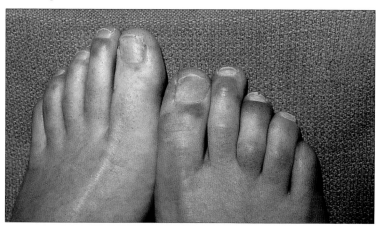

Chilblains/pernio

Acrocyanosis

Erythema multiforme

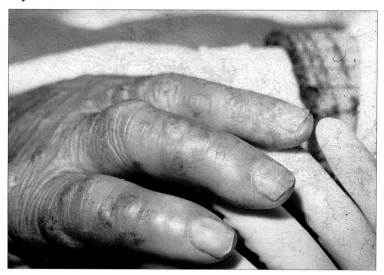

Bywater's lesions (rheumatoid arthritis)

PURPURA – FLAT (MACULES AND PATCHES, NON-INFLAMMATORY)

Trauma

Bites

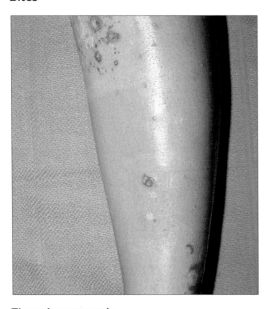

Thrombocytopenia
Idiopathic thrombocytopenic purpura (ITP)
Thrombotic thrombocytopenic purpura (TTP)
Bone marrow suppression secondary to chemotherapy
Lymphoma
Leukemia
Drugs (aspirin, NSAIDs)
Varicella
Streptococcus
Purpura fulminans secondary to infection
Rickettsial infections
Viral infections (measles)
Splenomegaly
Hereditary thrombocytopenia
Systemic lupus erythematosus (SLE)

Stasis dermatitis

Senile/actinic/solar pupura

Coagulation disorder

Corticosteroid related

Coumadin necrosis

Hemolytic–uremic syndrome

Post-transfusion

Drugs – anaphylactoid purpura
Cephalosporins
Allopurinol
Aspirin
NSAIDs
Penicillin
Phenytoin
Quinidine
Sulfonamides
Thiazides
Gold
Hydralazine
Coumadin
Cocaine

Cryoglobulinemia

Wegener's granulomatosis

Churg–Strauss syndrome

Pigmented purpuric eruption (Schamberg's, Majocchi's, lichen aureus, Gougerot and Blum)

Finkelstein's disease (hemorrhagic edema of infancy)

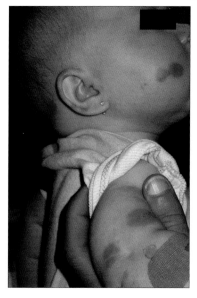

Disseminated intravascular coagulation (DIC)

Pupura fulminans (varicella, meningococcal meningitis, scarlet fever)

Parvovirus B19 (erythrovirus) (purpuric gloves and socks syndrome)

Diabetes mellitus

Waldenström's macroglobulinemia

Dysproteinemia

Scurvy (perifollicular purpura and petechiae)

Amyloidosis ('pinch purpura')

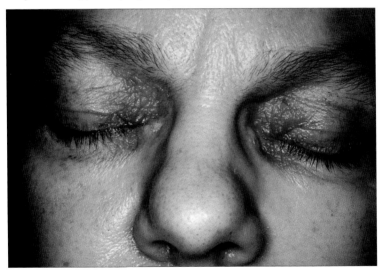

Polycythemia vera

Von Willebrand's disease

Hypercortisolism

Gardner–Diamond syndrome (autoerythrocyte sensitization)

PURPURA – FOLLICULAR

Scurvy/vitamin C deficiency

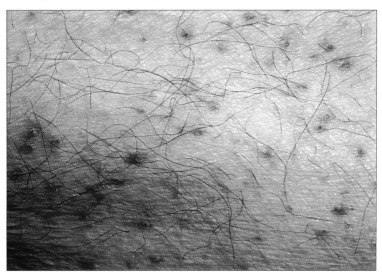

Cryoglobulinemia

Thrombocytopenia

PURPURA – PALPABLE: PAPULES AND PLAQUES (INFLAMMATORY)

Erythema multiforme
See page 484

Drug reaction

THE MOST COMMON DRUGS TO CAUSE A PURPURIC DRUG REACTION	
• Aspirin	• Phenothiazines
• Indomethacin	• Quinidine
• Sulfa drugs	• Iodide
• Thiazides	• Chloroquine
• Penicillin	• Phenylbutazone

Leukocytoclastic vasculitis

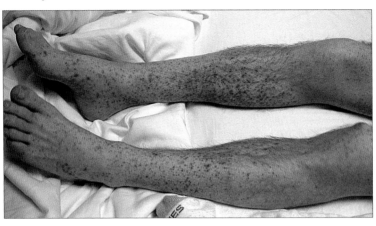

Description brown/red patches, papules and nodules (palpable purpura), may progress to hemorrhagic bulla or ulcerations, may also resemble urticarial plaques
Location lower legs
Characteristics females>males, children and adults, may resolve spontaneously vs. waxes and wanes chronically, asymptomatic vs. pruritic, ± fever, malaise, edema, arthralgias, may affect internal organ systems such as renal, GI or neurologic
Tests Histopathology: fibrinoid necrosis of small vessels with associated leukocytoclasis
Associated systemic disease can be associated with infections, drugs, malignancy or connective tissue diseases (*see box* p. 480)
Treatment pearls treat underlying disease, NSAIDs, antihistamines, dapsone, colchicine, oral corticosteroids, discontinue offending drug

Erythema nodosum
See page 252

Sweet's syndrome (acute febrile neutrophilic dermatosis)

Pityriasis lichenoides et varioliformis acuta (PLEVA)

Cholesterol emboli

CAUSES OF LEUKOCYTOCLASTIC VASCULITIS (LCV) AND LCV WORKUP

Drug reaction
Aspirin, NSAIDs, penicillin, phenothiazines, phenytoin, sulfonamides, sulfonylureas, iodides, radiocontrast dye, allopurinol, phenacetin, food dyes, OCPs, insulin, tamoxifen, quinidine, indomethacin

Connective tissue disease
Systemic lupus erythematosus, rheumatoid arthritis, Sjögren's syndrome, mixed connective tissue disease, polyarteritis nodosa, dermatomyositis

Allergic vasculitis
Henoch–Schönlein purpura, hypersensitivity vasculitis, urticarial vasculitis, Churg–Strauss syndrome

Cutaneous diseases
Erythema multiforme, erythema elevatum diutinum, PLEVA, Behçet's syndrome, Finkelstein's acute hemorrhagic edema of infancy

Bacterial and atypical mycobacterial infections
Streptococcus, *Neisseria meningitidis*, Staphylococcus, meningococcemia, gonococcemia, tuberculosis, leprosy

Viral infections
Hepatitis B, hepatitis C, influenza, EBV, CMV, HIV, Coxsackie, echovirus

Rickettsial infections
Rocky Mountain spotted fever

Fungal infections

Spirochete infections (syphilis)

Other infections

Inflammatory bowel disease
Crohn's disease, ulcerative colitis

Proteins
Serum sickness, hyposensitization, cryoglobulinemia, dysproteinemia

Malignancy
Hodgkin's lymphoma, myeloma, leukemia, lymphoma, other carcinomas including lung and colon

Chemical exposures
Insecticides, petroleum products

LCV workup
- History – medications, recent infections, family history, past medical diseases
- Labs – throat culture, hepatitis panel, cryoglobulins, ANA, urinalysis, complement levels, ESR
- Procedures – skin biopsy, CXR

PURPURA – RETICULATED

Heparin necrosis

Description purpuric patch with retiform/lacy border ± necrotic center
Location can occur at injection site or distant sites (even in CNS)
Characteristics occurs in patients on heparin usually within 5–10 days (sooner if previously sensitized, or can be delayed for up to 3 weeks), resolves with cessation of heparin; painful; platelet aggregation caused by antibodies leads to thrombosis
Tests check PTT, bleeding time, platelet count (can be decreased or normal); Histopathology: non-inflammatory platelet thrombi ('white clots') within vessels
Associated systemic disease none
Treatment pearls stop heparin

Atrophie blanche/livedo vasculopathy

See page 439

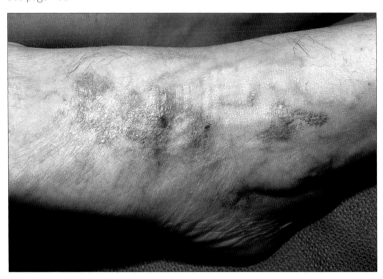

Degos' disease (malignant atrophic papulosis)

See page 438

Coumadin necrosis/protein C dysfunction

See page 486

Cutaneous calciphylaxis

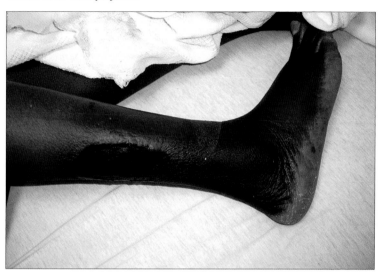

Description reticulated purpura which progresses to indurated hard, well-demarcated black retiform to solid patch ± necrosis and ulceration, ± bulla
Location lower extremities most common, but can occur anywhere
Characteristics female>male, adults, chronic course which may be fatal, very painful
Tests Histopathology: calcium within the walls of vessels
Associated systemic disease end stage renal disease (ESRD), diabetes, obesity
Treatment pearls supportive treatment, ± parathyroidectomy, low calcium dialysis solution, hyperbaric oxygen, oral corticosteroids

Myeloproliferative disease with thrombocytosis

Thrombotic thrombocytopenic pupura

Sickle cell disease

Anemia – hemolytic

Paroxysmal nocturnal hemoglobinemia

Cryoglobulinemia, cold agglutinins

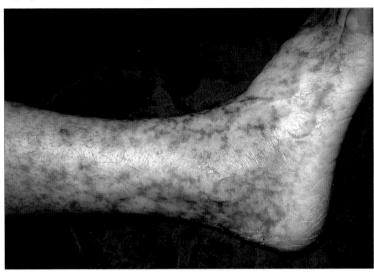

Paraproteinemia

Protein C or S deficiency

Lupus anticoagulant

Antiphospholipid antibody

Ecthyma gangrenosum (Pseudomonas)

Fungal – aspergillosis, mucormycosis

Disseminated strongyloidosis

Leprosy (Lucio phenomenon)

Cholesterol emboli

Septic emboli

Hypereosinophilic syndrome

Purpura fulminans secondary to infection

Sneddon syndrome

PURPURA – TARGETOID LESIONS
Erythema multiforme

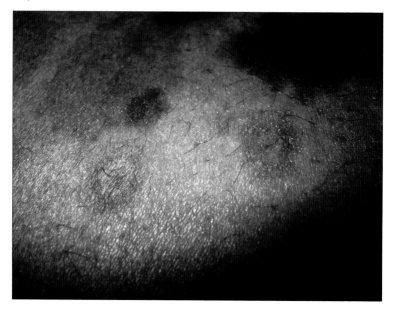

Description targetoid erythematous and/or purpuric macules and papules with central duskiness that may progress to bulla and erosions

Location dorsal hands, palms and soles, diffusely over body, only one mucous membrane involved – usually mild oral or genital erosions in over 50%.

Characteristics slight male>female, young adults (uncommon in children), usually self-limited and resolves in several weeks, +recurrences, abrupt onset of painful lesions typically without prodrome or fever

Tests Histopathology: normal epidermis with necrotic keratinocytes, perivascular infiltrate and spongiosis

Associated systemic disease HSV, orf, histoplasmosis, EBV

Treatment pearls antihistamines, local wound care, suppressive/chronic oral antivirals; avoid corticosteroids

CAUSES OF ERYTHEMA MULTIFORME

- Infectious:
  - a) Viral – herpes simplex (two-thirds of cases due to HSV), adenovirus, cat-scratch, Coxsackie, echovirus, hepatitis, EBV, influenza A, paravaccinia, psittacosis, ornithosis, orf, polio, vaccinia, variola
  - b) Bacterial – Mycoplasma pneumonia, BCG vaccine, diphtheria, gonorrhea, *Streptococcus hemolyticus*, leprosy, Pseudomonas, *Salmonella typhi*, Staphylococcus, syphilis, tuberculosis, tularemia, *Vibrio parahemolyticus*, Yersinia
  - c) Other – Trichomonas, fungus (coccidioidomycosis, dermatophytosis, histoplasmosis)
- Physical – cold, x-ray
- Endocrine – menses, pregnancy
- Drugs – allopurinol, antibiotics (esp. penicillin and sulfa), anticonvulsants (esp. phenytoin), antipyretics, analgesics, aspirin, corticosteroids, gold, hydralazine, mercury, nickel, NSAIDs, phenolphthalein, phenylbutazone, sulfonamides, sulfonylureas, tetracycline
- Neoplasia – internal malignancy, leukemia, lymphoma, multiple myeloma, myeloid metaplasia, polycythemia
- Connective tissue diseases – dermatomyositis, systemic lupus erythematosus, polyarteritis nodosa, rheumatoid arthritis, Wegener's granulomatosis
- Contact – fine sponge, poison ivy and oak, primula allergens
- Miscellaneous – beer drinkers, tooth extraction, food (margarine emulsifiers), Reiter's syndrome

Stevens–Johnson syndrome (SJS, erythema multiforme major)
See page 64

Pyoderma gangrenosum
See page 487

Sweet's syndrome
See page 447

Secondary syphilis
See page 401

Cryoglobulinemia

Rheumatoid vasculitis

Livedo vasculitis

Polyarteritis nodosa (PAN)

Wegener's granulomatosis

Churg–Strauss syndrome

PURPURIC PLAQUES AND ULCERS

Coumadin necrosis

Description well-demarcated erythematous patch that progresses to a hemorrhagic/necrotic area ± retiform purpura within the patch
Location fatty areas (breast, buttocks, upper legs)
Characteristics female>male, elderly, occurs within 2–5 days of starting coumadin without heparin, painful
Tests Histopathology: thrombus within dermal vessels with minimal surrounding inflammation
Associated systemic disease inherited protein C deficiency
Treatment pearls protein C concentrates

Factitial

Description erythematous/violaceous patch
Location in areas easily reached by the hands
Characteristics female>male, child/adolescent>adult, may resolve or wax and wane chronically
Tests Histopathology: traumatized epidermis with hemorrhage in dermis
Associated systemic disease may be associated with depression
Treatment pearls wound care, antidepressants, antianxiolytics

Vasculitis ulcer

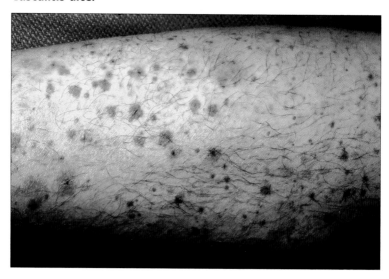

Description violaceous macules, papules and plaques (palpable purpura) that may progress to bulla and finally ulcers
Location lower legs most common but may progress to other areas including trunk and arms
Characteristics ± pain, may be associated with joint pain, fever and malaise
Tests Histopathology: inflammation of blood vessel walls with fibrinoid necrosis and leukocytoclasis (nuclear dust), + cultures to rule out infectious cause

Associated systemic disease may be associated with infections, drugs, malignancy or connective tissue diseases
Treatment pearls rest, elevation, colchicine, dapsone, oral corticosteroids; treat underlying condition, discontinue offending drug

Pyoderma gangrenosum

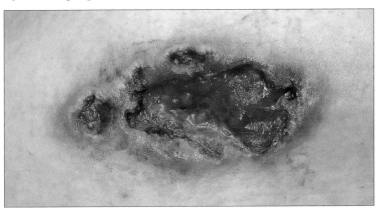

Description erythematous papule or pustule that quickly progresses to an ulcerated lesion with a necrotic base and a gray, undermined border
Location lower extremities most common, may also affect mucosa
Characteristics female>male, 20–50 years, worsens with trauma (pathergy), extremely painful, chronic and recurs, may occur with fever
Tests Histopathology: ulceration with necrosis and a surrounding neutrophilic inflammation
Associated systemic disease inflammatory bowel disease, arthritis, lymphoproliferative diseases
Treatment pearls high-dose oral corticosteroids, cyclosporine, treatment of underlying disease; avoid debridement

DISEASES ASSOCIATED WITH PYODERMA GANGRENOSUM

- Ulcerative colitis
- Crohn's disease
- Rheumatoid arthritis
- Spondylitis
- Osteoarthritis
- Congenital IgA deficiency
- Hypoglobulinemia/dysglobulinemia/dysproteinemia
- IgG, IgM or IgA gammopathy
- Myeloid leukemia
- Smoldering leukemia
- Multiple myeloma
- Hodgkin's lymphoma
- Hairy cell leukemia
- Myelofibrosis
- Polycythemia vera
- Solid tumors
- Takayasu's disease (Japan)
- Diabetes mellitus
- Hidradenitis suppurativa
- Diverticulitis
- Chronic active hepatitis
- Primary biliary cirrhosis
- Gastric and duodenal ulcers
- Wegener's granulomatosis
- Systemic lupus erythematosus (SLE)
- Sarcoid
- Necrotizing vasculitis
- Behçet's syndrome
- Lung abscess

Primary amyloidosis

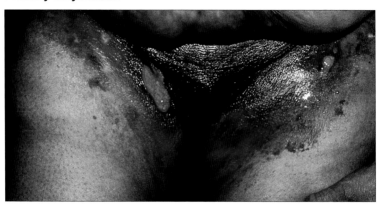

Description petechiae, 'pinch purpura', hemorrhagic bulla, waxy subcutaneous nodules, or blue/red papule or plaque

Location face (periorbital), can occur anywhere including mucosa

Characteristics adults, chronic and progressive, ± macroglossia, ± carpal tunnel syndrome

Tests SPEP or UPEP for paraproteinemia; +Bence-Jones protein in urine (λ light chains); bone marrow biopsy; Histopathology: amorphous pink material (AL amyloid) in dermis and within blood vessel walls, sparse to no inflammation, ± bulla, +plasma cells, +apple-green birefringence

Associated systemic disease paraproteinemia, amyloid deposits systemically which affect internal organs, up to 15% of cases are associated with multiple myeloma

Treatment pearls chemotherapy, oral corticosteroids

Infusion accident (extravasation of I.V. medications)

Pressure necrosis

Frostbite

Spider bite

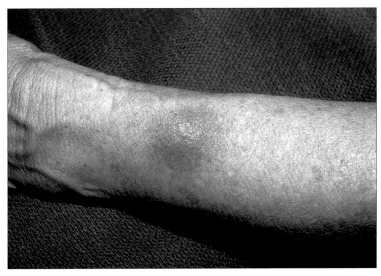

Dysglobulinemia

Malignancy

Sickle cell anemia

Trophic ulcers

Infection

PUSTULES

Acne
See page 39, Acne vulgaris

Insect bites
See page 120

Miliaria rubra
See page 337

Bacterial infection
Folliculitis
See page 333
Carbuncle/furuncle
Impetigo
Cellulitis (deep dermis and subcutaneous tissue)

Erysipelas (superficial dermis)
Staphylococcal scalded skin syndrome
Erysipeloid
Meningococcemia
Gonococcemia

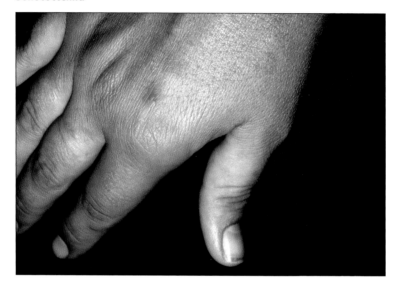

Anthrax
Ecthyma

Scabies
See page 52

Atypical mycobacterial infection

Fungal infection
Candidiasis
See page 145
Tinea corporis (dermatophytosis)
See page 86

Viral infection
Herpes simplex virus (HSV)
Varicella zoster virus (VZV)
Variola
Cowpox
Vaccinia

Pustular psoriasis
See page 58

Contact dermatitis
See page 189

Impetigo herpetiformis
See page 468

Pyoderma gangrenosum
See page 487

Drugs
Steroid acne
Lithium
Bromide
Iodide
Mercury

Eosinophilic folliculitis
See page 333

Sweet's syndrome
See page 447

Subcorneal pustular dermatosis

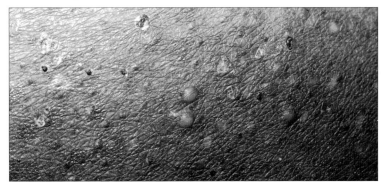

Swimmer's itch

Acrodermatitis enteropathica

Incontinentia pigmenti

Erythema toxicum neonatorum

Transient neonatal pustular melanosis

Acropustulosis of infancy

Hidradenitis suppurativa

PUSTULES – ACRAL

See page 57, Acral pustules

PUSTULES – NEWBORN

Acne neonatorum
Description tiny pustules and erythematous papules
Location face most common (especially cheeks)
Characteristics onset at 1–3 weeks old, resolves in weeks to months
Tests KOH may reveal Malassezia yeast forms
Associated systemic disease none
Treatment pearls no treatment necessary, topical tacrolimus if severe, ketoconazole cream

Erythema toxicum neonatorum
Description erythematous macules, tiny pustules, vesicles and papules
Location starts on face and progresses to trunk, buttocks and proximal extremities sparing palms and soles
Characteristics onset 24–48 h after delivery, resolves in days, exacerbated by rubbing
Tests scraping of a pustule reveals numerous eosinophils by Wright stain, rare peripheral eosinophilia; Histopathology: perifollicular subcorneal eosinophilic pustules with eosinophils perivascular as well
Associated systemic disease none
Treatment pearls no treatment necessary

Transient neonatal pustular melanosis
Description pustules with no surrounding erythema rupture leaving a collarette of scale and hyperpigmentation (if pustular phase occurs in utero, infant may only have hyperpigmented macules)
Location diffuse over body including palms and soles
Characteristics dark skin>light skin, pustules present at birth, resolves spontaneously over weeks to months with hyperpigmentation
Tests pustules are sterile; Histopathology: spongiosis, subcorneal neutrophilic pustules
Associated systemic disease none
Treatment pearls no treatment necessary

Miliaria rubra
See page 337

Bacterial infection (Staph or Strep)
Description tiny pustules, vesicles and erythematous macules
Location predominately in diaper area, can occur near umbilicus or elsewhere
Characteristics male>female, presents in first few weeks of life, resolves with treatment
Tests Gram stain reveals Gram+ cocci, bacterial culture
Associated systemic disease none
Treatment pearls topical or oral antibiotics

Candidiasis
See page 145

Herpes simplex infection
See page 116

Acropustulosis of infancy

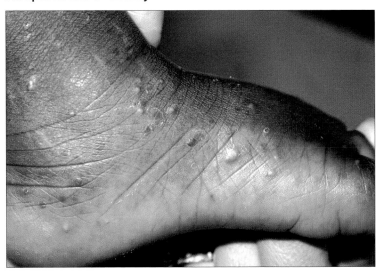

Description pustules and vesicles on an erythematous base that rupture and leave hyperpigmentation
Location palms and soles extending onto hands and feet to the wrists and ankles, ± scalp and trunk involvement
Characteristics male>female, dark skin>light skin, onset usually at 3–6 months but can occur earlier, recurs in crops every few weeks, improves with age and resolves by age 3, pruritic
Tests Histopathology: sterile pustule with neutrophils and eosinophils
Associated systemic disease none
Treatment pearls topical corticosteroids, antihistamines, dapsone if severe

Scabies
See page 407 – infant wrist with pustule

Nevus comedonicus

Pustular psoriasis

Eosinophilic pustular folliculitis of infancy (neonatal eosinophilic pustular folliculitis)

RETICULATED PAPULES

See page 331, Papillomatosis – reticulated

RETICULATED PIGMENTATION

See page 430, Pigmentation – reticulated

RETICULATED PURPURA

See page 481, Purpura – reticulated

SCALP LESIONS

Nevus sebaceus

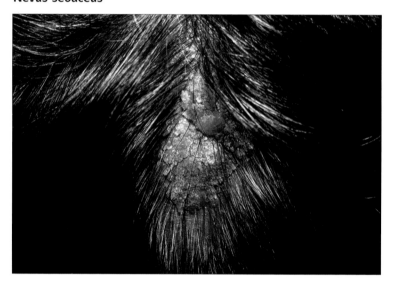

Description large yellow/orange/brown verrucous papule/plaque
Location scalp or face most common
Characteristics solitary, may be linear, present at birth but becomes more verrucous at puberty; BCC, syringocystadenoma papilliferum, or other epithelial neoplasms may develop within 10–30% of nevus sebaceus
Tests Histopathology: papillomatosis, hyperkeratosis, thickened dermis, sebaceous and apocrine glands present
Associated systemic disease none
Treatment pearls excise prior to puberty, rarely associated with internal abnormalities: CNS, renal, skeletal, ocular

Pilar cyst

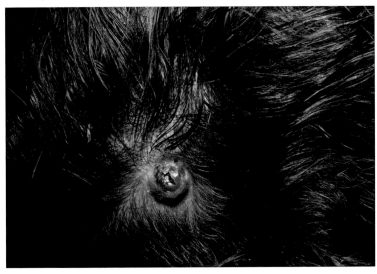

Lipoma

Folliculitis

Furuncle

Kerion

Dermatofibroma

Verruca vulgaris

Mastocytoma

Cylindroma

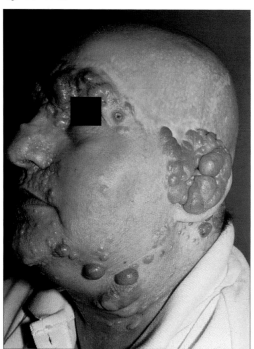

Spiradenoma
See page 362

Malignancy
Squamous cell carcinoma
Basal cell carcinoma
Melanoma
Keratoacanthoma
Malignant fibrous histiocytoma
Merkel cell carcinoma
Metastatic disease

Prurigo nodules

Angiosarcoma

Hemangioma

Nevus

SCALP – SCALY

Seborrheic dermatitis

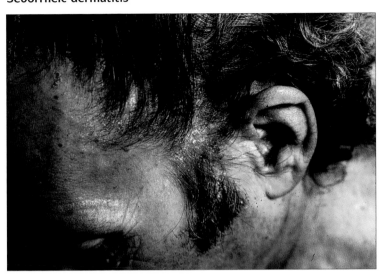

Psoriasis

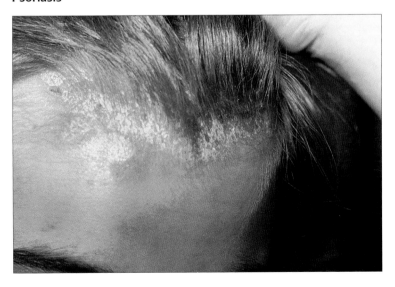

Tinea capitis
See page 74

Contact dermatitis

Atopic dermatitis

Pityriasis rubra pilaris

Pemphigus foliaceous

Sézary syndrome

SCALY RED PATCH (INCLUDING NUMMULAR PATCHES)

Nummular eczema

Description usually 1–3 cm, well-demarcated nummular (coin-shaped) erythematous, scaly patches and plaques but can be annular especially if partially treated

Location can occur anywhere, but common on extremities

Characteristics men>women, any age but more common at later age, pruritic

Tests KOH–; Histopathology: spongiosis, perivascular lymphocytic infiltrate

Associated systemic disease none

Treatment pearls emollients, topical corticosteroids, topical tacrolimus or pimecrolimus, phototherapy

Bowen's disease

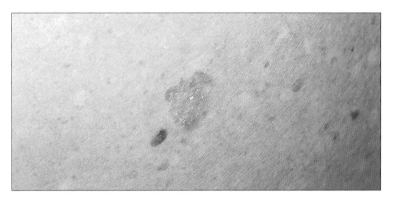

Description pink/erythematous well-demarcated scaly patch
Location can occur anywhere
Characteristics older adults, progressive, asymptomatic
Tests Histopathology: atypical keratinocytes involving the entire thickness of epidermis but not extending into dermis (squamous cell carcinoma in situ)
Associated systemic disease none
Treatment pearls electrodessication, excision, topical imiquimod, topical 5-FU

Xerotic eczema (eczema craquelé, asteatotic eczema)

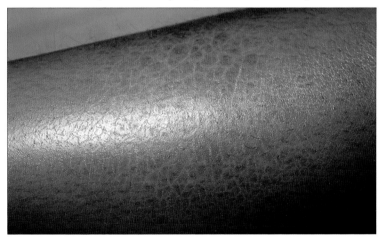

Description dry, erythematous, scaly patches confluent in some areas, ± linear 'dried river bed' appearance
Location lower legs, flanks and posterior axillary folds common, but can occur anywhere
Characteristics male>female, older adults most common, resolves with treatment, worse in winter or dry climate

Tests Histopathology: ± slight hyperkeratosis, mild perivascular infiltrate, mild spongiosis and parakeratosis

Associated systemic disease none

Treatment pearls emollients (especially humectants like lactic acid), decrease frequency of bathing, mild topical corticosteroids

Contact dermatitis

See page 189, Contact/irritant dermatitis

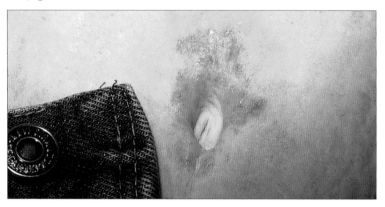

Seborrheic dermatitis

See page 398

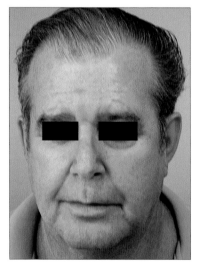

Actinic keratosis

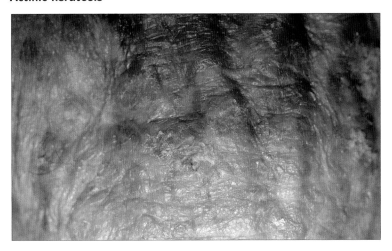

Description small, erythematous, scaly patch or plaque
Location sun-exposed areas
Characteristics older adults, small percentage may progress to squamous cell carcinoma if left untreated, asymptomatic
Tests Histopathology: atypical cells in basal layer of epithelium with overlying parakeratosis ± inflammatory infiltrate
Associated systemic disease none
Treatment pearls cryotherapy, topical 5-FU, topical imiquimod, topical retinoids, photodynamic therapy

Pityriasis rosea
See page 400

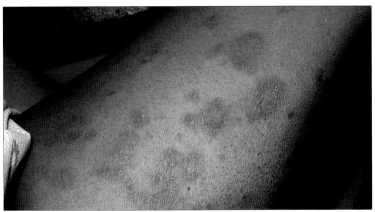

Tinea corporis (dermatophytosis)
See page 86

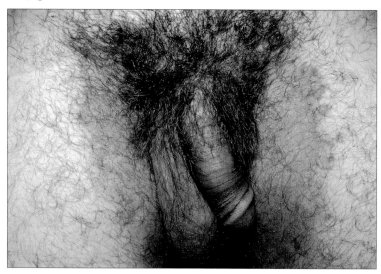

Cutaneous T-cell lymphoma (CTCL)
See page 402

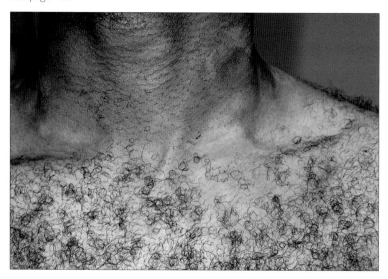

Superficial BCC
See page 366

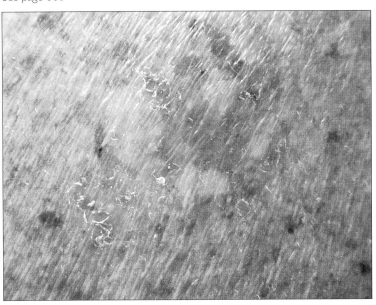

Lichen simplex chronicus
See page 201

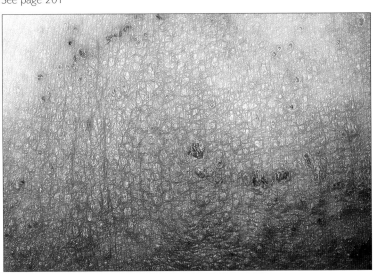

Atopic dermatitis
See page 141

Candidiasis
See page 145

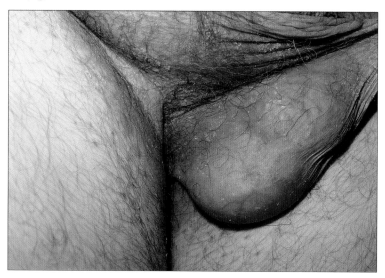

Psoriasis
See page 397

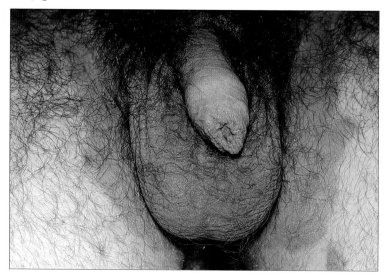

Systemic lupus erythematosus (SLE)
See page 425

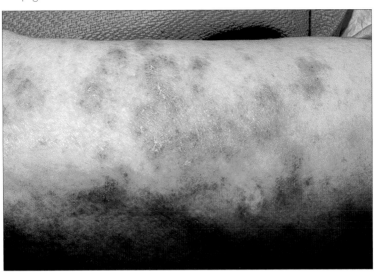

Dermatomyositis
See page 427

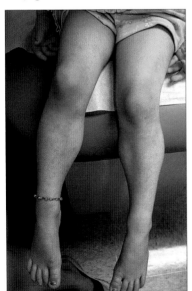

Pityriasis rubra pilaris
See page 159

Parapsoriasis
See page 409

Pityriasis lichenoides chronica (PLC)
See page 411

Secondary syphilis
See page 401

Drug reaction
See page 286

Poikiloderma vasculare atrophicans

Pigmented purpura of Doucas and Kapetanakis

Chronic mucocutaneous candidiasis

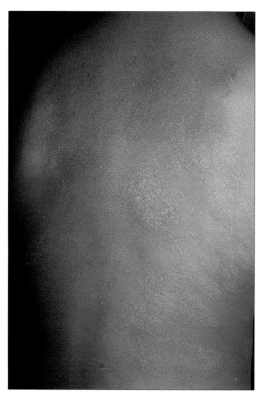

SCLERODERMOID CHANGES

Morphea
See page 99

CREST syndrome (Calcinosis cutis (CC), Raynaud's (R), esophageal dysmotility (E), Sclerodactyly (S), Telangiectasias (T)

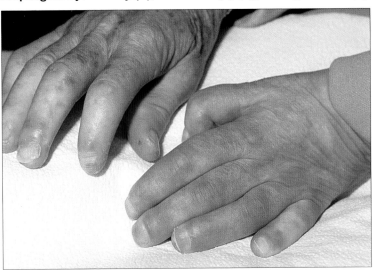

Description CC: white, firm papules and nodules; R: purple/white patches on digital tips; S: firm, tight, indurated skin on digital tips; T: telangiectatic mats
Location CC: most common on extremities near joints and distal, R and S: distal digits, T: face, lips, palms and trunk most common
Characteristics female>male, middle-age onset, chronic course
Tests ANA, anti-centromere antibodies
Associated systemic disease this is a systemic disease which can be associated with internal organ involvement
Treatment pearls supportive treatment

Scleroderma

Scleroderma (progressive systemic sclerosis)

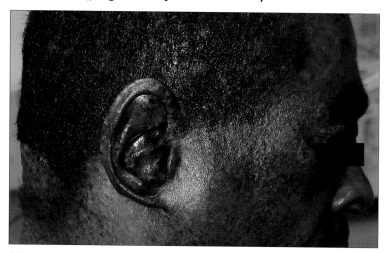

Salt and pepper mottled pigmentation

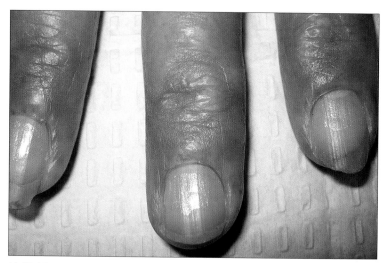

Nailfold telangiectasias

Description symmetric firm, tight, indurated, skin-colored to erythematous plaques; ± ulcerations on fingers; mottled hyper- and hypopigmented patches ('salt and pepper'); ± few telangiectatic mats, telangiectasias of proximal nail folds (90%)

Location most common in distal extremities and face but can progress to diffuse cutaneous involvement, hyperpigmented macules most common at waistline and upper trunk

Characteristics female>male, middle-age onset, chronic, usually shortens life span

Tests ANA, Scl-70 antibodies; Histopathology: normal epidermis, early lesions show perivascular infiltrate with plasma cells, thickened dermis with increased collagen and with blunt demarcation between dermis and thin subcutaneous fat, loss of adnexal structures

Associated systemic disease associated with Raynaud's phenomenon (90%) and internal organ involvement including pulmonary, kidney, heart and GI sclerosis (esophageal dysphagia)

Treatment pearls supportive treatment, can try PUVA, methotrexate or oral corticosteroids for cutaneous induration

Mixed connective tissue disease

Dermatomyositis

Overlap syndromes – other connective tissue diseases (SLE and DLE)

Lichen sclerosus et atrophicus

Porphyria cutanea tarda (sclerodermoid)

Scleredema

Scleromyxedema

Graft-versus-host disease
See page 290

Acrodermatitis chronica atrophicans (late stage of Lyme disease)

Lichen myxedematosus

Werner's syndrome

Carcinoid syndrome (especially on legs)

Bleomycin
Pulmonary fibrosis
Raynaud's phenomenon
Scleroderma skin changes
Dose dependent, reversible when off drug

Polyvinyl chloride exposure
Raynaud's phenomenon

Scleroderma skin changes
Osteolysis
Hepatic and pulmonary fibrosis

Phenylketonuria

SPLINTER HEMORRHAGES

Endocarditis

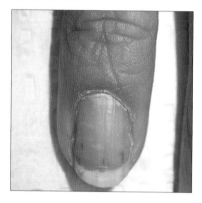

Trichinosis

Trauma

Connective tissue diseases
Systemic lupus erythematosus (SLE)
Scleroderma
Dermatomyositis

Microscopic polyarteritis

SPOROTRICHOID SPREAD

Sporotrichosis

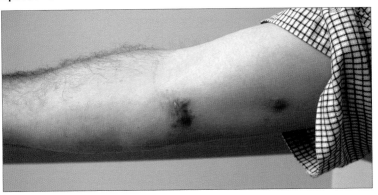

Atypical mycobacteria

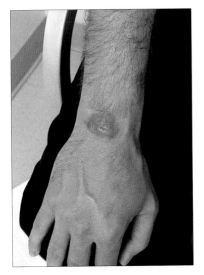

Cat scratch disease/bacillary angiomatosis

Tularemia

Bacterial infection with lymphatic involvement

Leishmaniasis

Cellulitis

SUBCUTANEOUS CORDS
Eosinophilic fasciitis

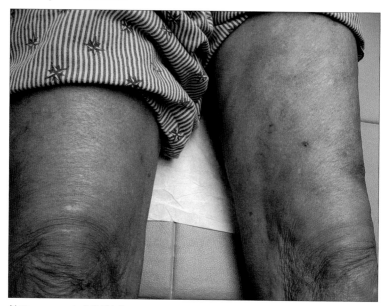

Note groove in left thigh

Thrombophlebitis

Panniculitis

Mondor's disease

Nephrogenic fibrosing dermopathy

SUBCUTANEOUS PAPULES AND NODULES
Erythema nodosum
See page 252

Dermoid cyst
See page 138

Deep granuloma annulare
See page 87, Granuloma annulare

Rheumatoid nodule
See page 183

Gout tophus

Thrombophlebitis

Deep fungal infection

Erythema induratum/nodular vasculitis

Polyarteritis nodosa (PAN)

Subcutaneous fat necrosis of the newborn

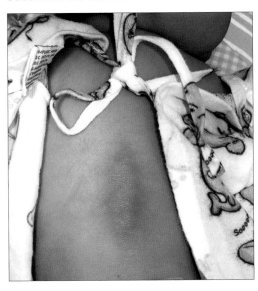

Lupus profundus

Tumid lupus

Pancreatic panniculitis

Metastatic disease

Sarcoid

Kaposi's sarcoma

Furuncle

Cutaneous T-cell lymphoma (CTCL)

Natural killer cell lymphoma

TELANGIECTASIAS – MATS

Scleroderma

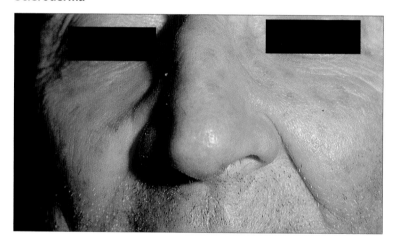

CREST syndrome

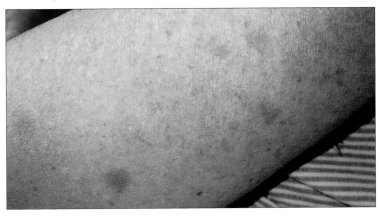

Dermatomyositis

Systemic lupus erythematosus (SLE)

Rheumatoid arthritis

Sjögren's syndrome

Osler–Weber–Rendu syndrome (hereditary hemorrhagic telangiectasias)

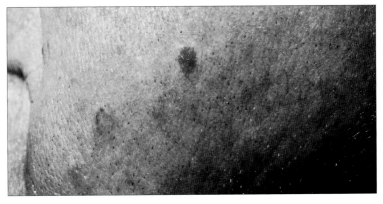

Essential telangiectasias
Mats in linear fashion, no mucous membrane involvement

Estrogens
Occurs with palmar erythema

Carcinoid syndrome

Mastocytosis (telangiectasia macularis eruptiva perstans variant)

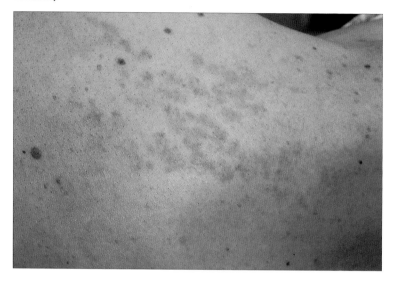

TELANGIECTASIAS – NON-MATTED/WIRY

Rosacea
See page 40

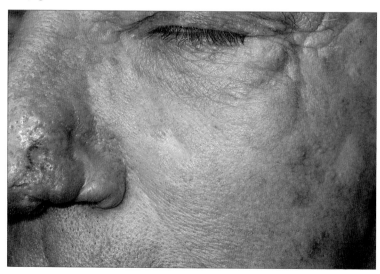

Drugs (estrogens, chronic topical or oral corticosteroids)

Poikiloderma of Civatte
See page 463

Essential telangiectasias

CREST syndrome
See page 507

Scleroderma
See page 508

Dermatomyositis
See page 427

Systemic lupus erythematosus (SLE)
See page 425

Radiation dermatitis

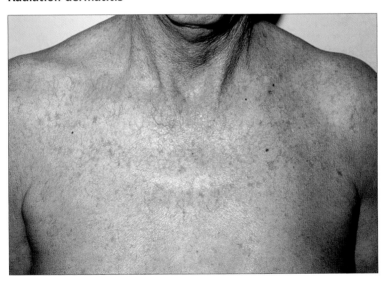

Involuting infantile hemangioma

Osler–Weber–Rendu syndrome (hereditary hemorrhagic telangiectasias)

Mastocytosis (telangiectasia macularis eruptiva perstans variant)

Cutaneous T-cell lymphoma (CTCL)
See page 402

Syndromes
Ataxia telangiectasia
Rothmund–Thompson syndrome
Bloom's syndrome
Werner's syndrome
Parkes–Weber syndrome
Hutchinson–Gilford syndrome
Cockayne syndrome
Xeroderma pigmentosum
Acrogeria

TONGUE LESIONS
Aphthous ulcer

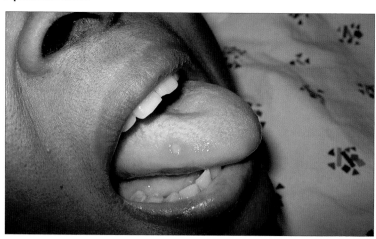

Mucocele

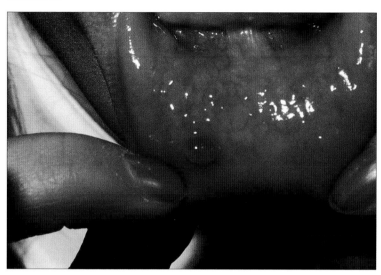

Black hairy tongue (secondary to antibiotics or bismuth)

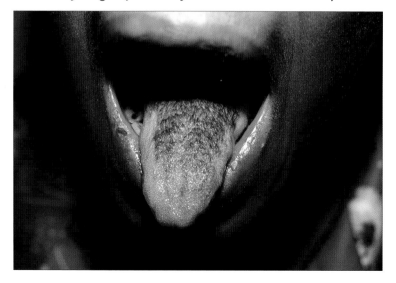

Fordyce granules

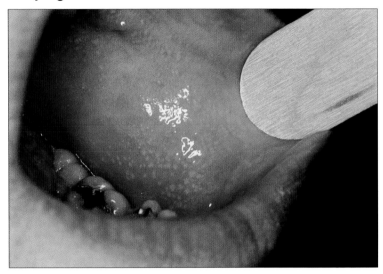

Geographic tongue

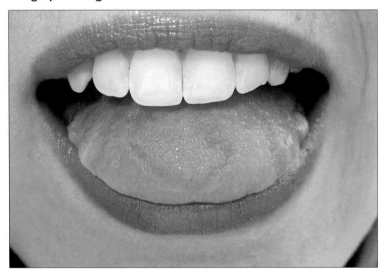

Scrotal (fissured tongue)

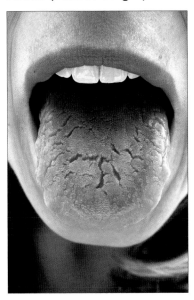

Lichen planus

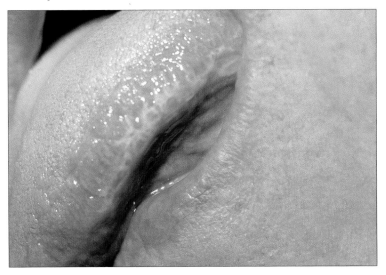

Sjögren's syndrome

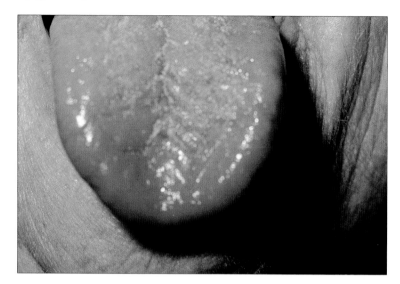

Granular cell tumor

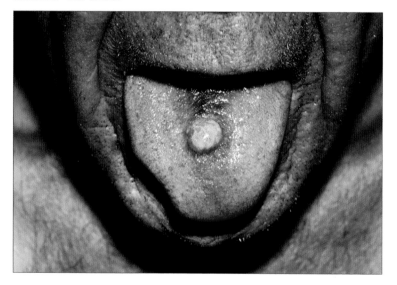

Cobblestoning (Cowden's, Crohn's, Darier's, lipoid proteinosis)

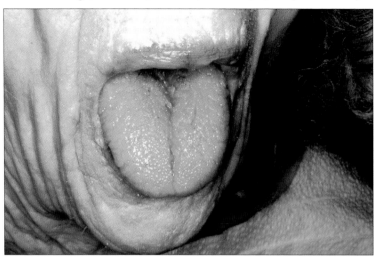

Macroglossia (secondary to amyloid)

Smooth (vitamin deficiency)

Squamous cell carcinoma

Herpes simplex virus

Hemangioma

Condyloma

Koplik spots (secondary to measles)

Syphilis (primary and secondary)

Oral hairy leukoplakia (white plaques on lateral tongue)

ULCER – GENITAL

Infectious

Herpes simplex virus
See page 116

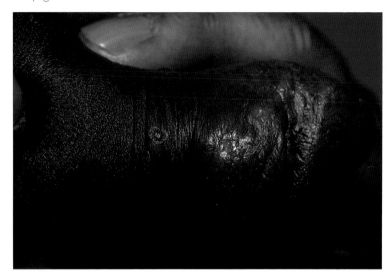

Bacterial infection (Staph and Strep common)
See page 492
Chancroid
See page 135
Primary syphilis (chancre)
See page 117
Lymphogranuloma venereum
Granuloma inguinale (donovanosis)
Gonorrhea
Fungal
  Dermatophytosis
  Candidiasis
  Histoplasmosis
  Cryptococcosis
Tuberculosis

Lichen planus
See page 257, Lichen planus (mucosal)

Fixed drug reaction

Erythema multiforme

Trauma
Factitial
Foreign body
Chemical or physical injury (postcoital)

Balanitis circinata

Lichen sclerosus et atrophicus

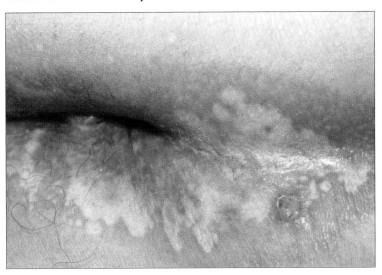

Lichen simplex chronicus

Extramammary Paget's disease

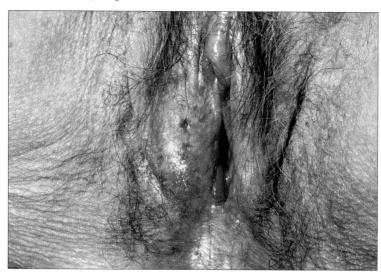

Plasma cell balanitis (Zoon's balanitis)

Behçet's syndrome

Pemphigus

Bullous pemphigoid

Malignancy
Squamous cell carcinoma
Basal cell carcinoma
Melanoma
Lymphoma
Leukemia

ULCER – LEGS

See page 248, Leg ulcers

ULCER – PAINLESS

Diabetes mellitus

Leprosy

Polyneuropathy

Necrotizing fasciitis

Syphilis ulcer secondary to tabes dorsalis

Syringomyelia

ULCER – SKIN

Traumatic (injury, pressure, heat, animal bite, factitial)

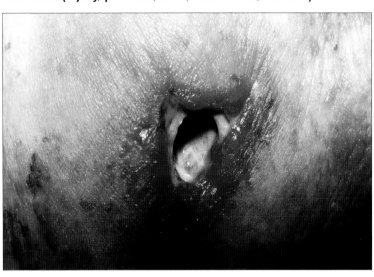

Neoplastic
Basal cell carcinoma

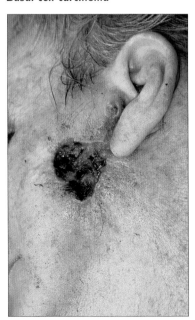

Squamous cell carcinoma
Melanoma
Metastatic
Cutaneous T-cell lymphoma (CTCL)

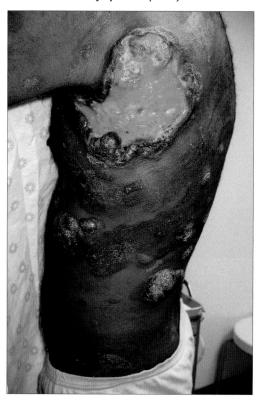

Lymphoma

Infectious
Fungal (actinomycosis, blastomycosis, coccidioidomycosis, chromoblastomycosis, sporotrichosis, histoplasmosis, cryptococcosis, fusarium)

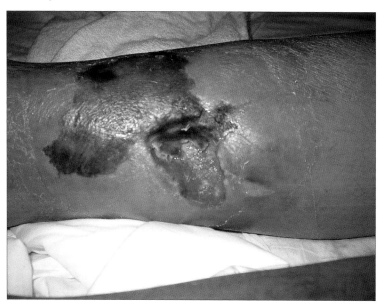

Bacterial (bacterial emboli, ecthyma, chancroid, anthrax, Pseudomonas, granuloma inguinale, botryomycosis, glanders)
Atypical mycobacteria (tuberculosis [lupus vulgaris, erythema induratum], leprosy, Mycobacterium marinum)
Parasitic (amebiasis, leishmaniasis)
Spirochete (syphilis, yaws)

Vascular
Venous stasis
Arteriosclerosis
Diabetes

Stasis

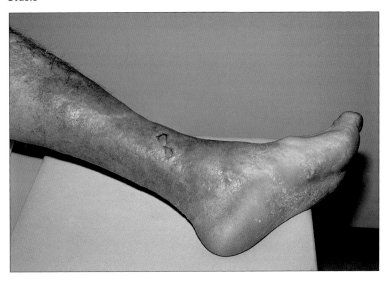

Infantile hemangioma

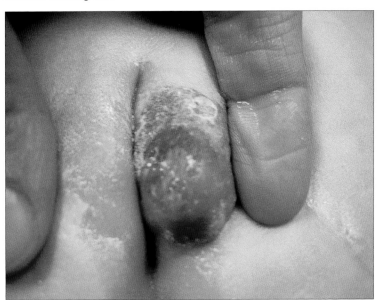

Raynaud's phenomenon
Thromboangiitis obliterans
Leukocytoclastic vasculitis

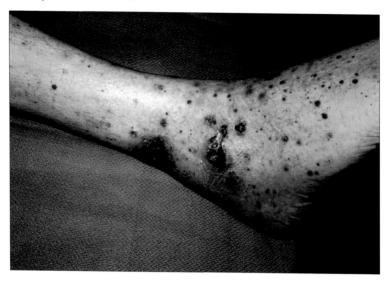

Hypertensive
Buerger's disease
Thrombophlebitis

Calcinosis cutis

Necrobiosis lipoidica diabeticorum (NLD)

Chilblains/pernio

Lymphedema

Atrophie blanche

Livedo vasculitis

Thrombotic thrombocytopenic purpura (TTP)

Cryoglobulinemia

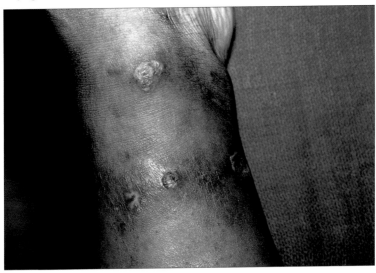

Sickle cell disease

Cholesterol emboli

Coagulopathy

Polycythemia vera

Decubitus secondary to pressure

Pyoderma gangrenosum

Insect bite (brown recluse spider, hobo spider)

Coumadin necrosis

Polyarteritis nodosa (PAN)

Scleroderma

Systemic lupus erythematosus (SLE)

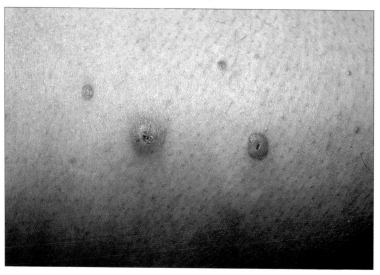

Rheumatoid vasculitis (Felty's syndrome)

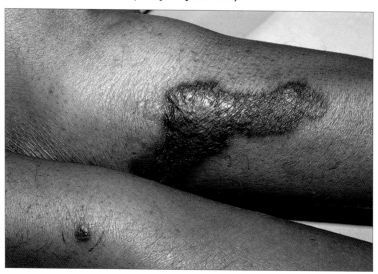

Wegener's granulomatosis

Prolidase deficiency

Werner's syndrome

URTICARIA

See page 88, Annular lesions/Urticaria

VASCULITIS

Small vessel vasculitis
See page 479, Leukocytoclastic vasculitis

Medium vessel vasculitis
Polyarteritis nodosa
Kawasaki's disease
Necrotizing vasculitis
    Polyarteritis nodosa
    Microscopic polyarteritis
    Churg–Strauss syndrome
    Wegener's syndrome
    Connective tissue diseases

Large vessel vasculitis
Giant cell/temporal arteritis
Takayasu's arteritis

Lymphocytic vasculitis
Pityriasis lichenoides et varioliformis acuta (PLEVA)
Drug-induced vasculitis
Arthropod bite
Some connective tissue diseases

VERRUCOUS LESIONS

Verruca vulgaris

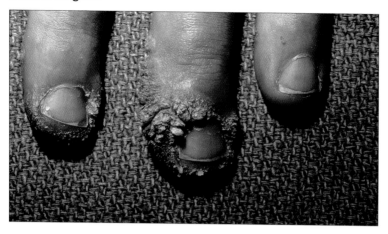

Seborrheic keratosis

Dermatosis papulosis nigra

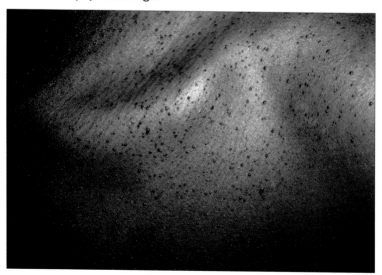

Condyloma

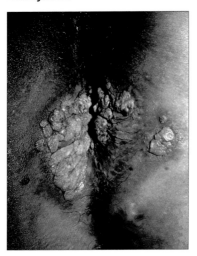

Warty dyskeratoma

Acanthosis nigricans

Epidermal nevus

Inflamed linear verrucous epidermal nevus (ILVEN)

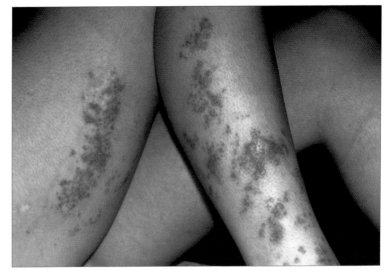

Chromoblastomycosis

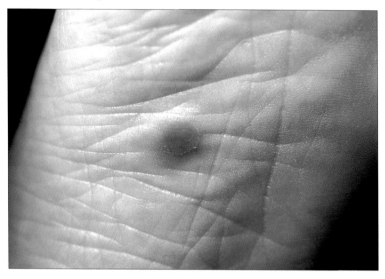

Lichen striatus
Nevus sebaceus
Incontinentia pigmenti
Tripe palm

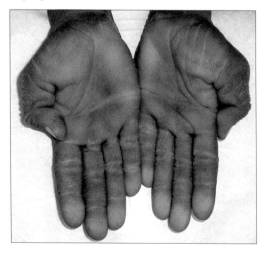

Pemphigus vegetans
Pyoderma vegetans

Arsenical keratoses

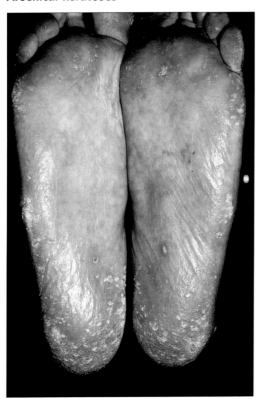

VULVA – PAPULES AND PLAQUES

Psoriasis
See page 397

Atopic dermatitis
See page 141

Seborrheic dermatitis
See page 398

Tinea corporis (dermatophytosis)
See page 86

Lichen planus (mucosal)
See page 257

Lichen simplex chronicus
See page 201

Lichen sclerosus et atrophicus
See page 100

Intertrigo
See page 145

Nevus
See page 379

Seborrheic keratosis
See page 381

Furunculosis

Hidradenitis suppurativa

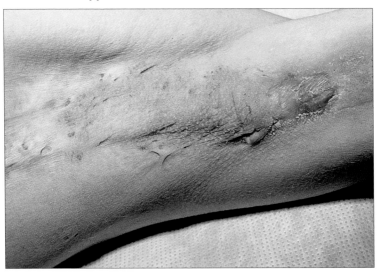

Molluscum contagiosum

Condylomata acuminata

Scabies

Pediculosis pubis

Hemangiomas

Achrochordon (skin tag, fibroepithelioma)

Melanoma

Pruritus vulvae

Herpes zoster

Erythema multiforme

Reiter's syndrome

VULVA – PRURITUS

Systemic causes
Diabetes mellitus
Anemia
Psychosomatic pruritus vulvae
Drug reaction
Jaundice conditions
Lichen planus
Plant dermatitis (Rhus)
Leukemia
Hypervitaminosis A

Local causes
Bacterial vaginitis
Candidiasis
See page 145
Tinea corporis (dermatophytosis)
See page 86
Lichen simplex chronicus
See page 201
Neurodermatitis
Scabies
See page 52
Pediculosis pubis
Contact dermatitis
Irritant dermatitis
Dermatitis medicamentosa
Molluscum contagiosum
Lichen sclerosus et atrophicus
Lichen planus
Pruritus ani
Atrophic vulvovaginitis
Carcinoma in situ
Fox–Fordyce disease

VULVA – ULCERS/EROSIONS

See page 524, Ulcer – genital

Achenbach's syndrome (paroxysmal hand hematoma) – acute palm hematoma, piercing pain, circumscribed edema, resolves rapidly within a few days.

Acquired generalized lipodystrophy (Lawrence syndrome, Seip–Lawrence syndrome) – marked loss of fat from face, body and limbs; usually begins in childhood by age 5 years or sometimes puberty; liver failure, variceal bleeds, diabetes mellitus, insulin resistance, increased triglycerides, early death. Female>male. One-third of cases with preceding autoimmune disease, connective tissue disease or infection.

Acquired partial lipodystrophy (Barraquer–Simons' syndrome) – progressive lipodystrophy beginning on face and moving to cephalothoracic area, then to thighs and buttocks, spares distal legs. Begins in childhood or puberty, may be preceded by febrile illness, ± diabetes mellitus and insulin resistance, increased triglycerides, 50% associated with renal changes/glomerulonephritis, retinitis pigmentosa, vasculitis. Female:male 3:1.

Acrodermatitis enteropathica – acral and periorificial dermatitis, alopecia, psoriasiform plaques over bony prominences, diarrhea, zinc deficiency. Begins 4–6 weeks after weaning breast-fed infants, occurs sooner in bottle-fed infants.

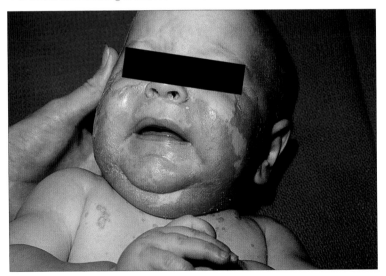

Adams–Oliver syndrome – large, irregular, deep aplasia cutis congenita causing distal transverse limb defects, associated with cutis marmorata or reticular capillary malformations, CNS and cardiac abnormalities. AD (rarely AR).

Addison's disease – hypocortisolism (adrenal gland insufficiency or hypopituitarism), bronze pigmentation, alopecia of pubic/axillary/scalp areas, longitudinal pigmented bands in nails, xerosis, anemia, muscular asthenia, GI abdominal pain and diarrhea.

Albinism (oculocutaneous albinism) – many types including disorders of melanin synthesis of hair, skin and nails; hypopigmentation or depigmentation at birth, ocular changes (photophobia, nystagmus, decreased visual acuity.) Types 1A and 1B: AR, tyrosinase defect, TYR gene; Type 2: AR, P-protein, P, PED genes; Type 3: AR, tyrosinase-related protein, TYRP1 gene; Type 4: AR, membrane-associated transporter protein, MATP gene.

Albright syndrome – *see* McCune Albright syndrome.

Albright's hereditary osteodystrophy – cutaneous ossification/osteoma cutis, brachydactyly, obesity, short stature, round face, ptosis, dimpling sign over knuckles when fist is clenched, short broad nails, basal ganglia calcification, mental retardation, hypocalcemia, pseudohypoparathyroidism. AD. GNAS1 gene.

Allezandrini syndrome – vitiligo on face, poliosis, unilateral degenerative retinitis ± deafness.

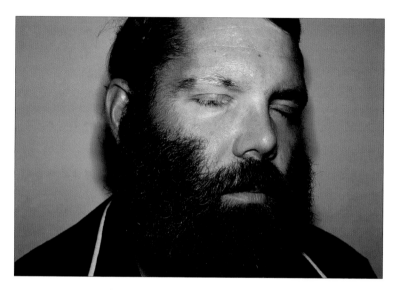

Alpha-1 antitrypsin deficiency – panniculitis, cutaneous vasculitis, urticaria, angioedema, COPD, low alpha-1 antitrypsin level, hepatitis, cutaneous vasculitis. AR.

Antiphospholipid syndrome/lupus anticoagulant syndrome – SLE, livedo reticularis, purpura, leg ulcers, multiple spontaneous thromboses, recurrent spontaneous abortions, thrombocytopenia, hypertension.

Apert's syndrome (acrocephalosyndactyly) – nail changes, seborrheic dermatitis, acne refractory to treatment, disfiguring synostosis of bones, hypopigmentation, cardiac anomalies, craniosynostosis, broad and flat face with beak-like nose. AD. FGFR2 gene.

Arndt-Gottron syndrome (scleromyxedema, lichen myxedematous-papular form) – diffuse red thick skin with underlying papules, papules may be linear and/or accentuated in skin folds, exaggerated facial ridges, ± limited finger flexion, ± IgG paraproteinemia, dysphagia, proximal muscle weakness, pulmonary disease, peripheral neuropathy.

Ascher's syndrome – upper eyelid edema, blepharochalasis, hyperplastic labial gland tissue, acquired 'double' lip, endocrine abnormalities (acromegaly, enlarged thyroid, irregular menses).

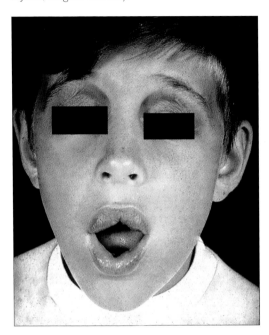

Ataxia telangiectasia (Louis-Bar syndrome) – granulomatous plaques on skin, acanthosis nigricans, vitiligo, hypo- and hyperpigmentation, café-au-lait macules, progeria, premature graying, oculocutaneous telangiectasias, cerebellar ataxia begins about age 2, peculiar eye movements, sinopulmonary infections, defective cell-mediated and humoral immunity (all immunoglobulins decreased), delayed/absent secondary sex characteristics with hypogonadism/ovarian agenesis, neoplasms, elevated serum alphafetoprotein, increased carcinoembryonic antigen. AR. Chromosome 11q22–23. ATM gene.

Auriculotemporal syndrome – *see* Frey's syndrome.

Autoerythrocyte sensitization (Gardner–Diamond) syndrome – painful ecchymoses, prodromal stinging or burning before lesion occurs, neurologic and psychiatric symptoms, abdominal pain, GI bleed, menometrorrhagia, muscle pain, adult women (95%). Etiology uncertain – possibly factitial or allergic sensitivity.

Bannayan–Riley–Ruvalcaba syndrome (Bannayan–Zonana syndrome) – acanthosis nigricans, facial papules, facial drooling, down-slanting palpebral fissures, lipomas, hemangiomas, systemic lipoangiomatosis, genital lentigines (spotted penis/vulva), oral papillomas, venous or lymphatic malformations, motor and speech delay, mental retardation, macrocephaly, GI polyps, myopathy, joint hyperextensibility. AD. PTEN and MMAC1 genes.

Barroquer–Simons' syndrome – *see* Acquired partial lipodystrophy.

Bart's syndrome – congenital absence of skin, dystrophic epidermolysis bullosa, shedding/dystrophic nails. Resolves by 12 months.

Bart–Pumphrey syndrome – knuckle pads, total leukonychia, sensorineural deafness.

Basal cell nevus syndrome (nevoid basal cell carcinoma, Gorlin's syndrome, Ward's syndrome) – multiple basal cell carcinomas (BCCs), milia, dyskeratosis of palms and soles with pitting, multiple odontogenic cysts of jaws, frontal bossing, hypertelorism, calcification of falx cerebri, skeletal changes (spina bifida, bifid ribs), ovarian and cardiac fibromas, cysts, carcinomas, medulloblastoma, mental retardation, short fourth digit and dimple (Albright's sign). PTCH and PTC genes.

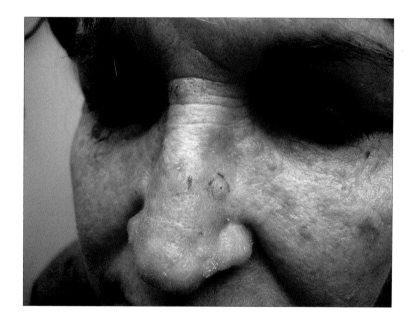

Battered child syndrome – bruising, bite marks, patterned burns (cigarettes, scalding, rope, irons), multiple fractures, sexual abuse, internal injuries.

Bazex syndrome (acquired) (acrokeratosis paraneoplastica) – violaceous, hyperkeratotic psoriasiform lesions over joints and ears, alopecia, keratoderma, nail changes, SCC in pulmonary/upper GI tract.

Bazex syndrome (inherited) (follicular atrophoderma and BCC syndrome) – multiple BCCs begin in adolescence, follicular atrophoderma, hypohidrosis, localized anhidrosis, hypotrichosis or pili torti, milia, skeletal defects. Presents at birth or soon after. X-linked dominant or AD.

Beckwith–Wiedemann syndrome (Wiedemann–Beckwith syndrome) – facial port-wine stain, macroglossia, exophthalmos, fine short lightly pigmented sparse hair, variable intelligence, hemihypertrophy including visceral, omphalocele, hypoglycemia, increased incidence of Wilm's tumor and possibly pancreatic cancer.

Behçet's syndrome – recurrent genital ulcers, aphthous lesions, ocular (uveitis, iridocyclitis or hypopyon), erythema nodosum-like lesions, pustular pathergy, leukocytoclastic vasculitis. CNS (meningoencephalitis or cerebral infarcts), thrombophlebitis or aneurysms, renal disease, arthritis, synovitis and immunologic abnormalities. Increased Middle Eastern and Japanese. HLA B51, also B5, B12, B27.

Beradinelli–Seip syndrome (congenital total lipodystrophy) – loss of fat diffusely from birth, acanthosis nigricans, xanthomas, increased genitalia and height, virilization, hepatosplenomegaly, hypertrophic cardiomyopathy, renal failure, increased triglycerides, insulin resistance, diabetes mellitus. AR. Chromosome 9q34, chromosome 11q13. Seipin gene.

Berlin syndrome – face like anhidrotic ectodermal dysplasia, delayed dentition, general mottled pigmentation, fine dry skin, hyperkeratosis of soles and palms, sparse pubic and axillary hair, telangiectasia of lips, normal nails, mental and physical retardation.

Birt–Hogg–Dube syndrome – fibrofolliculomas, acrochordons, multiple trichodiscomas, intestinal polyposis, carcinomas (thyroid, GI, renal). AD. BHD and FLCL genes.

Björnstad's syndrome – pili torti, cochlear-type deafness.

Blau syndrome – granulomas in skin (red papules), eyes (iritis, uveitis), joints (arthritis). AD.

Bloom's syndrome – primordial dwarfs, photosensitivity, café-au-lait spots, crusted bullous lesions on lips, telangiectatic erythema in malar areas (lupus-like butterfly pattern), short stature, high-pitched voice, hypogonadism, malignancy (leukemia, lymphoma, GI), abnormal immunity. Primarily males. AR. DNA helicase abnormalities. BLM and RECQ2 genes.

Blue rubber bleb nevus syndrome – bluish bladder-like cutaneous vascular malformations which empty with pressure, GI vascular malformations, nocturnal pain, supralesional sweating, GI bleeds with secondary anemia, onset at birth/early childhood. Sporadic or AD. Receptor tyrosine kinase TIE2 (endothelial). TIE2 and TEK genes.

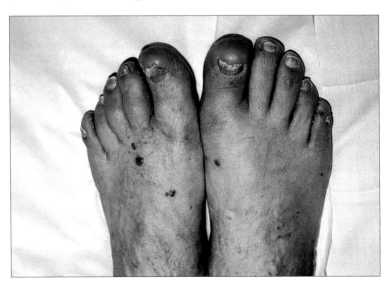

Bockenheimer's syndrome – progressive venous ectasia of one limb.
Bonnet–Dechaume–Blanc syndrome – *see* Wyburn–Mason syndrome.
Böök's syndrome – premature whitening of hair, premolar bicuspid aplasia, malocclusion, hyperhidrosis. AD.
Bourneville's syndrome – *see* Tuberous sclerosis.
Bowel bypass syndrome – pustular neutrophilic vasculitis usually in crops on upper abdomen, pathergy, fever, diarrhea, arthritis, myalgia.
Brooke–Spiegler syndrome (familial cylindromatosis) – multiple trichoepitheliomas and cylindromas. Can be associated with multiple basal cell adenomas of parotid glands, nevus sebaceus, milia, basal cell carcinomas and spiradenomas. AD. Chromosome 16q12–q13.

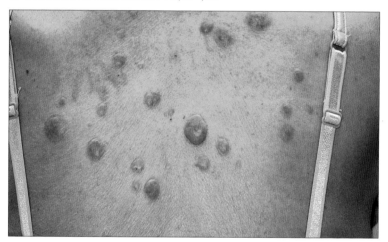

Brunauer syndrome – striate palmoplantar keratosis with islands of thickening over pressure points, abnormal teeth, sparse hair and eyelashes, pili torti, hypohidrosis, sensorineural deafness.
Brunsting–Perry syndrome (Brunsting–Perry cicatricial pemphigoid) – chronic head and neck red plaques with recurrent crops of herpetiform blisters which heal with atrophic scarring, severe burning and itching, mostly middle-aged/older males, no mucosal involvement. May represent a localized form of cicatricial pemphigoid.
Brushfield–Wyatt syndrome – extensive port-wine staining (unilateral nevus flammeus), hemiplegia, cerebral vascular malformation, mental retardation.
Burger–Grutz syndrome (idiopathic familial hyperlipemia) – xanthomas, hepatosplenomegaly, lipemia retinalis, recurrent abdominal pain. Gene map locus 8p22.

Buschke–Ollendorf syndrome (dermatofibrosis lenticularis disseminata) – asymptomatic cutaneous fibromas/connective tissue nevi mainly on trunk and lower extremities (dermatofibrosis lenticularis disseminata), osteopoikilosis. Increased desmosine content in skin with accumulation of interlacing elastic fibers in dermis. AD with variable expression.

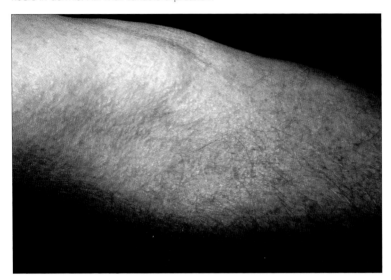

Cantu syndrome – punctate palmoplantar keratoderma, small reticulated hyperkeratotic and hyperpigmented macules on the face, arms, hands and feet. AD.

Carcinoid syndrome – peculiar flushing and episodic cyanosis, pellagra-like dermatitis, scleroderma-like changes on the lower extremities, periorbital edema, telangiectasias, asthma, diarrhea, syncope, cardiac (fibrosis of endocardium). Carcinoid tumors secreting serotonin, kallikrein, histamine.

Carney syndrome/complex (LAMB or NAME syndrome) – mucocutaneous 'spotty' lentigines, blue nevi, congenital nevi, schwannomas, atrial myxomas, mucocutaneous myxomas, endocrine abnormalities (overactivity), testicular tumors. CNC and PRKAR1A genes.

Cervico-oculo-acoustic syndrome (Wildervanck's syndrome) – stiff short neck (Klippel–Feil anomaly with fused cervical vertebrae), low implantation of hair, congenital perceptive deafness, abducens palsy with retractio bulbi (Duane syndrome). Nearly always females.

Chand's syndrome – curly hair, ankyloblepharon, nail dysplasia. AR form of ectodermal dysplasia.

Chediak–Higashi syndrome – oculocutaneous albinism and increased pigment in sun-exposed areas, silver-blonde hair, gingivitis, oral ulcerations, pan-immune dysfunction (decreased phagocytosis, decreased chemotaxis, decreased lysosomal transport), ocular changes (photophobia and pale fundi and decreased tears), hepatosplenomegaly, lymphadenopathy, recurrent pyogenic sinopulmonary and cutaneous infections, neurologic changes (abnormal gait, nystagmus, seizures, paresthesias), bleeding tendency. Early death from lymphoma. AR. Chromosome 1q. CHS1 and LYST genes.

CHILD syndrome – **C**ongenital **H**emidysplasia, **I**chthyosiform erythroderma, **L**imb **D**efects (digital hypoplasia, extremity agenesis), sharp midline demarcation of unilateral ichthyosis with contralateral patchy cutaneous involvement, face spared, unilateral alopecia, stippled epiphyses, other organ involvement (CNS, musculoskeletal, cardiac, visceral), teeth normal, claw-like dystrophy or ipsilateral onychorrhexis. Disorder of lipid metabolism with disturbed cholesterol synthesis. X-linked dominant, lethal in males. Defect on chromosome Xq28. NSDHL gene.

Chlorpromazine syndrome (purple people, skin–eye syndrome) – light brown, slate gray or violaceous discoloration of exposed areas, fine particulate star-shaped deposits in lens and cornea, cataracts.

Christ–Siemens syndrome (Christ–Siemens–Touraine, anhidrotic ectodermal dysplasia) – *see* Ectodermal dysplasia (hypohidrotic).

Chronic granulomatous disease – recurrent purulent and granulomatous infections to catalase-positive organisms (neonatal pustulosis, skin abscesses, recurrent pneumonia, lung abscesses), periorificial eczema, oral ulcers, lupus-like cutaneous lesions (female carriers), lymphadenopathy with drainage, short stature, diarrhea, nitroblue tetrazolium test low or negative, all immunoglobulins increased (hypergammaglobulinemia), decreased NADPH oxidase of phagocytes, leukocyte defect in production of superoxide anion. X-linked recessive or AR.

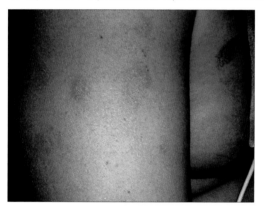

Churg–Strauss syndrome (allergic granulomatosis) – vasculitic red papules or nodules on scalp and extensor surfaces (can appear urticarial, purpuric, ulcers, erythema multiforme-like), livedo reticularis, severe asthma or allergic rhinitis, eosinophilia, pulmonary infiltrates, arthralgias, bloody diarrhea, febrile attacks, neuropathy, seizures, p-ANCA usually positive.

Clouston syndrome – *see* Ectodermal dysplasia (hidrotic).

Coat's syndrome – retinal telangiectasia and ipsilateral port-wine stain.

Cobb syndrome (cutaneous meningospinal angiomatosis) – kyphoscoliosis with vascular malformation, port-wine stain or angiokeratoma of spinal dermatome, neurologic signs consistent with cord compression/anoxia (sensory and motor changes, GI and GU problems, e.g. incontinence), vertebral angiomas, renal angiomas. Sporadic inheritance.

Cockayne syndrome – red scaly, photosensitive, lupus-like dermatitis, subcutaneous fat atrophy with sunken eyes, decreased and defective physical and mental development, ocular changes (salt and pepper retinal changes), progressive deafness, premature aging with short life span, microcephaly, enlarged hands, feet and ears, demyelination of CNS and peripheral nervous system, bone changes. Onset at 1–2 years of age. AR. DNA helicase abnormalities.

Cogan's syndrome – non-syphilitic interstitial keratitis, deafness, ataxia, tinnitus, vertigo, large-vessel arteritis (PAN – polyarteritis nodosa).

Conradi–Hünermann–Happle syndrome (X-linked dominant chondrodysplasia punctata) – scaly ichthyosiform generalized erythroderma with whorled or linear hyperkeratosis at birth replaced by linear or patchy follicular atrophoderma especially on hands, ice-pick scars, patchy scarring alopecia, epiphyseal stippling, dwarfing, stiff and contracted joints, congenital unilateral cataracts, few and rudimentary hairs (scalp, brows and lashes), frontal bossing, flat nasal bridge. Defect in cholesterol biosynthesis, mutations on short arm of X chromosome in some cases. Patterns may be X-linked dominant, EBP gene (Happle type, moderate) or AD (mild form), (cholesterol biosynthesis).

Cornelia de Lange syndrome (Brachmann–de Lange syndrome) – cutis marmorata and facial 'cyanosis', small hairline, 'beak' in upper lip with notch in lower lip, confluent eyebrows, long eyelashes, hypertrichosis, hemangiomas, depressed nose bridge with uptilted nose tip, primordial growth failure, skeletal abnormalities (small hands and feet, low-set thumbs, hypoplastic limbs, short broad first metacarpal), mental retardation, characteristic low-pitched and weak growling cry.

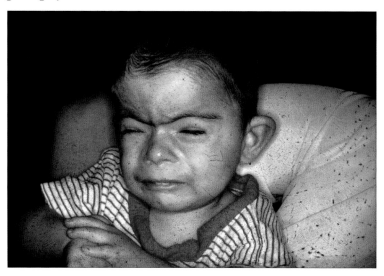

Cowden's disease/Cowden's syndrome – multiple trichilemmomas, facial papules, oral papillomatosis (cobblestoning of tongue), acral keratoses, epidermal cysts, lipomas, angiomas, neuromas, meningiomas, neurofibromas, multiple hamartomas, carcinoma of breast and thyroid, GI hamartomatous polyps, ovarian cysts, fibrocystic breast disease, bone cysts, craniomegaly, high palate. Associated with thyroid, breast and colon cancer. AD. PTEN and MMAC1 genes.

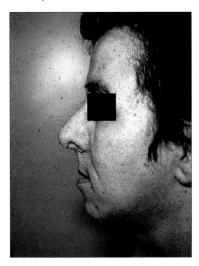

CREST syndrome – **C**alcinosis cutis, **R**aynaud's, **E**sophageal dysfunction, **S**clerodactyly, mat-like **T**elangiectasias, anti-centromere antibody positive, subset of scleroderma.

Cri-du-chat syndrome – high-pitched cat-like cry, cleft palate, premature graying, epicanthal folds, malformed ears with preauricular skin tags, hypertelorism, narrow forehead, simian (single palmar) crease, microcephaly, severe mental retardation, growth retardation. Partial deletion of chromosome 5.

Crigler–Najjar syndrome (familial non-hemolytic jaundice with kernicterus) – increased bilirubin retention, icterus, severe neurologic disease. Unconjugated hyperbilirubinemia occurs in association with otherwise normal liver function.

Cronkite–Canada syndrome – general alopecia, diffuse and spotty pigmentation, nail dystrophy with triangular nail plate and shedding, GI polyposis, diarrhea, neurologic symptoms.

Crow–Fukase syndrome – *see* POEMS syndrome.

Cushing's syndrome – hirsutism, acne, abdominal striae, moon face, buffalo hump, truncal obesity with slender limbs, mild insulin-resistant diabetes mellitus, arterial hypertension, osteoporosis, compression fractures.

Cutis laxa – different patterns can include: loose-hanging skin, inguinal and umbilical hernias, lung disease, aortic aneurysm, hyperlaxity, GI diverticula. Defect in elastic fibers. Types include: AD-dominant (elastin, ELN gene), AR (Fibulin-5, FBLNS and DANCE genes), AD-marfanoid (Laminin beta-1, LAMB1 gene) and X-linked recessive.

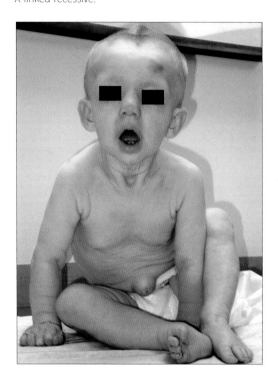

Cutis marmorata telangiectatica congenita (Van Lohuizen's syndrome) – congenital phlebectasia characterized by deeply erythematous, reticulate vascular network, increased mottling with crying, cold or increased activity. Can be general or regionalized. Often unilateral, segmental pattern on extremities, trunk, face, scalp. Most cutaneous vascular conditions improve over 2 years, but may have ulceration, varicosities, hypertrophy or atrophy of affected limb. Craniofacial abnormalities, neurologic abnormalities, GI (rectal), hyperplastic skin, aplasia cutis, syndactyly, hypospadias. 50% have associated port-wine stain.

Darier–Roussy syndrome – subcutaneous sarcoid nodules on trunk and extremities.
Degos' disease (malignant atrophic papulosis) – crops of crusted dome-shaped or umbilicated papules which progress to depressed atrophic scars, acute abdomen, fatal fulminating peritonitis, headache, ataxia, hypesthesia.
Dercum's disease – painful and symmetrical lipomas, ecchymoses, obesity, neuritis, mental depression and deterioration, more common in postmenopausal women.
DeSanctis–Cacchione syndrome – xeroderma pigmentosum, mental deficiency, stunted growth, neural deafness, progressive neurologic degeneration (ataxia, choreoathetosis), ± gonadal immaturity. Defect in DNA repair mechanism.

DiGeorge syndrome – seborrheic or atopic dermatitis, abscesses, hypoplastic or absent thymus, absence of T cells, increased infections (candida), cleft palate, cardiac anomalies, small ears, short palpebral fissures. AD in some.

Dilantin hypersensitivity syndrome – morbilliform, scarlatiniform, urticarial or exfoliative eruptions, fever, malaise, arthralgia, lymphadenopathy (especially cervical), splenic and/or hepatic enlargement, eosinophilia. Due to hypersensitivity to dilantin. Can occur with phenobarbital and other anticonvulsants.

Donahue syndrome (leprechaunism) – hirsutism (especially facial), retarded somatic and mental development with large genitalia.

Dowling–Degos' disease – axillary and groin reticulated hyperpigmentation. Adult onset.

Dowling–Mera syndrome – *see* Epidermolysis bullosa simplex.

Down's syndrome (trisomy 21) – skin soft and velvety in childhood, dry skin (ichthyosiform hyperkeratosis), premature wrinkling, atopic dermatitis, increased fungal infections, syringomas, angular cheilitis, vitiligo, alopecia areata, elastosis perforans serpiginosa, tongue protrusion, hypoplastic teeth, cataracts, mental retardation, brachycephaly, flat facies, epicanthal folds, single palmar (simian) crease, dysplasia of fifth finger mid-phalanx. Trisomy 21.

Dresbach's syndrome – *see* Sickle cell disease.

Dubin–Johnson syndrome – chronic icterus, greenish-black liver, conjugated hyperbilirubinemia, defect in bilirubin excretion.

Dubowitz's syndrome – eczematoid eruption, thick skin, sparse hair and lateral eyebrows, small stature, peculiar facies with high sloping forehead and asymmetry, epicanthal folds, low-set ears, immunodeficiency. AR.

Dury–van Bogaert syndrome – cutis marmorata, acrocyanosis, nail dystrophy, ± hypertrichosis, spastic diplegia, epilepsy, mental retardation.

Dyskeratosis congenita (Cole–Rauschkolb–Tocmy, Zinsser–Cole–Engman, Zinsser–Fanconi syndromes) – skin atrophy and pigmentation, nail and teeth dystrophy, oral premalignant leukoplakia, ± bullae, ocular (ectropion, blepharitis), hyperkeratosis, ± hyperhidrosis, bone marrow hypofunction. AR (telomerase RNA component, TR and TERC genes) and X-linked recessive (dyskeratin, DKC1 gene).

Dysplastic nevus syndrome – increased number of nevi, variable size of nevi, increased incidence of melanoma, risk of ocular melanoma. AD familial form, also sporadic.

Ectodermal dysplasia (hidrotic) (Clouston syndrome) – generalized hypotrichosis (sparse, fine, brittle, light-colored), nail changes (thickened, striated, slow growth), palmoplantar hyperkeratosis, normal teeth and sweating, mild mental retardation. French-Canadian inheritance, AD. Connexin 30, GJB6 and CX30 genes.

***Ectodermal dysplasia (hypohidrotic) (anhidrotic ectodermal dysplasia,
Christ–Siemens–Touraine syndrome)*** – hair changes (fine, sparse, light-
colored, twisted), nail changes (thin, brittle, ridged), frontal bossing, saddle
nose, large pointed ears, thick lips, atopic dermatitis, dental (hypodontia,
anodontia, conical incisors), absence of sweat glands (partial or complete), heat
intolerance, increased IgE, decreased cell-mediated immunity, loss of smell and
taste, decreased tears, increased infections (bronchitis, pneumonia, otitis media),
fever of unknown origin in infants, decreased salivary glands. AD: ectodysplasin
receptor, EDAR, DL genes; AR: ectodysplasin receptor, EDAR, DL genes or EDAR-
associated death domain (EDARDD); X-linked recessive: ectodysplasin A, EDA
gene.

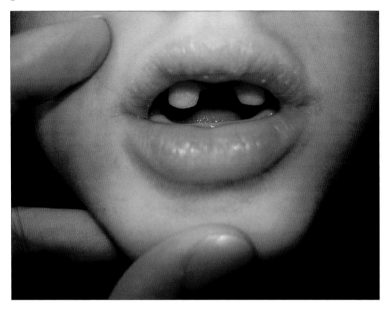

***Ectodermal dysplasia (hypohidrotic with immunodeficiency) (Zonana
syndrome)*** – as above with immunodeficiency. NF-kappa B essential modulator.
NEMO and IKBKG genes.

Ehlers–Danlos syndrome (cutis hyperelastica) – skin hyperelastic and friable, fragile blood vessels, papyraceous or atrophic scars, joint hyperextensibility, kyphoscoliosis, pseudotumors. 10 patterns with varied inheritance and genes.

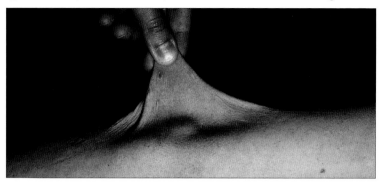

Ellis–van Creveld syndrome (chondroectodermal dysplasia) – ectodermal dysplasia of nails, hair and teeth, chondrodysplasia, short limbs, short ribs, polydactyly, congenital heart defect. AR. Gene map locus 4p16.

Eosinophilia–myalgia syndrome – myalgia, fatigue, weakness, eosinophilia (>2000/mm^3), respiratory changes, edema, hepatomegaly, arrhythmia, eosinophilic fasciitis, late stage scleroderma. L-tryptophan consumption.

Eosinophilic fasciitis (Shulman syndrome) – sudden onset of tender, painful, swollen face, extremities or abdomen, sparing hands; occurs after exercise or exertion, myalgia, arthritis, absent visceral changes, eosinophilia >1000/mm^3, responds to prednisone.

Epidermal nevus syndrome – epidermal nevi, hypochromatic nevi, café-au-lait macules, skeletal changes, ocular changes, CNS changes, developmental delay. Renal, cardiac, endocrine, and teeth malformations.

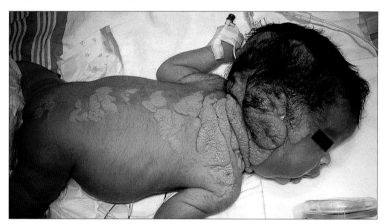

Epidermolysis bullosa
Epidermolysis bullosa dystrophica (EBD) – tense bulla and erosions especially acral, +Nikolsky sign, collagen 7 defect, heals with scarring, increased incidence of squamous cell carcinomas in scars. AD inherited: dominant dystrophic/Cockayne–Touraine (limited involvement), albopapuloid variant of Pasini, Bart's syndrome (good prognosis), transient bullous dermolysis of the newborn (heals by 4–12 months of age) and Weary–Kindler types. AR inherited: often fatal Hallopeau–Siemens (generalized with mitten deformity), localized and inverse types. COL7A1 gene.

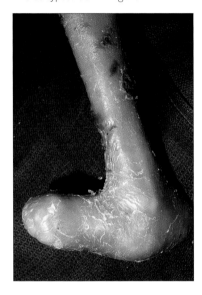

Epidermolysis bullosa junctional (EBJ) – bulla and erosions, especially acral with internal involvement of epithelium. AR inheritance: fatal Herlitz type (laminin 5; LAMC2, LAMB3 and LAMA3 genes), fatal type with pyloric atresia (integrin alpha-6 and beta-4; ITGA6 and ITGb4 genes) and non-Herlitz/ generalized atrophic benign (BPAg2/collagen 17; COL17A1 and BPAG2 genes) type.
Epidermolysis bullosa simplex (EBS) – bulla and erosions especially acral, no Nikolsky sign, keratin 5 and 14 defect in basal layer. Koebner (generalized), Weber–Cockayne (localized), Dowling–Mera (herpetiform), Ogna (hemorrhagic), and with mottled hyperpigmentation types inherited AD. KRT5 and KRT14 genes. With muscular dystrophy (plectin gene defect, PLEC1 and PLTN genes) inherited AR.

Epidermolytic hyperkeratosis of Brocq – *see* Ichthyosis: bullous congenital ichthyosiform erythroderma.
Erythermalgia/erythromelalgia – intense, burning pain with marked erythema of affected area secondary to paroxysmal vasodilatation. Primarily in feet, but can occur on hands, face, ears. Worsens with heat, improves with cold. Primary idiopathic in young children, must rule out hypertension. Secondary may be due to thrombocytosis, SLE, dermatomyositis, multiple sclerosis, polycythemia vera,

TTP. Aspirin therapy in secondary cases. Some families with AD pattern. Primary erythromelalgia localized to chromosome 2q.

Erythrokeratoderma variabilis (Mendes da Costa syndrome, Mendes da Costa's erythrokeratoderma) – bizarre geographic hyperkeratotic reddish-brown plaques, independent areas of erythroderma, lesions can occur over hours. Extensor limbs, buttocks, axillae, groin are favored locations. AD. GJB 3 and 4 and CX31 genes, connexin 31.

Fabry's syndrome (Fabry–Anderson syndrome, angiokeratoma corporis diffusum, Ruiter–Pompen syndrome, Ruiter–Pompen–Wyers syndrome) – angiokeratoma (bathing trunk distribution over trunk and lower extremities), pain in extremities, sweat secretion disturbances, hypertension, cardiomegaly, hypogonadism, ocular changes, stroke, seizure, weakness, albuminuria. Deficiency of lysosomal alpha-galactosidase A, ceramide trihexoside accumulates in blood vessels, causing lamellar bodies in endothelial cells. X-linked recessive.

Familial Mediterranean fever – erysipelas-like lesions on lower extremities, leukocytoclastic vasculitis, urticaria, intermittent fevers lasting 1–2 days, abdominal pain, pleurisy, arthritis, renal amyloidosis. AR.

Fanconi aplastic anemia (Fanconi's syndrome, Ehrlich–Fanconi syndrome) – generalized brown pigmentation of skin with areas of hypo- or hyperpigmented macules and café-au-lait spots, severe progressive refractory hypoplastic pancytopenia, hypoplasia of thumb, carpal bones, radius; short stature, renal abnormalities (aplasia, ectopia, horseshoe kidney, duplication), ear changes/deafness, congenital cardiac disease, mental retardation, microcephaly and microphthalmia. Defective DNA repair, increased rates of hepatocellular carcinoma, leukemia, squamous cell carcinoma of anus, vulvar and oral areas. AR.

Farber syndrome (ceramidase deficiency) – macula with cherry-red spots, periarticular cutaneous nodules, skin infiltrated around ears and occiput, joint abnormalities, voice changes, mental and motor retardation. AR.

Favre–Racouchot syndrome – senile atrophy of skin, elastoidosis, epidermal cysts and comedones in periorbital area, abnormal folds and wrinkles on face, neck and ears.

Felty's syndrome – leg ulcers, nodules, pigmentation of the skin, pyoderma gangrenosum, chronic deforming arthritis, splenomegaly, lymphadenopathy, leukopenia. Associated with rheumatoid arthritis.

Ferreira–Marques syndrome (lipoatrophia annularis) – painful bracelet swelling and loss of subcutaneous tissue in band-like area, often on arm. Arthralgias, may last up to 2 years. Female>male.

Fetal alcohol syndrome – hypertrichosis, hemangiomas, dysplastic nails, mental retardation, CNS/cardiac/renal malformations, skeletal abnormalities, microcephaly with elongated philtrum and maxillary hypoplasia, cleft palate, narrow palpebral fissure, ears with abnormal pinnae.

Focal dermal hypoplasia (Goltz syndrome) – linear/reticular hypo- and/or hyperpigmentation, round areas of skin thinning with adipose tissue herniation, papillomatosis of skin, mucus membranes and larynx; nail dystrophy; defects of bones (lobster claw of hand and osteopathica striata on leg x-ray); defects of teeth, eyes, heart, CNS; triangular facies, pointed chin, notched asymmetric nasal alae. X-linked dominant.

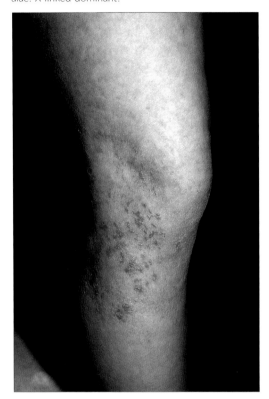

Fragile X syndrome – primary cutis verticis gyrata, hyperextensible velvety skin, abnormal palmar creases, autistic behavior, mental retardation, normal growth with developmental delay, hypotonia, scoliosis, hyperextensible joints, flat feet, long face with prominent forehead and jaw, pale-blue irides. Fragile sites on X chromosome at terminal site of long arm and chromosome 7.

***Franceschetti–Jadassohn syndrome (Naegeli–Franceschetti–Jadassohn
syndrome)*** – reticulate hyperpigmentation starting at age 2 and fading with
time, increased pigment on neck and axillae, nail dystrophy, hypohidrosis, absent
fingerprints, palmar–plantar keratoderma, dental enamel changes. AD.

Frey's syndrome (auriculotemporal syndrome) – vasodilatation, gustatory
hyperhidrosis, ± pain of cheek while eating after cranial nerve VI or VII damage,
typically unilateral. Often after parotid surgery or idiopathic in childhood.

Frolich's syndrome – lipoma, obesity, hypogonadism.

Gammel's disease (erythema gyratum repens) – figurate erythema (multiple
annular erythematous lesions that develop scale at edges and progress at a rapid
rate or up to one centimeter per day, may look like wood grain), usually
paraneoplastic (often lung cancer). Rash resolves with cancer resolution.

Gardner's syndrome (familial polyposis of the colon) – epidermal cysts and
lipomas of the face and trunk, multiple colon polyps, risk of GI (colon)
adenocarcinoma, bony exostoses/osteomas (especially jaw and face), soft tissue
tumors (leiomyomas), ovarian cysts, dental changes, congenital hypertrophy of
retinal pigment epithelium. AD. Increased beta-catenin, chromosome 5q21–22.
APC gene.

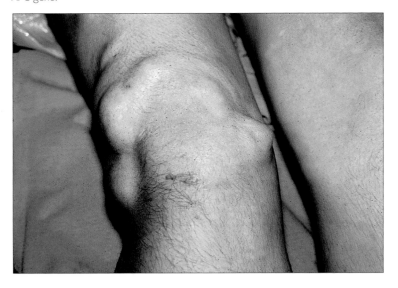

Gaucher's syndrome – Type I: diffuse yellow–brown hyperpigmentation of face,
hands, neck; easy tanning, petechiae, purpura, bone pain, hepatosplenomegaly
with secondary pancytopenia, lymphadenopathy, pingueculae. Type II (acute
neuropathic form): rigid neck, mental retardation, hepatosplenomegaly, bone
pain, pulmonary infections. Type III: hepatosplenomegaly, bone pain, lack of CNS
involvement. Type I with predisposition for Ashkenazi Jewish descent. No ethnic
predisposition in other types. Dysfunction of beta-glucocerebrosidase. Infantile
or childhood onset.

Gianotti-Crosti syndrome (papular acrodermatitis of childhood) – sudden onset of erythematous papular lesions on face, neck and extremities of children usually sparing trunk, respiratory or GI symptoms, lymphadenopathy, fever and malaise. Associated with EBV (most common), HBV, Coxsackie virus, echovirus, RSV, CMV, parainfluenza and polio virus.

Glucagonoma syndrome (necrolytic migratory erythema syndrome) – erythematous dermatitis with scaling and erosions primarily on abdomen, groin, buttocks; brittle nails, alopecia, candidal infections, anemia, glossitis, weight loss, conjunctivitis. Dermatitis resolves when tumor removed. Tumor of pancreatic alpha-cells causing hyperglucagonemia.

Godfried–Prick–Carol–Prakken syndrome (atrophoderma vermiculata) – von Recklinghausen's disease, atrophoderma vermiculatum, mongoloid facies, mental retardation, cardiac abnormalities.

Goldenhar's syndrome (oculoauriculovertebral dysplasia) – accessory tragus, hemifacial microsomia. May have cardiac, vertebral and CNS system defects. Gene map locus 14a32.

Goltz syndrome – *see* Focal dermal hypoplasia.

Gonococcal dermatitis syndrome – hemorrhagic vesiculopustular/vasculitic eruption with red halos, erythema nodosum, erythema multiforme, urticaria intermittent fever, arthralgias (pain and swelling of affected joint(s)). Disseminated gonococcal infection of *Neisseria gonorrhea*.

Gorham's syndrome – massive osteolysis ('disappearing bones') replaced by fibrous tissue usually occurring in long bones, ± venous or lymphatic malformations. Occurs in young children.

Gorlin syndrome – *see* Basal cell nevus syndrome.

Gorlin–Chaudhry–Moss syndrome (craniofacial dysostosis) – craniofacial dysostosis, hypertrichosis, hypoplasia of labia majora, dental and ocular abnormalities.

Gottron's syndrome (acrogeria) – vascular type Ehlers–Danlos, premature aging of extremities, short stature, small hands/feet, nail dystrophy, progressive acral erythema, lipoatrophy, increased bruising and scarring. AR.

Gougerot–Blum syndrome – *see* Pigmented purpuric eruptions/dermatoses.

Gougerot–Carteaud syndrome (confluent and reticulated papillomatosis) – verrucous hyperkeratotic papules or hyperkeratosis that become confluent in a reticulated pattern beginning on mid-trunk, ± endocrine dysfunction (diabetes, thyroid), dark-skinned females most common group.

Graham-Little syndrome (Graham-Little–Piccardi–Lassueur syndrome) – Triad of lichen planus (cutaneous or mucosal), acuminate follicular papules with plugging, and cicatricial alopecia.

Graves' disease – onycholysis, pretibial myxedema, diffuse hair loss, fine hair, palmar erythema, exophthalmos, hyperthyroidism. Autoantibodies to TSH receptors on thyroid cells resulting in increased T3 and T4 and decreased TSH level.

Greither syndrome (progressive palmoplantar keratoderma) – progressive diffuse thickening of palms and soles, warty keratoses on dorsa of hands, feet, arms and legs, poikiloderma of face, hands, feet, forearms and legs, sweat abnormalities, loss of teeth, spontaneous amputations, total alopecia. AD.

Griscelli syndrome – partial albinism, silver hair, neurologic changes, immune dysfunction. MYOSA or RAB27A genes.

Gunther's syndrome (congenital erythropoietic porphyria) – *see* Porphyria.

Haber syndrome – persistent rosacea-like facial eruption begins in childhood, intraepidermal epitheliomata of covered parts, pitted scars. AD.

Hallermann–Straiff syndrome (Francois) – brittle scalp hair, generalized hypotrichosis, skin atrophy, skull malformation, congenital cataracts, dental anomalies, small face with frontal bossing and narrow nose, micrognathia.

Hand–Schüller–Christian disease (chronic progressive multifocal histiocytosis) – a type of Langerhans' histiocytosis X; papules, pustules, and crusted patches especially in intertriginous areas, cutaneous xanthomas, stomatitis and gingivitis, increased otitis media, membranous bone defects, exophthalmos, diabetes insipidus.

Hartnup's syndrome – pellagra-like skin rash, intermittent cerebellar ataxia, aminoaciduria, photosensitive, onset 3–9 years of age. GI malabsorption of tryptophan causing decreased nicotinic acid.

Hashimoto–Pritzker syndrome (congenital self-healing histiocytosis) – a type of Langerhans' histiocytosis X; present at birth, spontaneous involution of diffuse papules usually over 1–4 years, no systemic involvement. Female>male.

Heerfordt syndrome – sarcoidosis, lacrimal and parotid enlargement, anterior uveitis, fever, cranial nerve palsies (usually facial nerve – cranial nerve VII).

Helwig–Larssen–Ludwigsen syndrome – congenital anhidrosis or severe hypohidrosis, neurolabyrinthitis in fourth to fifth decade. AD.

Hemochromatosis (bronze diabetes) – generalized hyperpigmentation. SLC11A3, TFR2, HFE genes; HFE2 and HAMP genes in juvenile forms.

Hemophagocytic syndrome – panniculitis, purpura, hepatosplenomegaly, lymphadenopathy, pancytopenia, high fevers. Associated with viral syndromes (CMV, EBV, VZV).

Henoch–Schönlein purpura – petechiae and palpable purpura (leukocytoclastic vasculitis) especially on legs and buttocks, subcutaneous tissue, joints; GI pain and hemorrhage, painful joint swelling, localized edema of hands and face, hematuria, ± proteinuria, ± IgA vasculitis. Occurs in children often after respiratory infection. Self-limited.

Hepatocutaneous syndrome – firm/reddish papules that leave slightly depressed atrophic scars, occurs with chronic active hepatitis, juvenile cirrhosis or primary biliary cirrhosis.

Hereditary benign intraepithelial dyskeratosis – soft, white asymptomatic thickenings of oral mucosa resembling leukoplakia (not precancerous), bulbar conjunctivitis or pterygium-like lesions. Gene map locus 4q35.

Hermansky–Pudlak syndrome – incomplete albinism with creamy skin color, yellow/red/brown hair, blue-gray to brown eyes; pseudohemophilia; nystagmus; fatal bleeding with aspirin intake, pulmonary changes, colitis. Tyrosinase-positive albinism. AR. HPS1, HPS2, HPS3, HPS4, and APB3B1 genes.

Hidrotic ectodermal dysplasia – see Ectodermal dysplasia (hidrotic).

Hines–Bannick syndrome (episodic hypothermia with hyperhidrosis) – intermittent bouts of low temperature and disabling sweating triggered by awakening or standing that last minutes to hours, diencephalic lesions or malformations.

Horner's syndrome (Bernard–Horner's syndrome, cervical sympathetic paralysis) – ptosis, miosis, ipsilateral anhidrosis of face and neck, increased tearing, enophthalmos, facial hemiatrophy. Can occur as a complication of cervicothoracic sympathectomy.

Howell–Evans syndrome – carcinoma of esophagus, palmoplantar keratoderma, oral leukoplakia. AD or sporadic.

Hunter syndrome (mucopolysaccharidosis type I) – milder than Hurler's syndrome, hypertrichosis, coarse facial features, plaques of confluent papules over scapula, CNS degeneration, hepatosplenomegaly. Increased dermatan sulfate and heparan sulfate in urine. Severe forms fatal by teens, mild form survives up to 60 years of age. X-linked recessive.

Huriez syndrome – scleroderma-like changes of fingers, atrophy of dorsal hands, palmar keratoderma, ± squamous epitheliomas in adolescence, hypohidrosis, internal malignancy, present at birth/early childhood. AD, Belgian ancestry.

Hurler's syndrome (mucopolysaccharidosis type II, gargoylism) – skin with specific papular and nodular lesions, thickening of skin of hands, hypertrichosis, enlarged tongue, dwarfism, bizarre skeletal deformities, hepatosplenomegaly, corneal clouding, mental retardation, deafness, increased dermatan sulfate and heparan sulfate in urine, fatal by age 10. AR.

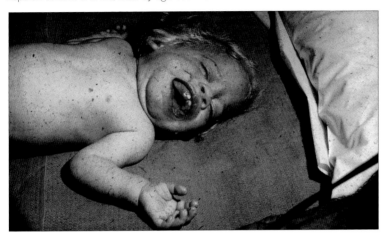

Hutchinson's triad – interstitial keratitis, VIIIth nerve deafness, characteristic incisors and molars. Seen in congenital syphilis.

Hutchinson–Gilford syndrome – *see* Progeria.

Hypereosinophilic syndrome – persistent idiopathic eosinophilia, urticaria, angioedema, dermatographism, fever, diarrhea, malaise, weight loss. Affects middle-aged males.

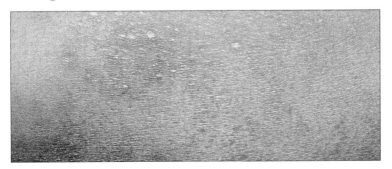

Hyperimmunoglobulin E syndrome (Job's syndrome) – extremely high IgE levels, atopic dermatitis-like eczematous eruption especially of scalp and flexural areas, dystrophic nail changes, red hair, blue eyes, hyperextensible joints, recurrent infections (pulmonary), eosinophilia, osteoporosis. Occurs in females. HIES gene.

Hypomelanosis of Ito – whorled or linear hypopigmentation following Blaschko's lines, secondary to mosaicism present at birth or early childhood; ± CNS, ocular or skeletal abnormalities. Sporadic inheritance.

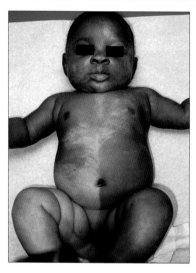

IBIDS syndrome – *see* Trichothiodystrophy.

Ichthyosis
Bullous congenital ichthyosiform erythroderma (epidermolytic hyperkeratosis of Brocq) – erythroderma at birth, then blisters and erosion, accentuated flexures and joints, ± erythroderma, ± palms/soles, odorous, pyogenic infections, postural changes. AD. Keratin 1 and 10. KRT1 and KRT10 genes.

Harlequin ichthyosis – born with thick, yellow–brown plate-like scale that 'encases' at birth; develop deep fissures, cracks; severe ectropion and eclabium, deformed ear, internal organ defects, sepsis, fluid problems, early demise after premature delivery. AR.

Ichthyosis bullosa of Siemens – born with blisters and erythroderma, hyperkeratosis over flexures, palms and soles not involved, skin 'molts'. AD. KRT2e gene.

Ichthyosis hystrix (Curth–Macklin syndrome) – variable palmoplantar keratoderma, verrucous changes over extremities and trunk, digital contractures. AD. KRT1 gene.

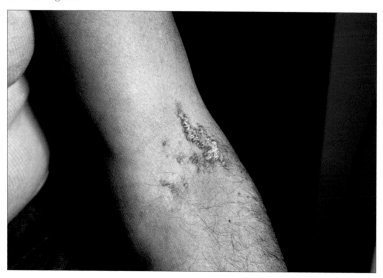

Ichthyosis vulgaris – fine adherent scale on extremities and trunk, spares flexures, hyperlinear palms and soles. AD.

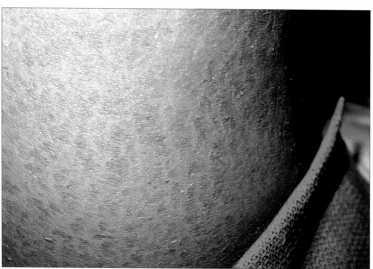

Lamellar ichthyosis – often collodion baby, generalized distribution; large, thick, plate-like, brown scale; absent or mild erythroderma, scarring alopecia, ectropion, heat intolerance. AR. TGM1 gene.

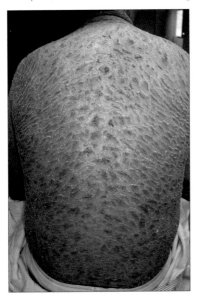

Non-bullous congenital ichthyosiform erythroderma (CIE) – frequent collodion baby; generalized fine, white scale; variable erythroderma, scarring alopecia, rare ectropion, heat intolerance. AR. TGM1, ALOXE3 and ALOX12B genes.
Syndromes with ichthyosis – *see* CHILD syndrome, Conradi–Hünermann–Happle syndrome, Erythrokeratoderma variabilis, KID syndrome, Refsum disease, Sjögren–Larsson syndrome and trichothiodystrophy.

X-linked recessive ichthyosis – fine to large, dark ('dirty') scale on extremities, trunk, neck and face, ± palms and soles, corneal opacities, cryptorchism. X-linked recessive. STS gene.

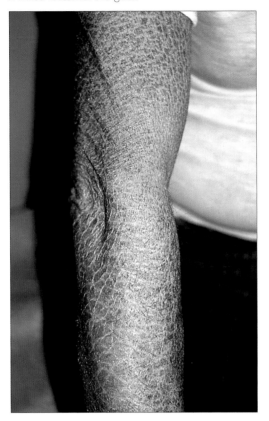

Incontinentia pigmenti (Block–Sulzberger syndrome) – irregular swirling blue/gray to brown pigmentation preceded by bullous and verrucous phases, peripheral blood eosinophilia during initial vesicular stage, skull abnormalities, neurologic changes, mental retardation, ocular changes, bony dental defects. X-linked dominant (short arm of X chromosome), lethal in males. NEMO and IKGKG genes.

Job's syndrome – *see* Hyperimmunoglobulin E syndrome.

Kallman syndrome – ocular albinism, hypogonadism, anosmia.
Kasabach–Merritt syndrome (hemangioma–thrombocytopenia) – giant vascular tumor (kaposiform hemangioendothelioma or tufted hemangioma), thrombocytopenia purpura, consumptive coagulopathy ± disseminated intravascular coagulation, recurrent internal bleeding, anemia. Begins in infancy. 30% mortality, usually self-limited.

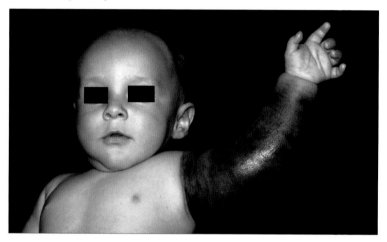

Kawasaki's disease – polymorphous exanthem, edema of hands/feet, erythema of palms/soles, periungual desquamation, acute non-suppurative lymphadenopathy, bilateral conjunctival injection, oropharynx inflamed, strawberry tongue, fever, cardiovascular changes (coronary artery dilatation or aneurysms, arrhythmias, valvular regurgitation), arthralgia, aseptic meningitis, uveitis, hepatic dysfunction.

KID syndrome (keratitis, ichthyosis, deafness) – **K**eratitis that can lead to blindness, **I**chthyosiform erythroderma usually at birth, neurosensory **D**eafness, follicular keratoses, verrucous plaques, nail changes, hypotrichosis, cutaneous infections, impaired sweating, mucosal neoplasms, progeria, short stature, ± mental retardation. AD or AR. GBJ2 gene, connexin 26.

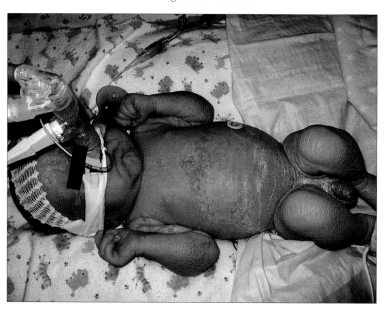

Kimura's syndrome – massive subcutaneous swelling of periauricular and submandibular areas, increased eosinophils, increased IgE, lymphadenopathy. Occurs in Asian females.

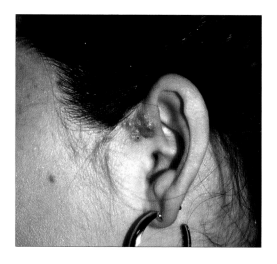

Kindler–Weary syndrome – congenital generalized poikiloderma with bulla that progress to atrophy, acral keratoses.

Kinky hair syndrome – *see* Menkes' syndrome.

Klippel–Trenaunay syndrome (angio-osteohypertrophy syndrome) – congenital vascular malformation of at least one extremity, present at birth as a port-wine stain; hypertrophy of underlying bone and soft tissue, varicosities, scoliosis, visceral venous malformation, ± lymphatic malformations; can be painful. With associated AVMs is referred to as Parkes–Weber syndrome.

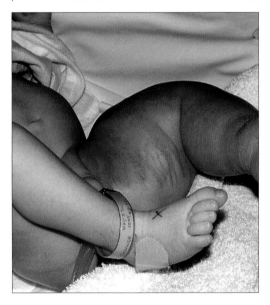

Köbberling–Dunnigan syndrome (congenital partial lipodystrophy) – normal at birth, at puberty loss of fat from extremities sparing face, acanthosis nigricans, hyperhidrosis, menstrual irregularities, increased triglycerides, diabetes mellitus. AD. Chromosome 1q21–22, LMNA mutation. Laminin A/C gene.

LAMB syndrome – *see* Carney syndrome.

Laugier–Hunziker syndrome – acquired pigmentation of nails, labial and buccal mucosa; no systemic associations.

Lawrence syndrome – *see* Acquired generalized lipodystrophy.

Leiner's disease (erythroderma desquamativa) – erythroderma and scaling in first weeks of life, diarrhea, failure to thrive, secondary bacterial infection. Complement (C3 and C5) dysfunction. Some consider it as a severe type of seborrheic dermatitis.

LEOPARD syndrome – **L**entigines, **E**KG changes, **O**cular telorism, **P**ulmonary stenosis, **A**bnormal genitalia, **R**etardation of growth, **D**eafness (sensorineural), low-set ears, dental changes, renal aplasia, webbed fingers. AD with variable expression. PTPN11 and SHP2 genes.

Leschke's syndrome – numerous brownish macules, growth retardation, mental retardation, weakness, hyperglycemia/diabetes, genital hypoplasia, hypothyroidism.

Lesch–Nyhan syndrome – hyperuricemia, severe mental retardation, choreoathetosis, spastic cerebral palsy, tophi on pinnae, self-mutilation, normal at birth, present by 6 months of age. Hypoxanthine guanine phosphoribosyl transferase (HGPRT) deficiency. X-linked recessive.

Leser-Trélat sign – multiple seborrheic keratoses which occur at once (eruptive), can be associated with internal malignancy.

Letterer–Siwe disease (acute disseminated histiocytosis) – type of Langerhans' histiocytosis X, hemorrhagic purpuric macules, papules or red plaques resembling seborrheic dermatitis, moist erosions and ulcers especially in intertriginous areas, hepatosplenomegaly, general lymphadenopathy, eosinophilic granuloma(s) of bone, oral changes, pulmonary involvement, diabetes insipidus, growth hormone deficiency. Onset by age 3.

Lhermitte-Duclos syndrome – abnormal neuronal proliferation of the cerebellum, increased cancers (squamous cell carcinoma, basal cell carcinomas, melanomas, Merkel cell carcinoma, trichilemmomal carcinoma.) AD. PTEN gene.

Libman–Sacks endocarditis – systemic lupus erythematosus, verrucous sterile endocarditis.

Lipoid proteinosis (Urbach–Wiethe disease) – hyaline infiltration into skin, oral cavity, larynx and internal organs; early disease has skin with hemorrhagic crusts, bullae and pustules; yellow papules/nodules on eyelids, face, neck, hands; skin thickening, alopecia, late disease with dark crusty lesions over joints; hoarseness starts in infancy; vocal cord nodules; coarse facies; thick tongue; parotitis; seizures; intracranial calcifications. AR.

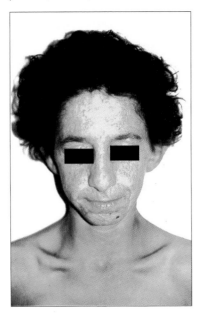

Lobstein's syndrome – *see* Osteogenesis imperfecta.

Löfgren syndrome – erythema nodosum, bilateral hilar lymphadenopathy, acute iritis, polyarthralgias, fever, anergy. Associated with Hodgkin's disease, sarcoidosis and psittacosis.

Loose anagen hair syndrome – loose anagen hairs. Hair exam shows 98–100% anagen hair. Thin, blonde hair. Affects girls aged 2–9 years.

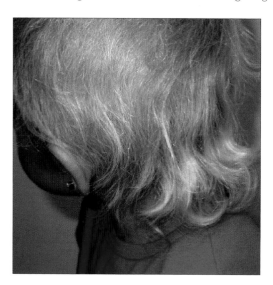

Lubersch–Pick disease (systemic amyloidosis) – amyloidosis with macroglossia, carpal tunnel syndrome, mucocutaneous lesions and visceral involvement.
Lyell syndrome – *see* Toxic epidermal necrolysis.

Madelung disease (multiple symmetric lipomatosis) – multiple large lipomas symmetrically around neck and upper body ('horse collar'), neuropathy. Associated with liver disease, alcoholism, diabetes, upper airway malignancy. AD.
Maffucci's syndrome (Beau–Maffucci syndrome, dyschondroplasia with hemangiomas, Kast–Maffucci syndrome, Kast syndrome) – typically unilateral multiple vascular malformations of skin, 'grape-like' hemangiomas on extremities, mucosae and internal organs, café-au-lait macules, ± vitiligo, bone lesions with frequent fractures, dyschondroplasia, endochondromas down extremities (deep subcutaneous nodules), normal at birth, risk of chondrosarcoma/sarcoma in 50%. Sporadic.
Mal de Meleda syndrome – progressive palmoplantar keratoderma starting shortly after birth with erythema and fissures, hyperkeratosis of elbows and knees, periorificial lesions, malodorous hyperhidrosis. AR. SLURP1 gene.
Malignant down – acquired hypertrichosis lanuginosa associated with internal carcinomas (lung, colon, gall bladder, prostate, uterine, lymphomas). Sudden profuse growth of non-medullated, non-pigmented hair in an adult (see p. 285).
Marfan's syndrome (arachnodactyly) – skin with striae, atrophy, elastosis perforans serpiginosa, subcutaneous fat deficiency; skeletal abnormalities (especially arachnodactyly), ocular lesions, cardiovascular disease (valves, aortic aneurysm), 'thumb sign' with projecting thumb when fist clenched.

kyphoscoliosis, pectus excavatum. AD with variable expression. Fibrillin-1, FBN1 gene.

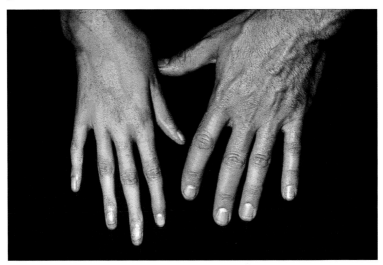

Marfan hand on left with normal hand on right for comparison

Margolis syndrome (Ziprowski–Margolis syndrome) – piebaldism, depigmented hair, heterochromic irides, congenital deafness. X-linked recessive.
Marie–Unna hypotrichosis syndrome – persistent widespread milia of infancy with hereditary trichodysplasia.
Marinesco–Sjögren syndrome – thin and brittle fingernails, cataracts, fine, short scalp hair deficient in pigment, cerebellar ataxia, mental and physical retardation, abnormal teeth, form of trichothiodystrophy. AR.
Maroteaux–Lamy syndrome (mucopolysaccharidosis type VI) – different from Hurler's, severe osseous changes, normal intellect, heart valve disease, increased dermatan sulfate in urine. AR.
Marshall's syndrome – cutis laxa and Sweet's syndrome with alpha-1-antitrypsin deficiency.
Marshall–White syndrome – Bier's spots (pale 1–2 cm macules on forearm or hand formed by occlusion of brachial artery), local palmar ischemia, periodic insomnia bouts, sinus arrhythmia/tachycardia, increased mottling or marbling when hands are lowered. Usually in white, middle-aged men.
Mastocytosis – reddish-brown macules, papules or nodules, Darier's sign (urticates with rubbing), hepatosplenomegaly, GI symptoms, headache, bony osteolytic or sclerotic changes, carcinoid-like symptoms. Types: solitary mastocytosis, urticaria pigmentosa, diffuse infiltrative mastocytosis, systemic mastocytosis, telangiectasia macularis eruptiva perstans (see p. 385).
McCune–Albright syndrome (Albright syndrome, polycystic fibrous dysplasia) – large, segmental café-au-lait macules with 'coast of Maine' border, polycystic fibrous dysplasia of long bones and facial bones often associated with the café-au-lait macules, precocious puberty, hyperthyroidism,

hyperparathyroidism, fractures and bowing of limbs, sclerosis of skull base, ovarian cysts. Female predominance. Sporadic inheritance.

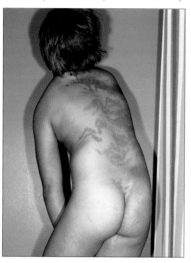

McKusick's syndrome (cartilage–hair hypoplasia) – dwarfism, fine and sparse hair, small nails, bowing of legs, immune incompetence (neutropenia and defective cell-mediated immunity). Amish and Finnish. AR.

Melkersson–Rosenthal syndrome (granulomatous cheilitis) – edema and granuloma formation of lips, recurrent facial paralysis or paresis (CN VII palsy), scrotal tongue, may have fever and malaise, may affect other cranial nerves.

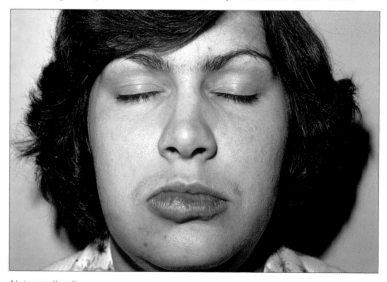

Note swollen lip

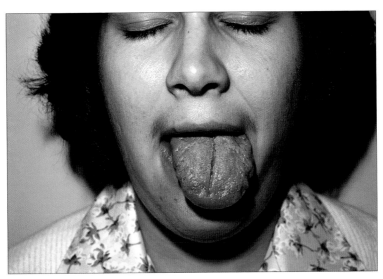

Scrotal tongue with deviation

Mendes da Costa syndrome (erythrokeratoderma) –
see Erythrokeratoderma variabilis.
**Mendes da Costa variant (epidermolysis bullosa simplex, Mendes da
Costa variant)** – epidermolysis bullosa simplex, tense bullae of trunk and limbs,
ocular, reticulate pigmentation with macular atrophy, alopecia, mental and
physical retardation, nails affected. Suprabasal split. X-linked recessive. EBM
gene.
Menkes' syndrome (kinky hair syndrome) – twisted and fractured stubby,
lusterless white hair; pili torti, diffuse hypopigmentation, small stature, severe
mental retardation, seizures, coarse facies, bladder diverticula, osteoporosis,
metaphyseal spurring, wormian skull bones, inconsistent aminoaciduria, low
serum copper and ceruloplasmin, decreased lysyloxidase activity. Early death.
X-linked recessive. Males. ATP7A gene.
Michelin tire baby syndrome – folded skin over body with underlying diffuse
lipomatous or smooth muscle hamartomas. May have other abnormalities of
limbs, face, teeth, and neurologic changes.
MIDAS syndrome – **M**icrophthalmia, **D**ermal **A**plasia, **S**clerocornea.
Mikulicz disease – bilateral painless enlargement of salivary and lacrimal glands,
xerostomia, decreased/absent lacrimation, parotitis. May be caused by
sarcoidosis.
Milroy syndrome – congenital lymphedema affecting legs and/or arms. AD.
Mondor's disease – superficial vein phlebitis in pectoral region, history of
trauma or association with breast cancer. More common in women. Can also
occur on penis.
Monilethrix syndrome – spindle/beaded hair formation primarily on scalp,
keratosis pilaris, koilonychias, dental changes, mild mental retardation, cataracts
Variable age of onset, usually in childhood. AD or AR.
Montgomery's syndrome – xanthoma disseminatum, benign and normolipemic
form of histiocytoxanthomatosis affecting skin and mucous membranes.

Hundreds of red–brown then yellowish papules that are symmetrical on trunk, face and proximal extremities coalescing into verrucous plaques. Dyspnea and dysphagia. Associated with diabetes insipidus, multiple myeloma and Waldenström's macroglobulinemia. Males more than females, usual onset before 25 years.

Morbihan's syndrome – solid facial edema with secondary distortion due to acne or rosacea.

Morgani–Stewart–Morel syndrome (Morgani syndrome) – symmetrical benign thickening of inner table of skull frontal bone, obesity, hirsutism, neurologic symptoms, progressive visual failure, primarily in women of middle age or elderly.

Morquio syndrome (mucopolysaccharidosis type IV) – differs from Hurler's, severe distinctive bone malformations and aortic regurgitation, thickened skin, café-au-lait macules, facial and limb telangiectasias, short stature, sternal protrusion, intellect normal to slightly retarded, urine with keratan sulfate. Fatal secondary to cervical spine complications. AR.

Morvan syndrome – recurrent painless finger/paronychial infections with perforating ulcers, progressive sensory loss, resorption of phalanges. Associated with syringomyelia or occasionally leprosy.

Moynahan syndrome – ectodermal dysplasia with xeroderma, dry and slow growing hair, teeth with enamel defects, nail dystrophy, hypohidrosis, skin blisters, photophobia, cleft palate, mild mental retardation. AD.

Mucha–Habermann syndrome (pityriasis lichenoides et varioliformis acuta, PLEVA) – fever, malaise, lymphadenopathy, macules, vesicles and papulonecrotic lesions, varioliform scars. May last months to years.

Muckle–Wells syndrome (hereditary familial amyloidosis) – recurrent urticaria, fever, progressive deafness, arthritis. One-third may progress to amyloidosis with cutaneous and renal involvement. Progressive, beginning in childhood. AD. Chromosome 1q. CIAS 1 gene.

Muir–Torre syndrome – multiple sebaceous gland neoplasms, multiple keratoacanthomas, thyroid disease, uterine fibroids, prostatic hyperplasia, renal cysts, carpal tunnel syndrome, malignancies (GI colon, GU, lungs). AD. MSH gene.

Multiple endocrine neoplasia syndromes – Type 1 (Werner syndrome) with pancreatic tumors, parathyroid hyperplasia/tumors, pituitary adenomas, adrenal adenomas, thyroid disease, thymomas, carcinoid tumors, lipoma, gastric polyps, schwannomas, AD, MEN1 gene. Type 2 or 2A (Sipple syndrome) with pruritic skin lesions over scapula, parathyroid hyperplasia or tumor, medullary thyroid cancer, pheochromocytoma, AD, RET gene. Type 3 or 2B (mucosal neuroma syndrome) with large, bumpy lips, café-au-lait macules, medullary thyroid cancer, pheochromocytoma, neuromas from lip to rectum, marfanoid body with joint laxity and kyphoscoliosis, early death from thyroid cancer, AD or sporadic, RET gene.

Multiple lentigines syndrome – see LEOPARD syndrome.

Myotonic dystrophy (Steinert's syndrome) – atrophy of skin, panniculus and musculature, hypogonadism, hypotrichosis, immobile face, scoliosis, tonic muscle spasms, heart conduction defects, cataracts, premature aging. AD with variable expression.

Naegeli–Franceschetti–Jadassohn syndrome – see Franceschetti–Jadassohn syndrome.

Nail–patella syndrome (congenital iliac horns, Fong's hereditary onycho-osteodysplasia) – onychodystrophy with triangular lunulae, usually spares toenails, absent or rudimentary patellae, iliac horns, congenital dislocation of head of radius, renal problems, skin laxity, Lester's iris (cloverleaf pigmentation). AD. LMX1B gene.

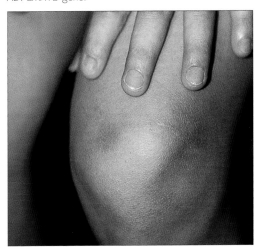

NAME syndrome – **N**evi (blue), **A**trial myxoma, **M**yxoid neurofibromas, **E**phelides. AD.
Naxos syndrome – diffuse non-epidermolytic palmoplantar keratoderma with wooly hair and cardiac myopathy.
Nelson's syndrome – diffuse hyperpigmentation caused by MSH-producing pituitary tumor.
Neonatal cold injury – feeding difficulty, lethargy, cold to touch, immobility, pitting edema, strikingly red hands/feet/cheeks, rectal temp <33°C. Rare in developed countries. Due to cold exposure in small neonates.
Netherton's syndrome – congenital ichthyosiform erythroderma, ichthyosis linearis circumflexa, 'bamboo' hair/trichorrhexis invaginata, atopy, short stature, elevated IgE, impaired cellular immunity, inconsistent aminoaciduria. AR.

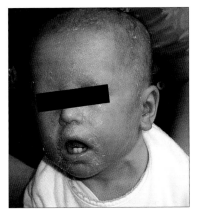

***Neurofibromatosis (four types with varied features, types 1 and 2 most
common)*** – café-au-lait macules, neurofibromas, axillary freckling (Crowe's sign),
endocrine changes, ocular changes (Lisch nodules), other dermal tumors, bone
changes. AD/sporadic. Diagnostic criteria for NF type 1 (von Recklinghausen
disease) – two or more of the following must be present: six or more café-au-
lait macules >5 mm prepubertal and >15 mm postpubertal; two or more
neurofibromas of any type or one plexiform neurofibroma; freckling in the axillary
region (Crowe's sign); optic gliomas; two or more Lisch nodules (ocular
hamartomas); osseous lesion (e.g. sphenoid wing dysplasia or thinning of long
bone cortex, with or without pseudoarthritis; and/or first-degree relative with
NF1 by the above criteria. NF1 gene (type 1) and NF2 gene (type 2).

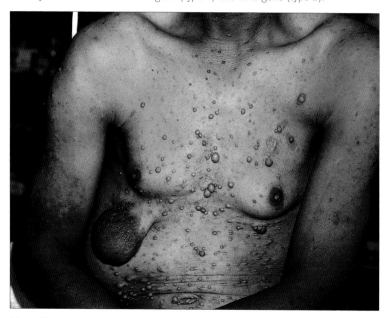

Neurofibromas

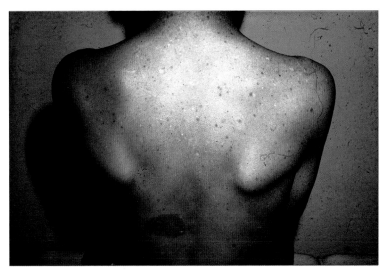

Multiple café-au-lait macules

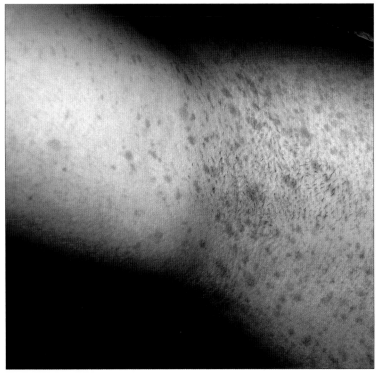

Axillary freckling – Crowe's sign

Nevus of Ito – blue-gray hyperpigmentation over supraclavicular and lateral brachial nerves.

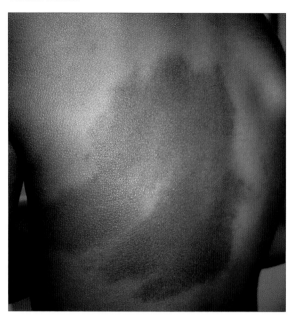

Nevus of Ota (oculocutaneous pigmentation) – benign blue-gray pigmentation of skin of face, ipsilateral eye and adnexa, distribution of first and second divisions of trigeminal nerve (see p. 434).
Nevus sebaceus syndrome – nevus sebaceus usually with extensive facial involvement, seizures, mental retardation, skeletal defects and ocular abnormalities.
Niemann–Pick disease – xanthomas, skin pigmentation, indurated skin, malnutrition and retarded development, hepatosplenomegaly, lymphadenopathy, ataxia, cherry-red retina. Sphingomyelinase deficiency. AR.
Nonne–Milroy–Meige syndrome – see Milroy syndrome.
Noonan syndrome – keratosis pilaris atrophicans, lymphedema, nevi, short stature, pterygium colli, abnormal facies, pulmonary valve stenosis and cardiac defects, skeletal and testicular defects. AD. PTPNII gene.

Oculocerebral hypopigmentation (Cross syndrome) – hypopigmentation resembling albinism with white to pink color, yellow metallic hair, ocular abnormalities, mental retardation, spastic, athetoid movement, growth retardation. AR. Tyrosinase-positive albinism.
Oculodentodigital dysplasia (ODD, Meyer–Schwickerath–Gruterich–Weyers syndrome) – microphthalmos, small nose, dental anomalies, hypotrichosis, fifth finger camptodactyly, syndactyly of fourth and fifth fingers, missing toe phalanges. Mutation in connexin-43 gene.
Ofuji's syndrome (eosinophilic pustular folliculitis) – sterile, eosinophilic pustules coalescing into papule or plaques, distribution face and upper trunk, eosinophilia, lymphadenopathy, steroid-responsive. Young males, Japanese or AIDS patients.

Oid-Oid disease – *see* Sulzberger–Garbe syndrome.

Ollier's syndrome – dyschrondoplasia with vascular malformation.

Olmsted's syndrome – severe mutilating palmoplantar keratoderma, digital constrictions, linear keratoses of limbs, nail changes, dental changes, growth retardation, hyperkeratosis periorally.

Omenn's syndrome – *see* severe combined immunodeficiency (SCID).

Oral–facial–digital (OFD) syndrome – Type I with widespread milia of infancy, abnormally developed frenuli, cleft lip and plate, skull malformations, abnormal tongue, mental retardation, syndactyly, patchy alopecia, granular facial skin appearance, polycystic kidneys. X-linked dominant (lethal in males) or AR. CXORF5 gene on chromosome Xp22.3–22.2.

Osler–Weber–Rendu syndrome (hereditary hemorrhagic telangiectasia) – telangiectasias (often mat-like) occur on face including lips, upper body, nail beds, mucosa, GI tract and retina; GI bleeds, epistaxis, CNS vascular anomalies, anemia, hepatomegaly and pulmonary AVMs. AD. Endoglin gene product. END gene.

Osteogenesis imperfecta (four types) – may include bone fragility, atrophic skin, bruising, joint laxity, blue sclerae, arcus senilis, otosclerosis, enamel defects, fine hair, short stature, mitral valve prolapse. Caused by defect in Type I collagen.

Pachyonychia congenita – Type I (Jadassohn–Lewandowsky syndrome): oral, nail and palmoplantar keratoderma, non-premalignant leukoplakia, Keratin 6a and 16 (KRT6A and KRT16 genes); Type II (Jackson–Lawler syndrome): natal teeth, steatocystoma multiplex, nail changes, and palmoplantar keratoderma, Keratin 6b and 17 (KRT6B and KRT17 genes); Type III (Schafer–Brunauer syndrome): like type I with addition of leukokeratosis of cornea; Type IV (pachyonychia congenita tarda/late onset): hyperpigmentation around neck, waist, axillae, thighs, flexures of knees/buttocks/abdomen.

PAPA syndrome – **P**yogenic **A**rthritis, **P**yoderma gangrenosum, **A**cne.

Papillon–Lefèvre syndrome – palmoplantar hyperkeratosis, periodontosis with tooth loss, skin pyodermas, hyperhidrosis, dura calcification. Onset in childhood. AR.

Papular–purpuric gloves and socks syndrome – pruritic erythema and edema of hands and feet, oral lesions, petechiae, purpura, fever, self-limiting. Associated with viral infection – including parvovirus B19 (erythrovirus) – and drugs.

Parinaud oculoglandular syndrome – granulomatous lesion of conjunctiva, usually unilateral, low grade fever, preauricular lymphadenopathy. Caused by cat-scratch disease, tuberculosis, tularemia, sarcoidosis, sporotrichosis or others.

Parkes–Weber syndrome – same as Klippel–Trenaunay syndrome with associated AVM.

Parkinson's disease – seborrheic dermatitis, muscular rigidity, immobile facies, tremor, salivation.

Parry–Romberg syndrome – progressive hemifacial atrophy of skin, fat, muscle; contralateral Jacksonian seizures; trigeminal neuralgia; eye and hair changes.

Peutz–Jeghers (periorificial lentiginosis) – lentigines in and around body orifices and on digits, general intestinal polyposis, abdominal pain with intussusception, ovarian tumors, clubbing of digits, carcinoma of GI and breast. AD. STK11, LKB1 and PJS genes.

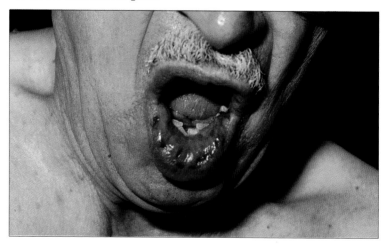

PHACE syndrome – **P**osterior fossa Dandy–Walker malformation, **H**emangioma, **A**rterial abnormalities, **C**ardiac abnormalities and coarctation of aorta, **E**ye abnormalities.

Phakomatosis pigmentovascularis – all types have nevus flammeus (PWS), increased in Asians, ± nevus anemicus, ± systemic abnormalities (CNS, visceral, ocular, hypertrophied limb). Type I with vascular malformations and epidermal nevus; Type II with vascular malformation and Mongolian spot; Type III with vascular malformation, nevus spilus and ± granular cell tumor; Type IV with vascular malformation, nevus spilus and Mongolian spot.

Phenylketonuria – generalized hyperpigmentation, blue eyes, blonde hair, eczema, sclerodermoid changes, urine with mousy odor, mental retardation, seizures, spastic reflexes. Present at birth. AR.

PIBIDS – *see* Trichothiodystrophy.

Pigmented purpuric eruptions/dermatoses

Ducas and Kapetanakis pigmented purpura – scaly and papular purpura distinguished by spongiosis on pathology.

Gougerot–Blum syndrome (pigmented purpuric lichenoid dermatosis) – minute, rust-colored lichenoid papules that can coalesce into plaques. May occur on legs, thighs, lower trunk.

Lichen aureus – sudden appearance of one or more golden or rust-colored patches of lichenoid papules. May be painful. No itch.

Majocchi's disease (purpura annular telangiectoides) – begins with asymptomatic bluish-red annular macules that fade with central involution and peripheral extension to concentric rings. Spreads symmetrically on lower extremities then to trunk and arms. May take a year to resolve.

Schamberg's disease – pinpoint, red puncta, 'cayenne-pepper', slow proximal extension that then fades over a few months.

Piebaldism – depigmented segmental macules especially on chest, upper extremities and forehead; poliosis (white forelock). AD. cKit defect, KIT gene.

Pierre Robin syndrome – micrognathia, glossoptosis, cleft palate, fine and light hair.

Pink disease (mercury poisoning) – pink tips of finger/toes/nose, painful hands/feet, pruritus, photophobia, paralysis, profuse salivation/sweating, elevated blood pressure, disorder of infancy/childhood. Fatal if not treated.

PLEVA syndrome – *see* Mucha-Habermann syndrome.

Plummer–Vinson syndrome (Paterson–Kelly syndrome) – atrophy of mucosa (mouth, pharynx, tongue, esophagus), dysphagia, thinning of lips and angular cheilitis, koilonychias, microcytic hypochromic anemia, risk of oral cancers. Middle-aged females.

POEMS syndrome (Crow–Fukase syndrome) – **P**olyneuropathy, **O**rganomegaly, **E**ndocrinopathy (diabetes, hypothyroid, increased prolactin), **M**onoclonal protein (plasma cell tumor), **S**kin changes (sclerodermatous, diffuse pigmentation, edema, clubbing, leukonychia, hypertrichosis, hyperhidrosis), ± associated cutaneous glomeruloid hemangioma.

Polycystic ovary syndrome (Stein–Leventhal syndrome) – dysfunctional ovaries with menstrual irregularities, hirsutism, acne, androgenetic alopecia, acanthosis nigricans, obesity.

Porokeratosis

Disseminated superficial actinic porokeratosis (DSAP) – superficial, annular, keratotic, red–brown macules with a ridged edge. Occurs in sun-exposed areas, particularly arms and legs. More common in women (see p. 90).

Linear porokeratosis – linear lesions that can present as erosions or ulcerations at birth. High risk of malignancy see p. 266.

Plaque type (Mibelli) – chronic, progressive with slightly atrophic macules and patches with an elevated border. Occurs on hands, feet, ankles, scalp, face, buccal mucosa, glans penis.

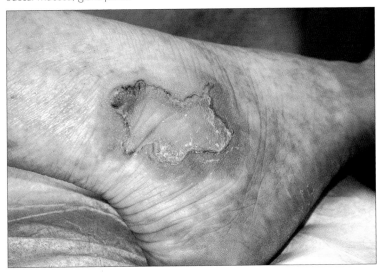

Porokeratosis palmaris plantaris et disseminata – lesions begin on palms and soles then progress over body. Often begins in twenties.

Porphyrias
Acute intermittent porphyria (AIP) – no skin lesions; acute periodic attacks of GI pain, paralysis and psychiatric changes. AD. Porphobilinogen deaminase defect.
Congenital erythropoietic porphyria (CEP, Gunther's disease) – presents at birth, severe burning and bulla of skin immediately upon sun exposure, red urine, red abnormal teeth, ectropion, diffuse hypertrichosis, scarring, anemia, thrombocytopenia, gallstones, brittle bones. AR. Uroporphyrinogen III cosynthase defect. UROS gene.
Erythropoietic protoporphyria (EPP) – immediate burning of skin on exposure to sunlight, chronic 'weathered skin', red edematous wheals, plaques and purpura. Child or adult onset. AD and AR. Ferrochelatase defect. FECH gene.
Hepatic erythropoietic porphyria (HEP) – infant with dark urine and vesicles in sun-exposed distribution. Hypertrichosis, scarring, sclerodermoid skin changes, ectropion and nail changes. Coral red fluorescence of teeth. AD. Uroporphyrinogen decarboxylase defect. UROD gene.
Hereditary coproporphyria (HCP) – some photosensitivity, GI and neurologic symptoms (a mix between AIP and VP). AD. Coproporphyrinogen oxidase defect. CPO gene.
Porphyria cutanea tarda (PCT) – bulla, sun-exposed distribution, hypertrichosis of face, scars with milia, sclerodermoid skin changes, alopecia. Associated with liver disease, SLE, HIV, hepatitis, OCP and hemochromatosis; coral red fluorescence of urine with Wood's light. Sporadic, familial or acquired. Uroporphyrinogen decarboxylase deficiency (see p. 46).
Variegate porphyria (VP) – bulla in sun-exposed distribution with neurologic and GI symptoms. Hypertrichosis, scarring and sclerodermoid changes. AD. Protoporphyrinogen oxidase defect. PPOX gene.

Postphlebitic syndrome – ulcer (often painless), pigmentation with characteristic stasis-like dermatitis, induration/lymphedema especially above internal malleolus. Occurs soon or decades after pelvic, thigh or leg DVT; development of collateral veins.
Pretibial fever (leptospirosis, Fort Bragg fever) – anicteric leptospirosis, with high fever, nausea, vomiting and headache that lasts 3–7 days, then fever decreases and erythematous exanthem appears on shins for 4–7 days.
Pringle's syndrome – see Tuberous sclerosis.

Progeria (Hutchinson–Gilford syndrome, premature senility) – dwarfism, alopecia of head, brows, and lashes; scleroderma-like skin and pinched facies, premature aging, high-pitched voice, micrognathia, small dystrophic nails. Live to age 10–15 years. AR or sporadic.

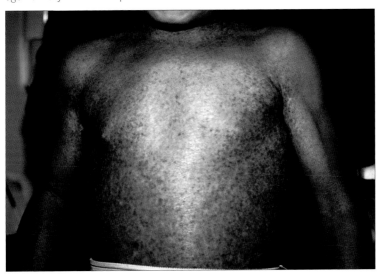

Proteus syndrome – asymmetrical overgrowth of body parts with cerebriform hyperplasia of skin especially over plantar surfaces, epidermal nevi, vascular malformation (port-wine stain), lipomas, ocular changes, skeletal changes, normal mental status, testicular tumors, linear or whorled hyper- or hypopigmentation.

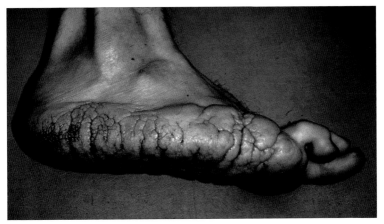

Pseudoxanthoma elasticum (Grönblad–Strandberg syndrome) – disorder of elastic tissue, six types which can include lax skin, yellow papules, vascular abnormalities, ocular abnormalities, strokes, hypertension, loose joints. AD or AR. AR type with gene map locus MRP6 and ABCC6 (see p. 387).

Ramsay Hunt syndrome (herpes zoster oticus) – herpes zoster affecting the external auditory canal with edema and swelling of cranial nerve VIII (auditory) and pressure on cranial nerve V (facial) resulting in facial palsy which can be permanent; vertigo, tinnitus, deafness, changed taste sensation in anterior two-thirds of tongue.

Red man syndrome – diffuse erythematous morbilliform eruption, red skin/urine/feces/sweat, pruritus, hypotension, tachycardia, respiratory discomfort. Histamine-induced flushing secondary to rapid infusion or overdose of rifampin or vancomycin.

Refsum disease – ichthyosiform eruption with small, white scales covering extremities and trunk; can have thicker scales or hyperkeratosis on palms and soles, chronic polyneuritis, atypical retinitis pigmentosa with night blindness, progressive nerve deafness, cerebellar ataxia, EKG changes. CSF with elevated protein content, cannot degrade phytanic acid secondary to deficiency of phytanic acid oxidase. AR. PHYH and PAHX genes.

Reiter's syndrome (urethro-oculo-synovial syndrome) – psoriasiform changes, lesions like erythema multiforme or keratoderma blennorrhagica (scales on palms, soles, glans penis), nails with oil-drop changes, polyarthritis (primarily sacroiliac and lower extremities), conjunctivitis, non-specific urethritis, circinate balanitis. Primarily in young men. Seronegative for rheumatoid factor. Associated with enteritis or venereal disease, especially HIV.

Reye's syndrome (acute encephalopathy with fatty degeneration of liver) – erythematous, ± papular or vesicular eruption, sudden vomiting, fever, seizures, coma. Often associated with varicella in children, particularly when given aspirin. Occurs 2–7 days after onset of eruption.

Richner–Hanhart syndrome (tyrosinemia type II, oculocutaneous tyrosinemia) – painful punctate palmoplantar keratoses appear early in life, prepatellar keratoses, herpetiform corneal dystrophy, glaucoma, photophobia, progressive mental retardation, growth failure. AR. Hepatic tyrosine aminotransferase deficiency, increased in Italians. TAT gene.

Riley–Day syndrome (familial autonomic dysfunction, familial dysautonomia) – intermittent erythematous patches while eating or with excitement, excessive sweating/drooling in infancy, failure to tear with crying, impaired esophageal and pharyngeal motility, absent corneal and deep tendon reflexes, delayed growth, acrocyanosis of hands and feet, absence of tongue papillae, abnormal histamine test with no flare. Most common in Ashkenazi Jewish descent. AR.

Riley–Smith syndrome – subcutaneous and cutaneous hemangiomas, macrocephaly without hydrocephaly, pseudopapilledema, respiratory infections. AD.

Robert's syndrome – facial port-wine stain, hypomelia, hypotrichosis, growth retardation, cleft lip.

Rombo syndrome – atrophoderma vermiculatum, milia, hypotrichosis, multiple trichoepitheliomas and BCCs, peripheral cyanosis. AD.

Rosenthal–Kloepfer syndrome – corneal leukomata, acromegaloid face, hands and feet, cutis verticis gyrata starting in fourth or fifth decade, large hands and feet.

Rothmann–Makai syndrome – spontaneous circumscribed panniculitis on trunk and extremities, afebrile, no systemic association. Most common in children.

Rothmund–Thomson syndrome (poikiloderma congenitale) – infantile poikiloderma, juvenile cataracts, short stature and congenital bone defects, disturbances of hair growth with sparse fine hair, nail dystrophy, photosensitivity, hyperkeratosis of palms/soles/hands/wrists/ankles, hypogonadism, predisposition to squamous cell cancers. Normal life span. AR with female predominance. DNA helicase abnormality.

Rowell syndrome (Rowell–Beck–Anderson syndrome) – discoid lupus-like or erythema multiforme-like lesions, chilblains.

Rubella syndrome (congenital rubella syndrome, blueberry muffin baby) – erythematous or violaceous infiltrated macules and papules (dermal erythropoiesis) within first two days of life, deafness, cataracts, cardiac defects, IUGR, growth failure, mental retardation, cutis marmorata, seborrhea. Due to fetus contracting rubella before 20th week of life.

Rubenstein–Taybi syndrome – broad thumbs and great toes, facial abnormalities, mental and psychomotor retardation, port-wine stains, GU anomalies, cardiac anomalies, hypertrichosis, highly arched palate, down-slanting palpebral fissures, crowded teeth, beak nose, long eyelashes and heavy brows.

Rud syndrome – ichthyosis, hypogonadism, mental deficiency, seizures. (Some feel that disease is not well defined and its spectrum is consistent with steroid sulfatase deficiency/X-linked recessive ichthyosis.)

Russell–Silver syndrome – café-au-lait macules, diffuse pigmentation, short stature, congenital asymmetry, premature sexual development, normal intelligence, frontal bossing, triangular face, excess sweating, GU anomalies. Sporadic inheritance.

Sanfilippo syndrome (mucopolysaccharidosis type III, subtypes A–D) – differs from Hurler's, somatic effects mild, CNS effects severe, coarse blond hair, hypertrichosis, develop normally to age 3–4 then miss developmental milestones, behavior problems, macrocephaly. Urinary heparan-N-sulfate. AR.

Sarcoidosis (Schaumann's syndrome) – erythema nodosum, papules and/or nodules (perinasal and periocular two common areas), other cutaneous lesions (annular, psoriasiform, subcutaneous), lesions in scars, lupus pernio (sarcoid of face and nose), ocular changes (uveitis, conjunctivitis, lacrimal gland enlargement), bilateral hilar adenopathy, lymphadenopathy, osteitis, hypercalcemia, hypercalciuria, CNS involvement, arthritis, cardiac changes (arrhythmia, heart block), renal changes, increased ACE levels (see also Heerfordt syndrome, Löfgren syndrome and Mikulicz disease).

Savill's syndrome (epidemic exfoliative dermatitis) – dry or moist exfoliative dermatitis of face, scalp and upper extremities, epidemics in institutions.

Scheie syndrome (mucopolysaccharidosis type IS) – differs from Hurler's, stiff joints, aortic regurgitation, intellect normal/decreased, corneal opacities, onset by age 5. Urine with dermatan sulfate and heparan sulfate. AR. Alpha-L-iduronidase deficiency.

Schnitzler's syndrome – urticarial vasculitis, increased IgM, fever, bone pain.

Schopf–Schulz–Passarge syndrome – multiple hydrocystomas of eyelids, hypotrichosis, hypodontia and nail abnormalities.

Seip–Lawrence syndrome – see Acquired generalized lipodystrophy.

Senear–Usher syndrome (pemphigus erythematosus) – variant of pemphigus foliaceous, crusted, red malar plaques, ± crusted bullous lesions (impetigo contagiosa-like) on chest and extremities, seborrheic or eczema related changes, positive Nikolsky sign, photosensitive, can be induced by penicillamine. May be associated with myasthenia gravis or thymoma.

Setleis syndrome – round, bitemporal aplasia cutis congenita (focal dermal dysplasia), abnormal eyelashes and upward slanting eyebrows, leonine faces. AD.

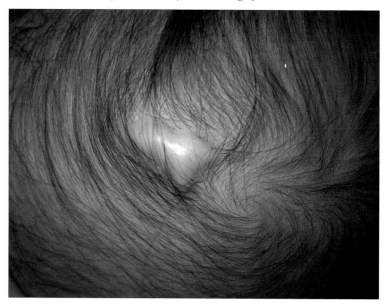

Severe combined immunodeficiency (SCID, Omenn's syndrome) – seborrheic dermatitis or eczema, cutaneous infection, erythroderma, alopecia (can include eyebrows and eyelashes), morbilliform eruption, graft-versus-host disease, pneumonia, diarrhea, failure to thrive. Abnormal thymus. Marked T- and B-cell deficiencies. RAG 1 and 2 gene.

Sézary syndrome – general exfoliative erythroderma, intense pruritus, pigmentation, benign lymphadenopathy, monocytosis, alopecia, splenomegaly, palmoplantar keratoderma, onychodystrophy, hepatomegaly. Peripheral blood with 10% or more Sézary cells (atypical cells with cerebriform nuclei).

Sheehan syndrome (post-partum pituitary necrosis) – increasing lassitude/lethargy, decreased appetite, wasting, alopecia, wrinkled skin, onycholysis with ridging and brown discoloration of nail plate, loss of axillary and pubic hair. May be associated with discoid lupus erythematosus.

Shell nail syndrome – shell-like nail deformities (like clubbed nail but with nail bed atrophy), associated with bronchiectasis.

Shoulder–hand syndrome – painful shoulder disability (usually on left side) that occurs with erythema, sweat, tenderness, pain, hand immobility. Vasomotor changes with hand swelling cause later dystrophic changes of hands and fingers.

Shulman syndrome – see Eosinophilic fasciitis.

Sickle cell disease (Dresbach's syndrome, Herrick's syndrome) – chronic hemolytic anemia, chronic leg ulcers, green sclerae, bone and joint pain, 'pain crisis' (extremity swelling, fever, pallor), weakness and dyspnea, acute abdominal pain attacks, recurrent hand and foot swelling, jaw deformities, osteomyelitis, jaundice, splenomegaly, hyposthenuria (inability to concentrate urine). Howell–Jolly bodies in RBCs.

Siemens syndrome (keratoderma palmoplantaris striata) – striate palmoplantar keratoderma, may extend onto body, deafness. Hair, teeth and mucous membranes normal. AD.

Silver syndrome – *see* Russell–Silver syndrome.

Sjögren syndrome (Sicca syndrome) – dry skin/mucous membranes/conjunctiva, rheumatoid arthritis, anemia, ± scleroderma-like changes, alopecia, telangiectasias, swelling of lacrimal/salivary glands, Schirmer test (lack of tearing). Associated with rheumatoid arthritis, lupus erythematosus, scleroderma. Anti-Ro (SSA) and/or anti-La (SSB) positive.

Sjögren–Larsson syndrome – congenital ichthyosiform erythroderma or collodion baby, mental deficiency, central spastic diplegia, degenerative retinitis, dry hair, palmoplantar hyperkeratosis, short stature, skeletal changes, dental changes. Fatty alcohol:NAD deficiency causing fat accumulation in cells. AR. FALDH and ALDH3A2 genes.

Sneddon syndrome – livedo reticularis, occlusive vascular disease, transient hypertension, CNS symptoms (stroke, TIA, headache). Young to middle age, progressive, ± antiphospholipid antibody, negative ANA.

Sneddon–Wilkinson syndrome (subcorneal pustular dermatosis) – sterile pustules in annular or gyrate groups favoring abdomen, groin or axillae; subcorneal neutrophilic abscesses, lesions dry or crust within few days; ± IgA paraproteinemia. Favors women aged 40–50.

Spannlang–Tappeiner syndrome – palmoplantar keratosis, partial or total alopecia, tongue-shaped corneal opacities related to lipid infiltration of cornea, hyperhidrosis.

Sphenopalatine syndrome – chronic and intermittent facial edema, lacrimation on affected side, ± occasional rhinitis, paroxysms of swelling alternating with erythema on side of bridge of nose

Staphylococcal scalded skin syndrome (SSSS, Ritter's disease) – initial widespread erythema and edema, extensive loosening of skin with/without bullae, desquamation with raw, red, oozing skin; vomiting, diarrhea, sore throat, conjunctiva, fever, pain. Neonatal mortality. Caused by exfoliative toxin of *Staphylococcus aureus*, Gram stain negative.

Stein–Leventhal syndrome – *see* Polycystic ovary syndrome.

Stevens–Johnson syndrome (SJS, erythema multiforme major) – targetoid, vesicobullous, petechial, hemorrhagic widespread lesions (erythema multiforme); fever and severe constitutional symptoms, including diarrhea; involvement of at least two mucosal surfaces (oral, genital, ocular, anal, rectal); onycholysis; renal involvement. Etiologies include HSV, drug, infection, other. (Some now refer to SJS-TEN complex because of overlapping features.)

Stewart–Treves syndrome – angiosarcoma arising in lymphedema due to edematous upper extremity following radical mastectomy.

Stiff-skin syndrome (congenital facial dystrophy) – rock hard skin, mild hirsutism, joint stiffness, lung dysfunction. AD.

Still's disease (juvenile rheumatoid arthritis) – eruption of macules/papules with irregular margins and pallor on trunk and extremities appearing at midday with high fever, subcutaneous nodules, arthritis, acute onset in childhood, chronic iridocyclitis, splenomegaly, lymphadenopathy.

Sturge–Weber syndrome (encephalotrigeminal angiomatosis, Sturge–Kalischer–Weber syndrome) – (1) vascular malformation of leptomeninges (often over parietal and occipital lobes) causing seizures, contralateral deafness and paralysis; (2) ipsilateral port-wine stain along superior and middle branches of trigeminal nerve (40% may have PWS); (3) mental retardation; (4) ocular changes (glaucoma, retinal detachment, blindness);

(5) vascular malformations of viscera. Train-track calcifications of peripheral cerebral cortex seen on imaging.

Sudeck's atrophy – occurs with reflex sympathetic dystrophy, acute pain, atrophy of skin/subcutaneous tissue/bone. Changes occur at site of minor injury.

Sulzberger–Garbe syndrome (Oid-Oid disease) – chronic exudative discoid and lichenoid dermatitis, severe nocturnal pruritus. Occurs in middle-aged Jewish males.

Superior vena cava syndrome – marked facial and eyelid edema, band of dilated blood vessels around lower chest wall, gynecomastia. Obstruction of superior vena cava/main tributaries.

Sweet's syndrome (acute febrile neutrophilic dermatosis) – raised painful violaceous plaques or nodules on limbs/face/neck, sterile pustules, fever, variable headache, vomiting, abdominal pain and prostration, increased PMNs. Histopathology shows neutrophils, not true vasculitis. Middle-aged women most common group. Associated with leukemia, lymphoma, ulcerative colitis, carcinoma, cellulitis, URIs.

Takahara's syndrome (acatalasemia) – progressive ulcers/gangrene of gingiva and alveolar bone, exfoliation of teeth, blood turns dark brown with H_2O_2 contact (no foaming). AR. Defect of blood and catalase activity.

TAR syndrome – **T**hrombocytopenia, **A**plasia of radius, **P**ort-wine stain.

Tetralogy of Fallot – group of congenital cardiac defects (pulmonary stenosis, dextroposition of aorta, VSD, RV hypertrophy), cyanosis of lips and nail beds, finger clubbing, gums red and swollen, ± cheek telangiectasia, squatting posture, hyperpnea, dyspnea on exertion.

Thrombotic thrombocytopenic purpura – thrombocytopenia, purpura, fever, hemolytic anemia (jaundice, pallor), CNS disturbance (headaches, confusion), renal changes.

Thyroid acropachy – triad of digital clubbing, soft tissue swelling of hands/feet and new periosteal bone formation. Increased thyroidism with exophthalmos, pretibial myxedema, clubbing, and usually painless hyperosteoarthropathy.

Tietz's syndrome – albinism, deaf mutism, eyebrow hypoplasia, no ocular changes.

Tooth and nail syndrome (Witkop syndrome) – absent or very small, thin, spoon-shaped nails, missing teeth (second molars, mandibular incisors and maxillary canines), lack of other ectodermal defects/associated disease. MSX1 gene.

TORCH syndrome – cutaneous changes (petechiae, purpura, vesicles, icterus), small for gestational age, neurologic changes, ocular changes, cardiac defects, hepatosplenomegaly, pneumonitis. Intrauterine infections with **T**oxoplasma, **O**ther (*Treponema pallidum*), **R**ubella, **C**ytomegalovirus, **H**SV.

Torre–Muir syndrome – see Muir–Torre syndrome.

Touraine–Solente–Gole syndrome (pachydermoperiostosis) – cutis verticis gyrata of scalp/forehead/face, finger and toe clubbing, hypertrophic skin changes begin at puberty, sebaceous hyperplasia, hyperhidrosis, periosteal lesions and long bone hypertrophy, mental retardation. Primary form is AD.

Toxic epidermal necrolysis (TEN, Lyell syndrome) – entire epidermis becomes necrotic, begins with inflammation of eyelids/conjunctiva/mouth/genitalia, tender/erythematous skin, positive Nikolsky sign, affects internal organs, fever, malaise, anorexia. High mortality rate, can leave scars and loss of hair/nails. Etiology: drug, graft-versus-host disease, idiopathic. (Some now refer to SJS-TEN complex because of overlapping features.)

Toxic shock syndrome – hand and foot edema, macular erythroderma, lack of discrete lesions, negative Nikolsky sign, eruption lasts about 3 days then desquamates 10–21 days after onset, hyperemia of mucous membranes, Beau's lines and telogen effluvium occur months later. Fever up to 2 weeks, hypotension, shock, myalgia, GI, renal, cardiac, pulmonary, hematologic (thrombocytopenia, DIC) dysfunction, elevated hepatic function tests, disorientation. Due to *Staphylococcus aureus* (TSS toxin 1) or *Streptococcus pyogenes*.

Treacher Collins syndrome – malar hypoplasia, partial/total absence of lower eyelashes, coloboma of eyelids, down-slanting palpebral fissures, extension of scalp hair on cheeks, occasional circumscribed scarring alopecia, hearing loss, skin tags between ear and mouth angle, cleft palate.

Trichorhinophalangeal syndrome (two types) – hypotrichosis, pear-shaped nose, multiple cone-shaped epiphytes of digits of hands and feet. TRPS1 gene.

Trichothiodystrophy (sulfur-deficient brittle hair, BIDS/IBIDS/PIBIDS, Tay's syndrome) – photosensitivity, ichthyosiform erythroderma, brittle hair (short and sulfur deficient), intellectual impairment, decreased fertility, short stature, dental caries, dystrophic nails, cataracts, microcephaly, deafness. Hair under polarized light shows pili torti, bands of light/dark ('tiger tail'), trichoschisis, trichorrhexis nodosa. AR. DNA repair enzyme defect. ERCC3 and XPB, or ERCC2 and XPD genes.

Trigeminal trophic syndrome – neurotrophic ulceration after minor trauma in anesthetic skin in trigeminal area usually begins in nasal ala area (ulcer of nose), paresthesia, nose tip spared, psychologic problems. Anesthesia may be due to infarct, tumor, degeneration.

Trisomy 13 (Patau syndrome) – malformed brain with holoprosencephaly/microcephaly, cutis aplasia of scalp, vascular malformations, cutis laxa of neck, narrow fingernails, deafness, rocker-bottom feet, cardiac abnormalities (ventricular septal defects), cleft lip/palate, bulbous nose.

Trisomy 18 (Edwards syndrome) – loose skin folds with typical dermal patterns, horizontal palmar creases and downy hair, dermatoglyphic abnormalities, poor subcutaneous tissue, clenched hand with overlapping, rocker-bottom feet, multiple congenital abnormalities, small chin, low-set ears, cleft lip/palate, neck webbing, cutis marmorata, vascular malformations, hypertrichosis, nail hypoplasia.

Trisomy 21 – *see* Down's syndrome.

Tropical anhidrotic asthenia – anhidrosis with keratin plugs in sweat pores, miliaria, bouts of pruritus, severe systemic symptoms, collapse.

Tuberous sclerosis (Bourneville's syndrome, Pringle's syndrome, epiloia) – adenoma sebaceum, shagreen patch, collagen nevi, angiofibroma, subungual fibromas, oral fibromas, skin tags, collagen nevi, phakomas, tumors (visceral and skeletal, fibrous and muscular), café-au-lait macules/patches, white macules (ash-leaf, confetti, polygonal, dermatomal), poliosis, tooth enamel pits, bone cysts, brain fibromas (tubers), seizures, mental retardation, increased lymphangiomas or lipomatosis (renal and pulmonary). AD or sporadic. Gene product – hamartin (TSC1 gene) or tuberin (TSC2 gene).

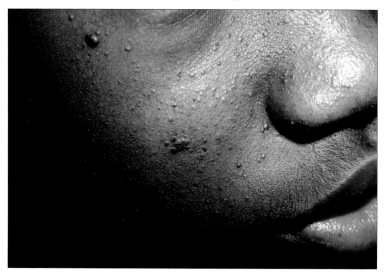

Adenoma sebaceum

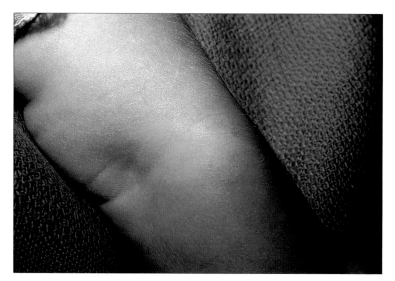

Ash leaf macule

Turner syndrome (Bonnevie–Ullrich syndrome, Ullrich–Turner syndrome) – webbed neck, lymphangiectatic edema of hands and feet at birth, cutis laxa and hyperelastica, multiple congenital anomalies, wide-spaced nipples on shield chest, increased nevi, keloid tendency, narrow nails, low occipital hairline, mental and physical retardation, amenorrhea. XO chromosome pattern or mosaic forms.

Ullrich–Turner syndrome – *see* Turner syndrome.
Uncombable hair syndrome – unmanageable silvery-blonde hair, slow hair growth. Hair: pili trianguli et canaliculi with longitudinal grooves in hair shafts and triangular cross-sections. AD.

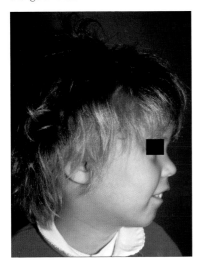

Unna–Thost syndrome (diffuse palmoplantar keratoderma) – diffuse palmoplantar keratoderma, painful fissures, not on extensor surfaces, keratosis of knees and elbows, palmoplantar hyperhidrosis, normal hair/teeth, oral leukoplakia (not premalignant), tendency to dermatophytosis. Begins in childhood. AD.
Urbach–Wiethe disease – *see* Lipoid proteinosis.

Van Den Bosch's syndrome – acrokeratosis verruciformis, mental deficiency, anhidrosis, skeletal deformity. X-linked recessive.
Van Lohuizen's syndrome – *see* Cutis marmorata telangiectatica congenita.
Vogt–Koyangi–Harada syndrome (uveomeningitis syndrome) – alopecia (alopecia areata or diffuse), vitiligo, poliosis, halo nevi, bilateral uveitis, iritis, glaucoma, retinochoroidal detachment, meningeal irritation with pleocytosis, dyscrasia, ± deafness.
Vohwinkel syndrome (keratoma hereditaria mutilans) – diffuse palmoplantar keratoderma honeycombed by small depressions, starfish-like keratoses on dorsa of hands and feet, irregular linear keratoses of knees and elbows, constricting fibrous bands on fingers and toes, cicatricial alopecia, deafness. AD or AR.
Von Hippel–Lindau syndrome (Lindau disease, angiomatosis retinae et cerebelli syndrome) – angiomatosis of retina and cerebellum, tumor and cysts of various organs, rarely vascular nevi of face, renal cell carcinoma, pheochromocytoma. Onset in third decade. AD.
Von Recklinghausen disease – *see* Neurofibromatosis type 1.

Von Zumbusch syndrome (acute generalized pustular psoriasis) – sheets of erythema and pustules involving flexural area, oral mucosa involvement, thick nails with underlying pus, telogen effluvium, fever, malaise, hepatic dysfunction, hypocalcemia, hypoalbuminemia, malabsorption.

Vörner disease/syndrome – epidermolytic palmoplantar hyperkeratosis beginning in childhood, may have diffuse keratoderma. Associated with ovarian and breast carcinomas. AD. Keratin 1 and keratin 9. KRT1 and KRT9 genes.

Waardenburg syndrome (Waardenburg–Klein syndrome) – pigment changes including albinism, white forelock and partial or complete heterochromia iridium, congenital deafness, fused thick eyebrows, broad nasal root and lateral displaced inner canthi, congenital megacolon (in type IV). AD. Genetic defects: PAX 3 (types I and III), MITF (type IIA), WS2B (type IIB), WS2C (type IIC), and SOXIO, EDN3 and EDNRB (type IV).

Waldenström macroglobulinemia – relapsing non-thrombocytopenic purpura, rarely infiltrated cutaneous and mucous membrane nodules and plaques, lymphocytoma cutis, vasculitis, Raynaud's phenomenon, xerostomia and xerophthalmia, hepatosplenomegaly and lymphadenopathy, mild anemia, increased ESR, marked increase in IgM. Associated with SLE, Sjögren's disease, multiple myeloma.

Waterhouse–Friderichsen syndrome – adrenal hemorrhagic infarct, cyanosis, purpuric maculas/diffuse purpura secondary to meningococcal or other septicemia, shock, fever.

Watson's syndrome – multiple café-au-lait macules, pulmonary vascular stenosis, decreased intellect, intertriginous freckling, short stature. AD. May be allelic variant of NF1.

Weber–Christian disease (relapsing febrile nodular non-suppurative panniculitis) – localized inflammatory, recurrent non-suppurative subcutaneous nodules (panniculitis), subcutaneous atrophy at sites of cutaneous disease, recurrent abdominal pain/fever/malaise/arthritis, can have systemic disease. Self-limiting. Idiopathic.

Weber–Cockayne syndrome – epidermolysis bullosa simplex limited to hands and feet.

Wegener's granulomatosis – symmetrical papulonecrotic lesions of extremities, widespread vesicular or urticarial lesions, oral ulcerations, gingivitis, severe sinopulmonary inflammation, general necrotizing angiitis of lungs/respiratory tract, ocular involvement, parotid glands with granulomas, asthma, arthritis, renal insufficiency due to glomerulonephritis. May be associated with pyoderma gangrenosum or erythema elevatum diutinum. 80% c-ANCA+.

Weill–Marchesani's syndrome – short stocky well-developed stature, thick skin and hair, spade-like hands with stubby fingers, ocular abnormalities. AR form on chromosome 19, similar syndrome AD form caused by mutation in fibrillin-1 gene on chromosome 15.

Well's syndrome (eosinophilic cellulitis) – recurrent erythematous indurated plaques (similar to cellulitis), persistent urticaria, eosinophilia (peripheral and bone marrow), skin lesions can be painful or pruritic.

Werner syndrome (progeria of the adult) – premature graying and loss of hair, atrophy of skin and subcutaneous tissue with loss of subcutaneous fat, poikiloderma and sclerodermatous changes; cataracts, endocrine abnormalities, thin extremities, bird-like face with narrow nose, dystrophic teeth. Onset in teens, life expectancy of 40–60 years. DNA helicase abnormalities.

Whipple disease (intestinal lipodystrophy syndrome) – arthritis, abdominal symptoms that worsen with eating, purpuric asthenia, patchy brown pigmentation of the skin, erythema nodosum, purpura, steatorrhea, cough, weight-loss, fever, lethargy, dementia. Systemic bacterial infection by *Tropheryma whipplei* (Whipple bacillus).

Wiedemann–Beckwith syndrome – *see* Beckwith–Wiedemann syndrome.

Wilson's disease (hepatolenticular degeneration) – Kayser–Fleischer rings of cornea, azure (blue) lunulae of nails, pretibial hyperpigmentation, frequent behavior disorders, liver cirrhosis, brain degenerative changes. Copper metabolism abnormalities causing deposition. AR.

Wiskott–Aldrich syndrome (Aldrich syndrome) – thrombocytopenic purpura, chronic eczema, recurrent purulence, petechiae, epistaxis, bloody diarrhea, intracranial bleeds, sinopulmonary infections, arthritic or renal autoimmune disease. Immunologic abnormalities. Increased risk of leukemia, lymphoma, Hodgkin's disease. X-linked recessive. WAS gene.

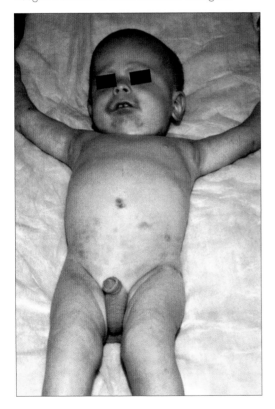

Witkop syndrome – *see* Tooth and nail syndrome.

Wolf syndrome – piebaldism and deafness.

Wyburn–Mason syndrome – congenital midbrain AVM with ipsilateral AVM and ipsilateral port-wine stain of face, telangiectatic nevus in region of affected eye, mental retardation, seizures. May be associated with Sturge–Weber syndrome.

Xeroderma pigmentosum – skin cancers, lentigines, hypopigmentation, ocular changes, neurologic abnormalities, sensorineural deafness, oral neoplasms. Defective repair of UV radiation damage due to DNA pyrimidine dimmers and reduced NK cell activity. Onset between 6 months and 3 years. AR.

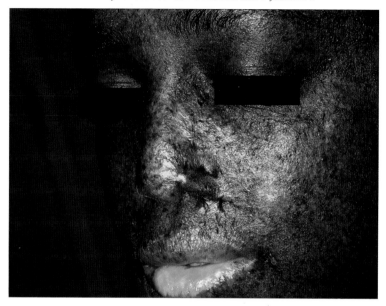

Yellow nail syndrome – thick and slow-growing yellow nails, onycholysis, loss of cuticles and lunulae, lymphedema of face/extremities, recurrent pulmonary abnormalities or pleural effusions. Associated with malignancy, nephritic syndrome, hypothyroidism, AIDS and D-penicillamine therapy.

Ziprkowski–Margolis syndrome – piebald-like hypomelanosis with hyperpigmented areas, congenital deafness. X-linked recessive. ADFN gene.

GLOSSARY OF ACRONYMS

5-FU	5-fluorouracil
8-MOP	8-methoxypsoralen
ACE	angiotensin converting enzyme
ACTH	adrenocorticotropic hormone
AD	autosomal dominant
AFB	acid-fast bacilli
AIDS	acquired immunodeficiency syndrome
AIP	acute intermittent porphyria
AML	acute myelogenous leukemia
ANA	antinuclear antibodies
APACHE	acral pseudolymphomatous angiokeratoma
AR	autosomal recessive
AST	aspartate aminotransferase
AVM	arteriovenous malformation
BCC	basal cell carcinoma
BMZ	basement membrane zone
CARP	confluent and reticulated papillomatosis
CBC	complete blood count
CEP	congenital erythropoietic porphyria
CGD	chronic granulomatous disease
CIE	congenital ichthyosiform erythroderma
CK	creatine kinase
CLL	chronic lymphocytic leukemia
CML	chronic myelogenous leukemia
CMV	cytomegalovirus
COPD	chronic obstructive pulmonary disease
CREST	**C**alcinosis, **R**aynaud phenomenon, **E**sophageal dysmotility, **S**clerodactyly, **T**elangiectasia [syndrome]
CTCL	cutaneous T-cell lymphoma
CXR	chest x-ray
DEJ	dermoepidermal junction
DF	dermatofibroma
DFA	direct fluorescent antibody
DFSP	dermatofibrosarcoma protuberans
DHEAS	dehydroepiandrosterone
DIC	disseminated intravascular coagulation
DIF	direct immunofluorescence
DIP	distal interphalangeal [joint]
DLE	discoid lupus erythematosus
DMSO	dimethyl sulfoxide
DNCB	dinitrochlorobenzene
DSAP	disseminated superficial actinic porokeratosis
DVT	deep venous thrombosis
EBA	epidermolysis bullosa acquisita
EBD	epidermolysis bullosa dystrophica
EBJ	epidermolysis bullosa junctional
EBS	epidermolysis bullosa simplex
EBV	Epstein–Barr virus
ED&C	electrodesiccation and curettage
EED	erythema elevatum diutinum

EPP	erythropoietic protoporphyria
EPS	elastosis perforans serpiginosa
ESR	erythrocyte sedimentation rate
ESRD	end stage renal disease
FSH	follicle stimulating hormone
FTA-ABS	fluorescent treponemal antibody absorption
GA	granuloma annulare
GI	gastrointestinal
GM-CSF	granulocyte-macrophage colony-stimulating factor
GU	genitourinary
GVHD	graft-versus-host disease
H&E	hematoxylin and eosin
HAART	highly active antiretroviral therapy
HBV	hepatitis B virus
HCP	hereditary coproporphyria
HEP	hepatic erythropoietic porphyria
HGPRT	hypoxanthine guanine phosphoribosyl transferase [deficiency]
HHV	human herpes virus
HIV	human immunodeficiency virus
HSV	herpes simplex virus
HZV	herpes zoster virus
Ig	immunoglobulin
IIF	indirect immunofluorescence
ILVEN	inflamed linear verrucous epidermal nevus
ITP	idiopathic thrombocytopenic purpura
IUGR	intrauterine growth retardation
IVIG	intravenous immunoglobulin
JXG	juvenile xanthogranuloma
KA	keratoacanthoma
LAD	lymphadenopathy
LCV	leukocytoclastic vasculitis
LFTs	liver function tests
LGV	lymphogranuloma venereum
LH	luteinizing hormone
LSC	lichen simplex chronicus
MCTD	mixed connective tissue disease
MHA-TP	microhemagglutination-Treponema pallidum
MR	miliaria rubra; multicentric reticulohistiocytoma
MS	multiple sclerosis
NAD	nicotinamide adenine dinucleotide
nbUVB	narrow band UVB [ultraviolet B phototherapy]
NF	neurofibroma, neurofibromatosis
NK	natural killer
NLD	necrobiosis lipoidica diabeticorum
NSAID	non-steroidal anti-inflammatory drug
OCP	oral contraceptive pill
ODD	oculodentodigital dysplasia
OFD	oral–facial–digital [syndrome]
OTC	over-the-counter
PABA	para-aminobenzoic acid
PAN	polyarteritis nodosa
p-ANCA	perinuclear anti-neutrophil cytoplasmic antibody
PAS	periodic–acid Schiff [stain]

PCN	penicillin
PCR	polymerase chain reaction
PCT	porphyria cutanea tarda
PCV	polycythemia vera
PIPA	postinflammatory pigmentary alteration
PLC	pityriasis lichenoides chronica
PLEVA	pityriasis lichenoides et varioliformis acuta
PMLE	polymorphous light eruption
PMN	polymorphonuclear leukocyte
PPD	purified protein derivative
PRP	pityriasis rubra pilaris
PSS	progressive systemic sclerosis
PTH	parathyroid hormone
PTT	partial thromboplastin time
PTU	propylthiouracil
PUPPP	pruritic urticarial papules and plaques of pregnancy
PUVA	psoralen and ultraviolet radiation
PWS	port-wine stain
PXE	pseudoxanthoma elasticum
RBC	red blood cell
REM	reticulated erythematous mucinosis
RF	rheumatoid factor
RMSF	Rocky Mountain spotted fever
RPR	rapid plasma reagin
RSV	respiratory syncitial virus
RV	right ventricle/ventricular
SCC	squamous cell carcinoma
SCID	severe combined immunodeficiency
SCLE	subacute cutaneous lupus erythematosus
SLE	systemic lupus erythematosus
SPEP	serum protein electrophoresis
SSSS	staphylococcal scalded skin syndrome
Staph	staphylococcus
Strep	streptococcus
TCN	tetracycline
TEN	toxic epidermal necrolysis
TIA	transient ischemic attack
TMEP	telangiectasia macularis eruptiva perstans
TMP	4,5',8-trimethylpsoralen
TSH	thyroid-stimulating hormone
TSS	toxic shock syndrome
TTP	thrombotic thrombocytopenic purpura
UPEP	urine protein electrophoresis
URI	upper respiratory tract infection
UTI	urinary tract infection
UV	ultraviolet
VDRL	venereal disease research laboratory
VP	variegate porphyria
VSD	ventricular septal defect
VZV	varcilla zoster virus
WBC	white blood cell count

BIBLIOGRAPHY

In compiling this text, much of our work came from the lists we had each compiled over the years. Below are listed sources we used in completing the text.

Bolognia J, Jorizzo J, Rapini R et al. Dermatology. St Louis: Mosby, 2003

Champion R, Burton J, Ebling F. Rook/Wilkinson/Ebling Textbook of Dermatology, 5th edn. Oxford: Blackwell Scientific, 1995

Freedburg I, Eisen A, Wolff K, Austen KF, Goldsmith L, Katz S. Fitzpatrick's Dermatology in General Medicine, 6th edn. London: McGraw-Hill, 2003

Goldman L, Ausiello D. Cecil Textbook of Medicine, 22nd edn. Philadelphia: Saunders, 2003

Mallory S. An Illustrated Dictionary of Dermatologic Syndromes. New York: Parthenon Publishing, 1994

NIH-OMIM website: http://www.ncbi.nlm.nih.gov/entrez/query.fcgi?db=OMIM

Odom R, James W, Berger T. Andrews' Diseases of the Skin: Clinical Dermatology, 9th edn. Philadelphia: Saunders, 2000

Schachner L, Hansen, R. Pediatric Dermatology, 3rd edn. St Louis: Mosby, 2003

Spitz J. Genodermatoses. Baltimore: Lippincott, Williams and Wilkins, 1996

INDEX